Diabetic Retinopathy

Diabetic Retinopathy

Edited by

O Paul van Bijsterveld MD PhD

Oogcentrum Houten
The Netherlands

MARTIN DUNITZ

First published in the United Kingdom in 2000 by

Martin Dunitz Ltd
The Livery House
7–9 Pratt Street
London NW1 0AE

A CIP record for this book is available from the British Library.

ISBN 1-85317-625-7

Distributed in the United States by:
Blackwell Science Inc.
Commerce Place, 350 Main Street
Malden, MA 02148, USA
Tel: 1-800-215-1000

Distributed in Canada by:
Login Brothers Book Company
324 Salteaux Crescent
Winnipeg, Manitoba, R3J 3T2
Canada
Tel: 204-224-4068

Distributed in Brazil by:
Ernesto Reichmann Distribuidora de Livros, Ltda
Rua Coronel Marques 335, Tatuape 03440-000
Sao Paulo, Brazil

Composition by Scribe Design, Gillingham, Kent, UK
Printed and bound in Spain by Grafos, S.A. Arte Sobre papel

Contents

Contributors

Francesco Bandello MD
Associate Professor of Ophthalmology
Department of Ophthalmology
University of Udine
Udine
ITALY

Jan D Banga MD PhD
Consultant in Vascular Medicine
University Medical Center, Utrecht
Division of Internal Medicine
3508 GA Utrecht
THE NETHERLANDS

Toke Bek MD PhD
Associate Professor of Ophthalmology
Århus University Hospital
DK-8000 Århus C
DENMARK

O Paul van Bijsterveld MD PhD
Oogcentrum Houten
Achterom 16B
3995 EB Houten
THE NETHERLANDS

Rosario Brancato MD
Professor of Ophthalmology and
Chairman, Department of Ophthalmology
and Visual Sciences
Scientific Institute San Raffaele Hospital
University of Milan
Milan 20132
ITALY

Chris Canning FRCOphth FRCS FCP(SA) MRCP
Consultant Vitreoretinal Surgeon
Southampton Eye Unit
Southampton General Hospital
Tremona Road
Southampton SO16 6YD
UK

Louis MT Collum FRCS FRCSI FRCOphth EBOD
Professor of Ophthalmology and
Consultant Ophthalmic Surgeon
Royal College of Surgeons in Ireland and
Royal Victoria Eye and Ear Hospital
Adelaide Road
Dublin 2
REPUBLIC OF IRELAND

Gabriel Coscas MD
Ophtalmologiste des Hôpitaux de Paris
Clinique Ophtalmologique
Universitaire de Créteil
94010 Créteil
FRANCE

José Cunha-Vaz MD PhD
Professor and Chairman
Department of Ophthalmology, University
Hospital and
Center of Ophthalmology
Institute of Biomedical Research on Light
and Image
University of Coimbra
PORTUGAL

Jonathan Dowler FRCS FRCOphth
Consultant Ophthalmic Surgeon and
Chairman, Diabetic Retinopathy Screening
Moorfields Eye Hospital
City Road
London EC1V 2PD
UK

Isobel Ford BSc MIBiol PhD
Research Fellow
Department of Medicine and Therapeutics
University of Aberdeen
Aberdeen
UK

Arnd Gandorfer MD
Augenklinik
Ludwig-Maximilians-Universität
Mathildenstraße 8
D-80336 München
GERMANY

Michael Greaves MD FRCP FRCPath
Professor of Haematology
Department of Medicine and Therapeutics
University of Aberdeen
Aberdeen
UK

Philip G de Groot PhD
Laboratory Center
Section of Hemostasis and Thrombosis
Research, University Medical Center
Utrecht
THE NETHERLANDS

A M Peter Hamilton FRCS FRCOphth
Consultant Ophthalmic Surgeon
149 Harley Street
London W1N 2DE
UK

Ellen C La Heij MD PhD
Faculty member
University Eye Institute Maastricht
PO Box 5800
6202 AZ Maastricht
THE NETHERLANDS

Fred Hendrikse MD PhD
Professor and Chairman
University Eye Institute Maastricht
PO Box 5800
6202 AZ Maastricht
THE NETHERLANDS

Jan P Hoops MD
Department of Ophthalmology
Ludwig-Maximilians-Universität
Mathildenstraße 8
D-80336 München
GERMANY

Anselm Kampik MD
Professor of Ophthalmology
Direktor der Augenklinik
Ludwig-Maximilians-Universität
Mathildenstraße 8
D-80336 München
GERMANY

Nynke Klaassen-Broekema MD PhD
Oogcentrum Houten
Achterom 16B
3995 EB Houten
THE NETHERLANDS

Jean-Jacques De Laey MD PhD
Professor and Chairman
Department of Ophthalmology
University Hospital
Ghent
BELGIUM

Isabelle Meunier MD
Ophtalmologiste des Hôpitaux de Paris
Clinique Ophtalmologique
Universitaire de Créteil
94010 Créteil
FRANCE

Gisèle Soubrane PhD MD
Ophtalmologiste des HÙpitaux de Paris
Clinique Ophtalmologique
Universitaire de Créteil
94010 Créteil
FRANCE

David R Tomlinson BSc PhD DSc
Professor of Neuropharmacology
School of Biological Sciences
University of Manchester
Stopford Building
Oxford Road
Manchester M13 9PT
UK

Michael W Ulbig MD
Lecturer, Department of Ophthalmology
Ludwig-Maximilians-Universität
Mathildenstraße 8
D-80336 München
GERMANY

Bruno Vincke MD
Department of Ophthalmology
University Hospital
Ghent
BELGIUM

David E Wallace FRCSI(Ophth)
Specialist Registrar in Ophthalmology
Dublin
REPUBLIC OF IRELAND

Preface

It is often forgotten that the risk of blindness as a result of diabetic retinopathy expanded 15-fold after the introduction of insulin as this therapy increased life expectancy without significantly inhibiting the microvascular angiopathy. Little wonder, then, that interest in ocular complications of diabetes has increased exponentially over the last few decades. In the study of diabetic retinopathy researchers of various medical specialties across many areas of basic science are participating and the knowledge generated covers a wide field.

Much of the early medical knowledge of the ocular complications of diabetes sprang from clinicians with an interest in this metabolic disease. The more recent advances in the conceptual and scientific perception of the intricacies of diabetic retinopathy have their origin in general medicine and basic science. This information has only slowly become available to ophthalmologists as the flood of countless reports of highly specialized research seems to be directed mainly to experts of their own group and so only a few ophthalmologists are able to grasp more than a fraction of the available knowledge.

I have been fortunate to obtain the assistance of ranking experts in diabetic retinopathy of many countries, to overcome this ever widening gulf of information from medical and basic science specialists and to clarify the interdisciplinary complexities. Their contributions cover all modern clinical and fundamental aspects of diabetic retinopathy. Also, I hope the topics presented here will stimulate and encourage new ideas on diabetic retinopathy which remains one of the most challenging fields in all of medical research.

O Paul van Bijsterveld
Houten, The Netherlands, 2000

1 Clinical features of diabetic retinopathy

Jonathan Dowler and AM Peter Hamilton

The concept that diabetic retinopathy progresses through a sequence of recognizable stages is of fundamental importance. The scientific basis for this concept is provided by the Early Treatment Diabetic Retinopathy Study,[1] in which a small number of clinical signs indicative of the likelihood of retinopathy progression was statistically abstracted from a much larger number incorporated in the modified Airlie House Classification of Diabetic Retinopathy.[2] These few signs were used to formulate a hierarchy of levels of retinopathy severity, the Final Retinopathy Severity Scale.[1] Application of this scale provides the basis for assessment of retinopathy progression in many clinical contexts, epidemiological studies, and interventional trials.[3]

It is important, however, to recognize the limitations inherent in a simplified hierarchy of this type. Statistical analysis of long-term prospective studies may underplay the importance of less common or more transient signs indicative of retinopathy progression. Furthermore, retinopathy progresses in a unique fashion in each eye, at a non-uniform rate which may differ between areas of retina, and between eyes. A variety of influences affect the rate of progression between and within individuals; with more rapid progression, levels in the hierarchy may be skipped. Certain patterns of maculopathy and retinopathy in specific groups of diabetics can be recognized, and have distinct prognostic significance. Thus, although the use of a retinopathy severity scale is of considerable value, retinopathy levels must be interpreted in the context of the overall clinical picture.

The first part of this chapter is devoted to the development of models of retinopathy progression and the evolution of maculopathy, the

Critical signs: major parameters of the Early Treatment Diabetic Retinopathy Study Final Retinopathy Severity Scale.[1]

Non-proliferative retinopathy
Haemorrhages and/or microaneurysms
Intraretinal microvascular abnormalities
Venous beading
Cotton wool spots

Proliferative retinopathy
New vessels elsewhere (NVE)
New vessels on the optic disc (NVD)

Fibrous proliferation elsewhere
Fibrous proliferation on the optic disc

Preretinal haemorrhage
Vitreous haemorrhage

Retinal detachment

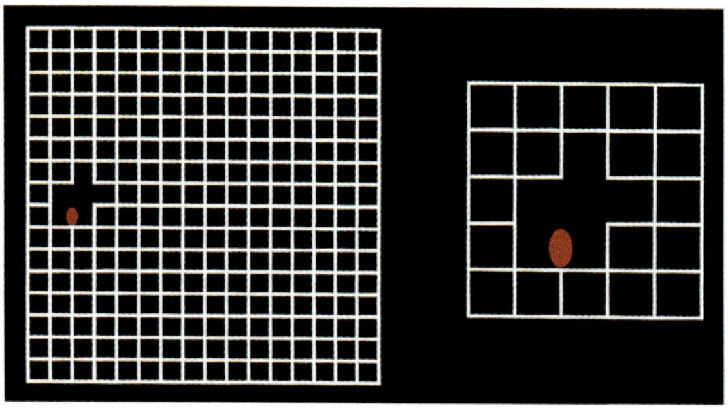

(a)

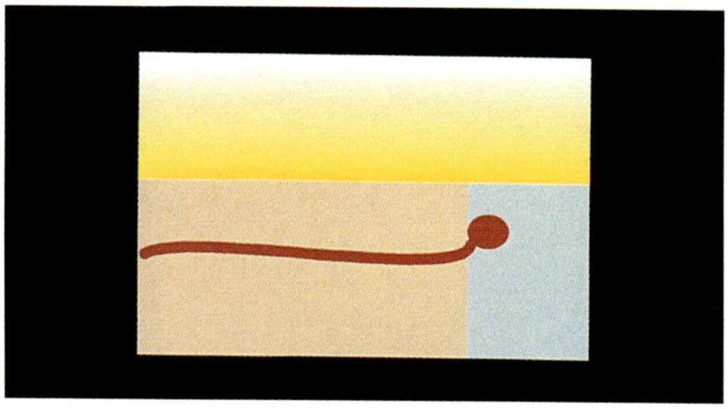

(b)

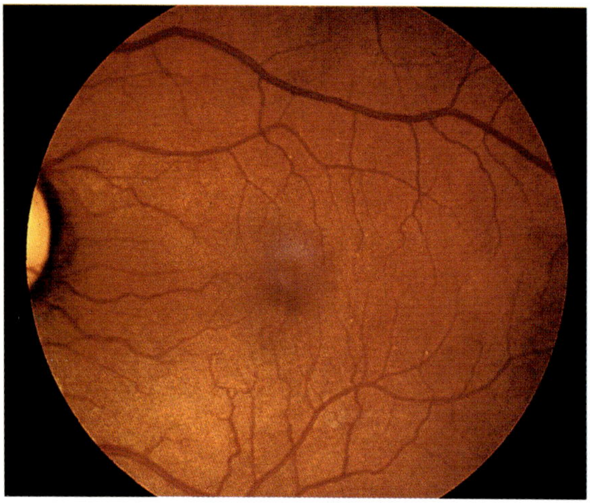

(c)

Figure 1.1
(a) Diagram of retinal capillary network (white) as seen on ophthalmoscopy, with one small area of capillary non-perfusion and associated microaneurysm (red). (b) Diagram of retina seen in cross-section showing vitreous (yellow), perfused retina (orange), non-perfused retina (grey) and microaneurysm (red) at junction between perfused and non-perfused retina. (c) Microaneurysms adjacent to fovea; to locate, see source of hyperfluorescence on angiogram (*Fig. 1.8b*).

second to the clinical signs of retinopathy, and the third to patterns of retinopathy in two specific patient groups.

MECHANISTIC MODELS

Model of retinopathy progression

The earliest ophthalmoscopically visible sign of diabetic retinopathy is the microaneurysm, which represents a localized endothelial cell proliferative response to a small area of retinal capillary non-perfusion, presumably mediated by growth factors produced by the ischaemic area (*Fig. 1.1a,b,c*). Microaneurysms are thus markers of capillary non-perfusion, and the microaneurysm count whether angiographically or ophthalmoscopically determined is a measure of the likelihood of retinopathy progression.[4] Another indication of the presence of capillary non-perfusion is the cotton wool spot, which represents arrest of axoplasmic flow in the retinal nerve fibre layer at the margin of a microvascular infarct. There is some correlation between numbers of cotton wool spots and the risk of progression to proliferative retinopathy.[1]

With occlusion of larger vessels producing more extensive areas of capillary non-perfusion, or confluence of smaller areas of non-perfusion, the microaneurysm count typically falls and the

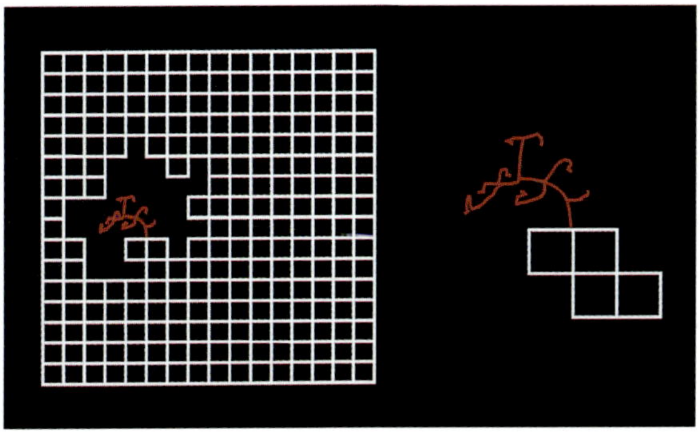

(a)

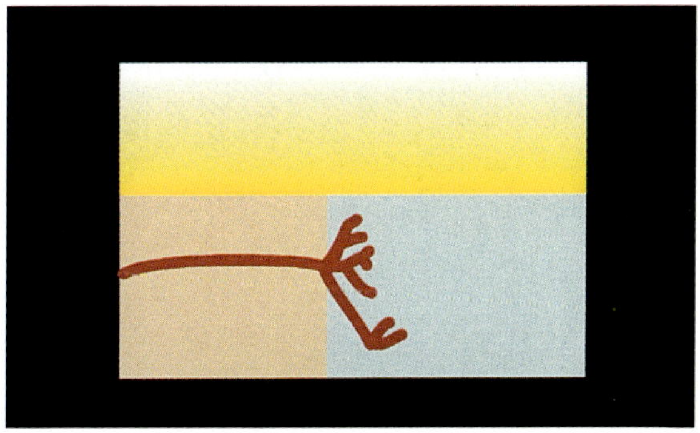

(b)

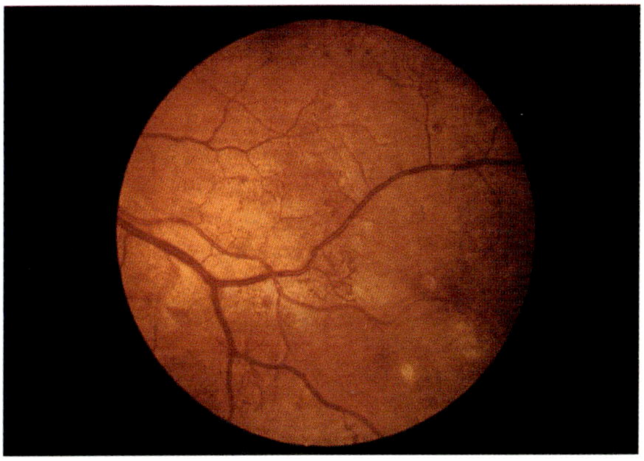

(c)

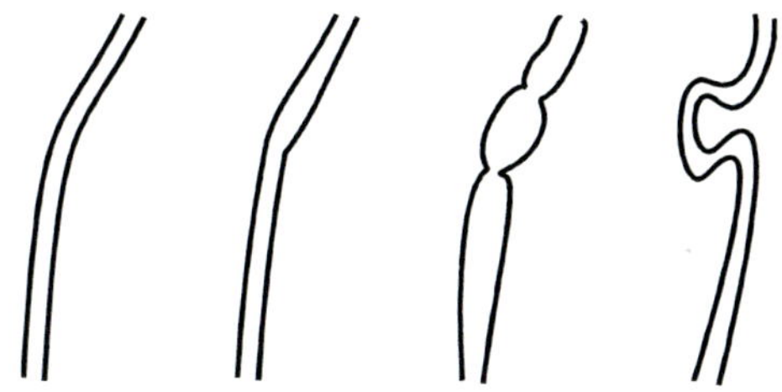

(d)

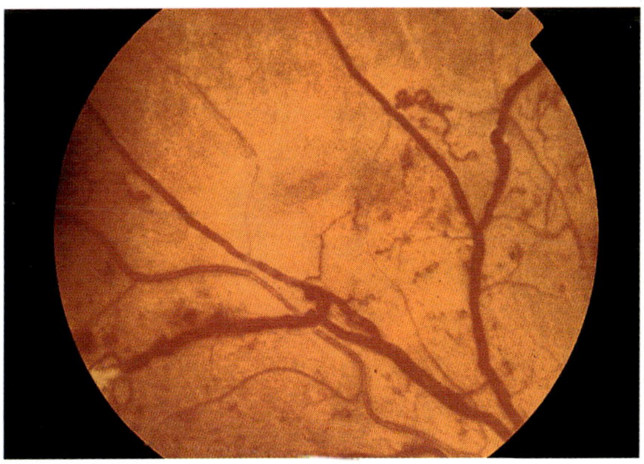

(e)

Figure 1.2
(a) Diagram of retinal capillary network (white) as seen on ophthalmoscopy, with a larger area of capillary non-perfusion and associated intraretinal microvascular abnormality (red); (b) diagram of retina seen in cross-section showing vitreous (yellow), perfused retina (orange), non-perfused retina (grey) and intraretinal microvascular abnormality (red) at junction between perfused and non-perfused retina; (c) fundus photograph showing intraretinal microvascular abnormalities as abnormally branching structures adjacent to veins; (d) range of venous abnormalities; (e) fundus photographs showing extensive venous beading and segmentation.

nature of the marginal endothelial cell proliferative response changes, being characterized by irregularly branching structures termed intraretinal microvascular abnormalities (IRMAs) (*Fig. 1.2a,b,c*). This may be because as the area of capillary non-perfusion rises, the ratio of unit circumference to area also rises, resulting in delivery of a higher marginal dose of vasoproliferative

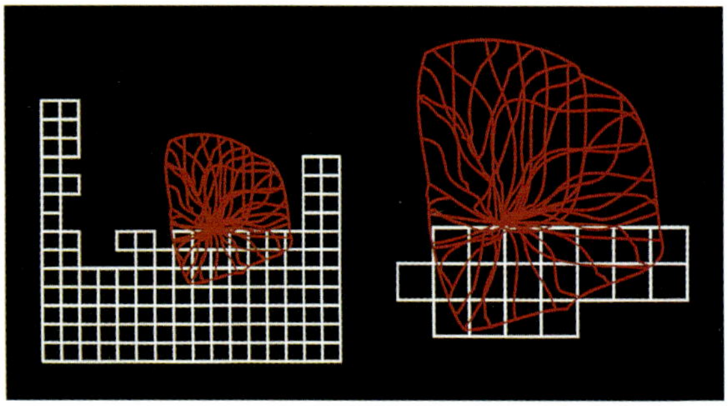

(a)

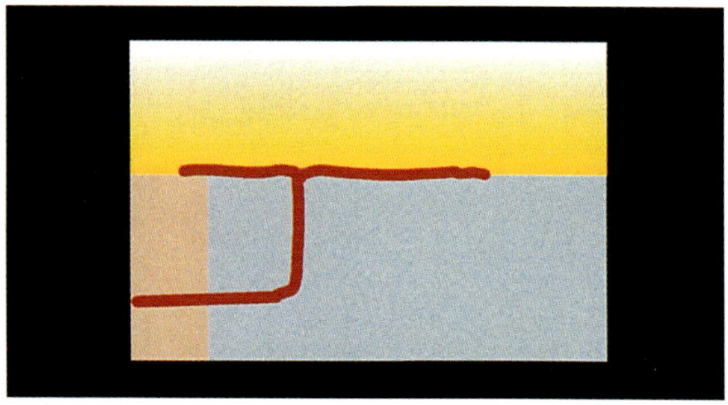

(b)

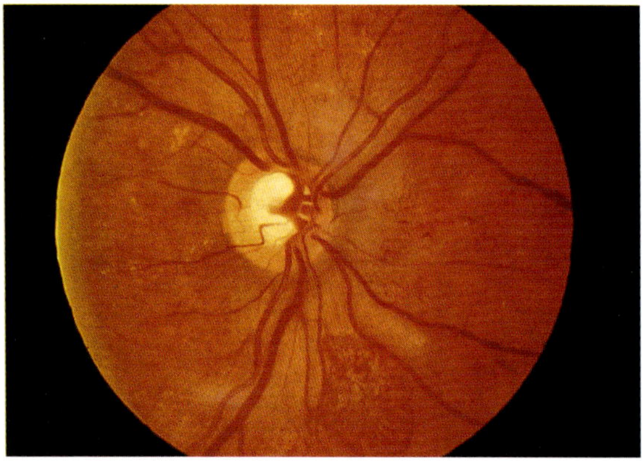

Figure 1.3
(a) Diagram of retinal capillary network (white) as seen on ophthalmoscopy, with a very large area of capillary non-perfusion and associated retinal neovascularization (red); (b) diagram of retina seen in cross-section showing vitreous (yellow), perfused retina (orange), non-perfused retina (grey) and retinal new vessels (red) arising at junction between perfused and non-perfused retina; (c) retinal new vessels arising in a net-like form on the retinal surface.

growth factor. IRMAs mainly represent intraretinal neovascularization and their irregular structure arises from the density of the inner retinal matrix through which they proliferate. The severity of IRMAs is strongly correlated with the risk of progression to proliferative retinopathy.[1]

If capillary non-perfusion extends up to major veins, secondary changes are induced in the vein wall resulting in irregularity of venous calibre, termed venous beading, or in its more severe form, venous segmentation (*Fig. 1.2d,e*), where the vein takes on the appearance of a string of sausages. The severity and extent of venous beading is the best single predictor of the likelihood of progression to proliferative retinopathy.[1]

With yet more extensive capillary non-perfusion, and higher vitreous concentrations of vasoproliferative growth factors, intraretinal neovascularization may become so exuberant as to break out of the retina through the internal limiting membrane on to the retinal surface, or more commonly, neovascularization may arise de novo on the retinal surface of veins (*Fig. 1.3a,b*). This extraretinal neovascularization, which unlike the intraretinal variety, is not constrained by the dense inner retinal matrix, may grow rapidly and form characteristic net-like structures which may be seen to overlie existing retinal vasculature and signal the presence of proliferative retinopathy. With increasing area of capillary non-perfusion, these may appear on the retina and/or optic disc.

The arborization on the posterior hyaloid face of proliferating endothelial cells may induce changes in the configuration of vitreous collagen resulting in localized detachment of the vitreous from the retina, and vitreous contraction (*Fig. 1.4a,b*). This may result in haemorrhage either

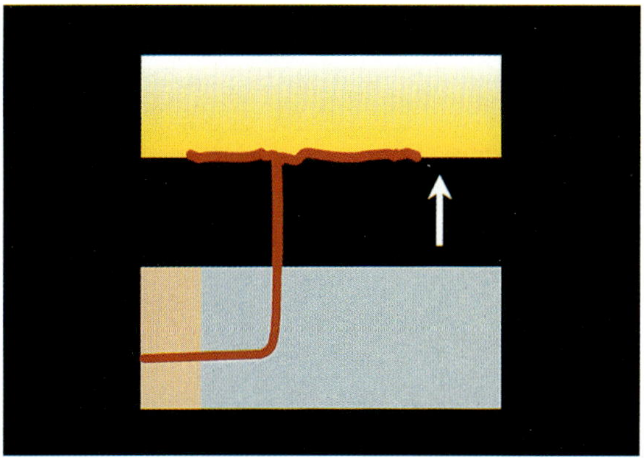

(a)

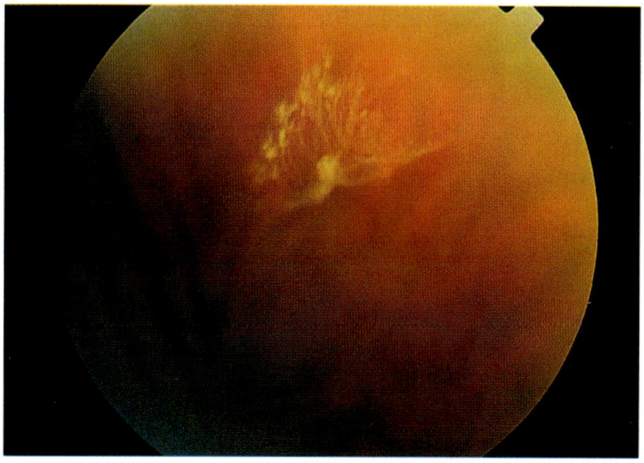

(b)

Figure 1.4
(a) Diagram of retina seen in cross-section showing perfused retina (orange), non-perfused retina (grey) and retinal new vessels (red) at junction between perfused and non perfused retina. Retraction (white arrow) of the vitreous (yellow) is drawing the new vessels attached to its posterior surface forward. (b) New vessels attached to the posterior surface of the vitreous and branching from the central stalk.

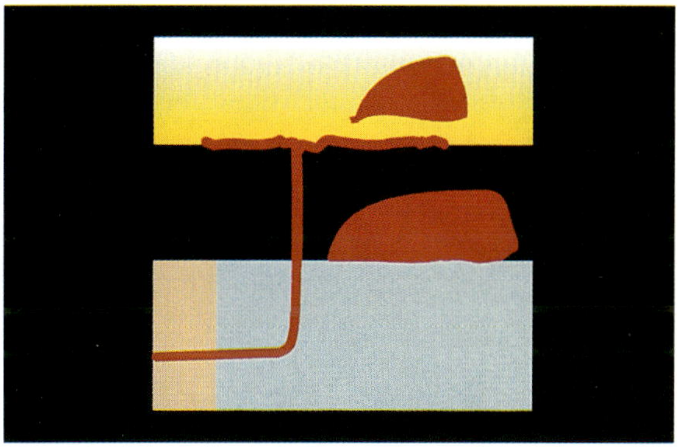

(a)

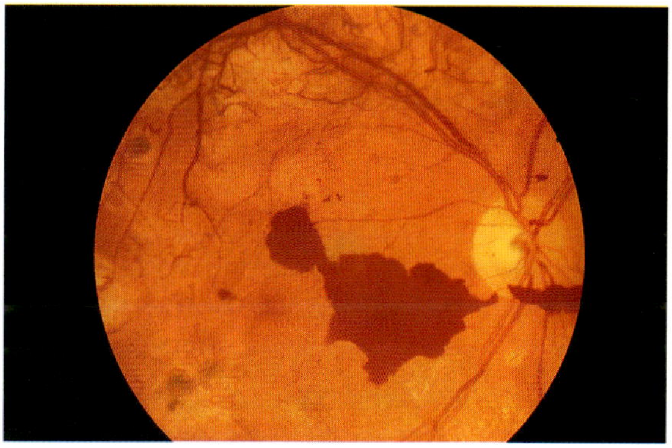

(b)

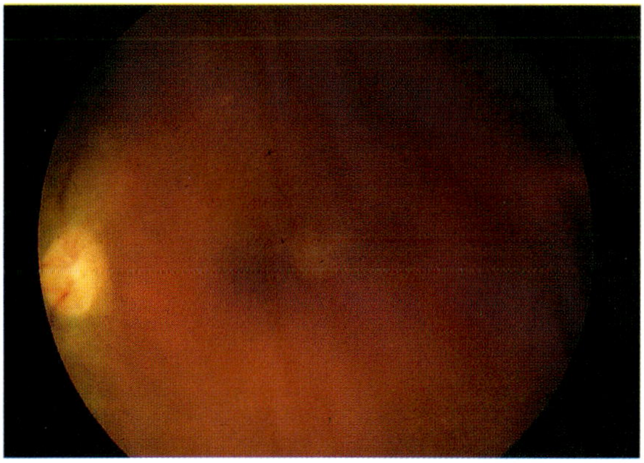

(c)

Figure 1.5
(a) Diagram of retina seen in cross-section showing perfused retina (orange), non-perfused retina (grey) and retinal new vessels (red) at junction between perfused and non-perfused retina. Retraction of the vitreous (yellow) has produced haemorrhage between retina and vitreous (preretinal haemorrhage) and within the vitreous (vitreous haemorrhage); (b) preretinal haemorrhage; (c) vitreous haemorrhage.

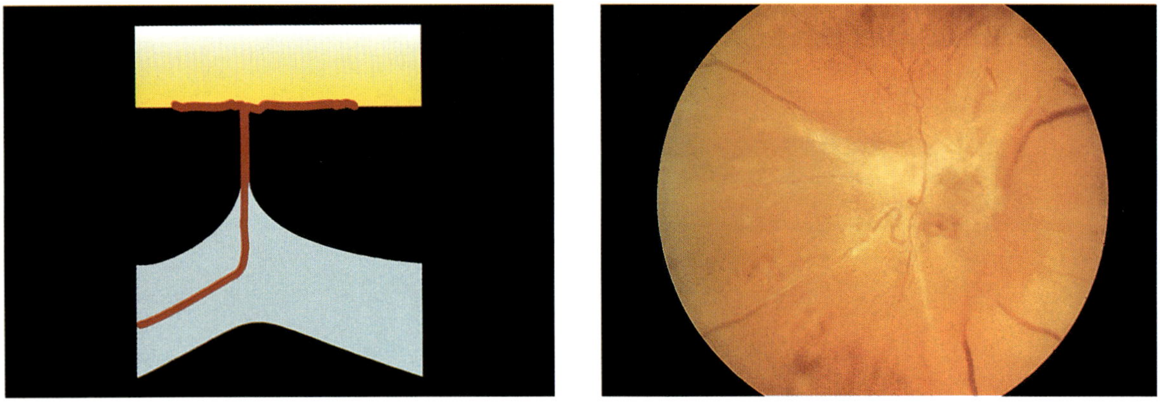

(a) (b)

Figure 1.6
(a) Diagram of retina seen in cross-section. Continued vitreous retraction and fibrosis of the connection between retina (grey) and vitreous (yellow) has drawn the retina up into a concave tractional retinal detachment. (b) Traction retinal detachment.

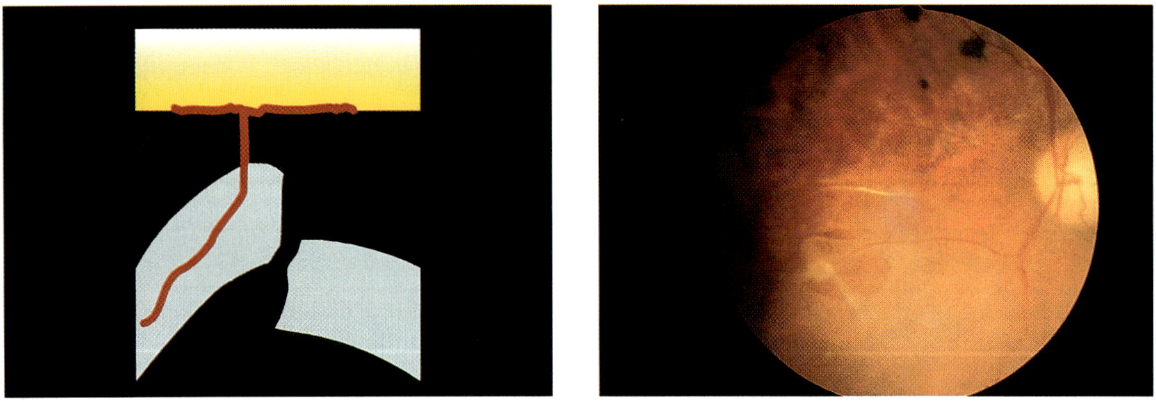

(a) (b)

Figure 1.7
(a) Diagram of retina seen in cross-section. Contraction of the vitreous (yellow) has torn the retina (grey) producing a convex traction rhegmatogenous detachment. (b) Traction rhegmatogenous retinal detachment.

between retina and posterior hyaloid face (preretinal or retrohyaloid haemorrhage) or within the vitreous (intragel haemorrhage) (*Fig. 1.5a,b,c*). Such haemorrhages may obscure the neovascularization causing them, but the presence of haemorrhage overlying retinal vessels suggests preretinal processes and proliferative disease.

Increasing recruitment of fibrous elements into the connection between vitreous and retina may result in a mechanically robust link which

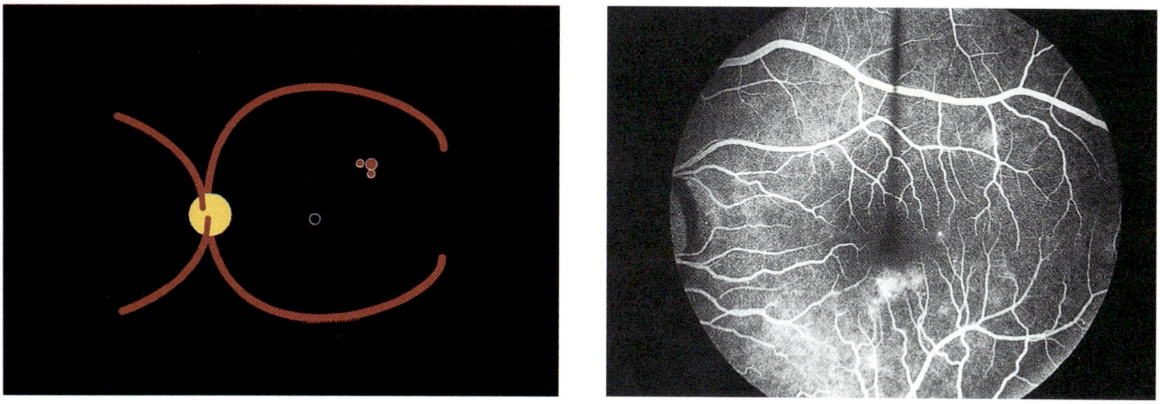

(a) (b)

Figure 1.8
(a) Diagram of retina as seen ophthalmoscopically. Localized leakage from microvascular abnormalities. (b) Fluorescein angiogram of focal leakage (white area below marker) adjacent to the fovea. Same eye as *Fig. 1.1c*.

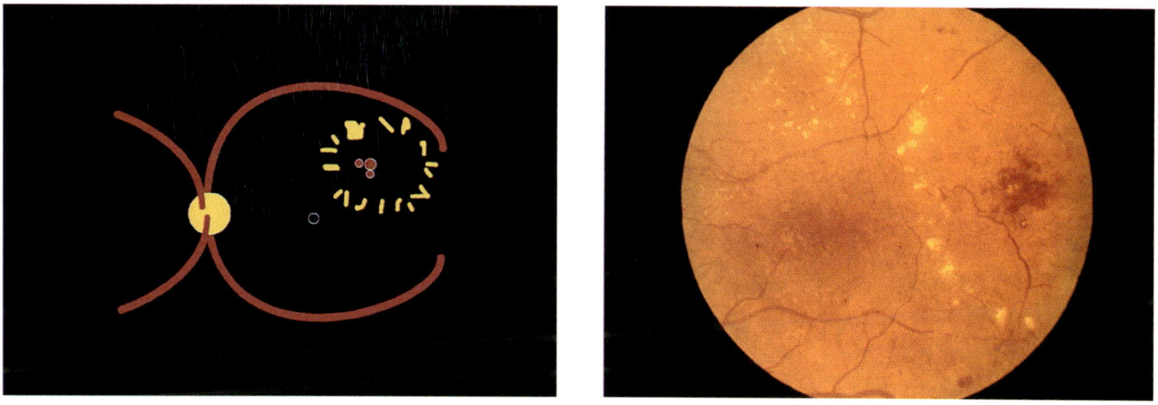

(a) (b)

Figure 1.9
(a) Diagram of retina as seen ophthalmoscopically. Chronic localized leakage from microvascular abnormalities has resulted in precipitation of lipoprotein exudate at junction between thickened and non-thickened retina. (b) Small, and partial large ring of exudate around localized leaking microvascular abnormalities.

with further vitreous contraction may avulse the retinal vessel from the retina, with the risk of haemorrhage. Alternatively, the retina may become elevated in a traction retinal detachment, which typically adopts a concave configuration (*Fig. 1.6a,b*). The retina may tear at the site of traction, producing a full-thickness retinal hole, which may result in a traction-rhegmatogenous retinal detachment, which typically adopts a convex configuration (*Fig. 1.7a,b*).

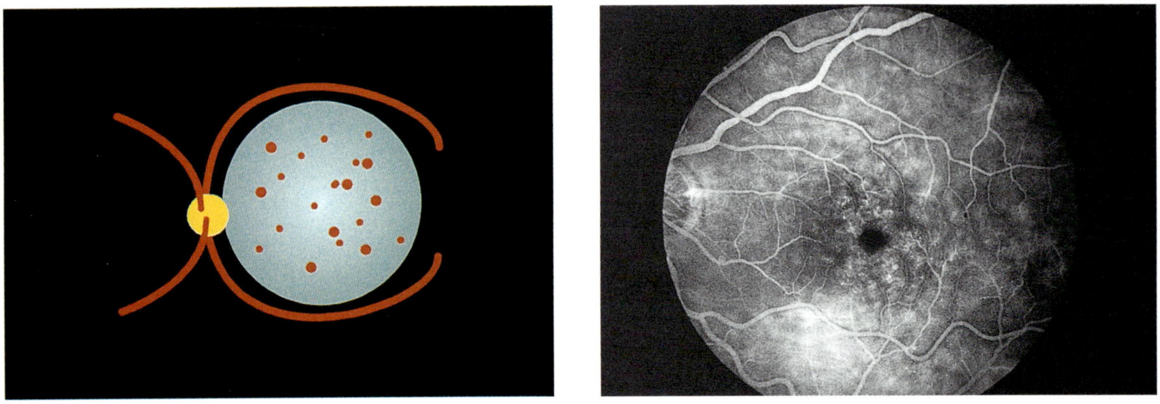
(a) (b)

Figure 1.10
(a) Diagram of retina as seen ophthalmoscopically. Diffuse leakage from multiple microvascular abnormalities. (b) Fluorescein angiogram showing diffuse leakage from microvascular abnormalities–central white areas.

Model of maculopathy

If retinopathy is present, it may involve the macula. The mildest form of maculopathy is manifest as a localized microvascular abnormality, leakage from which results in thickening of the surrounding retina (*Fig. 1.8a,b*). With short-term leakage from a small microvascular abnormality, the ratio of circumference to area of thickened retina is sufficient to permit clearance of lipoprotein from the margin of the area, but with more extensive or chronic leakage, lipoprotein may be deposited at the junction of thickened and non-thickened retina in the form of exudate, and a circinate ring forms around the microvascular abnormality–focal maculopathy (*Fig. 1.9a,b*). If permeability is increased throughout the majority of the macular microvasculature, the macula becomes diffusely thickened (*Fig. 1.10a,b*), and in the absence of surrounding normal retina, exudate may be absent. With increases in the area of macular capillary non-perfusion, a mixed maculopathy may result (*Fig. 1.11a,b*), with leakage from the margins but not the centres of non-perfused areas. In a more extreme form, ischaemic maculopathy, capillary closure precludes leakage and the retina ultimately becomes thinned and atrophic (*Fig. 1.12a,b*).

CLINICAL SIGNS

Microaneurysms

Microaneurysms are visible ophthalmoscopically as round intraretinal lesions ranging from 10 to 100 μm in size, red or occasionally white in colour, which may be associated with intraretinal haemorrhage or retinal thickening (*Fig. 1.1c*). They occur most frequently at the posterior pole, especially in the area temporal to the macula. Fluorescein angiography usually demonstrates microaneurysms as hyperfluorescent spots at the margins of small areas of capillary non-perfusion (*Fig. 1.8b*). Dye may leak from them into the surrounding retina. Approximately twice as many

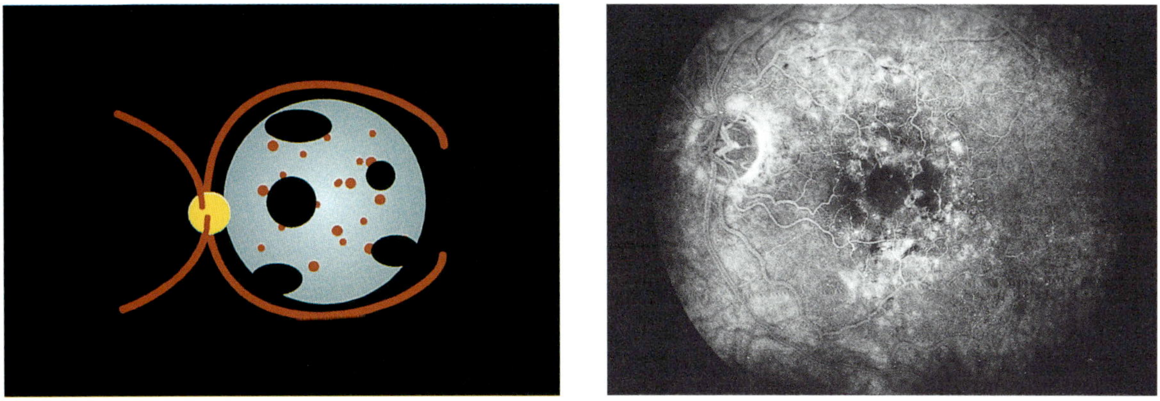

(a) (b)

Figure 1.11
(a) Diagram of retina as seen ophthalmoscopically. Diffuse leakage from multiple microvascular abnormalities interspersed with areas of capillary non-perfusion. (b) Fluorescein angiogram of mixed maculopathy with leakage–white areas and non-perfusion–dark areas.

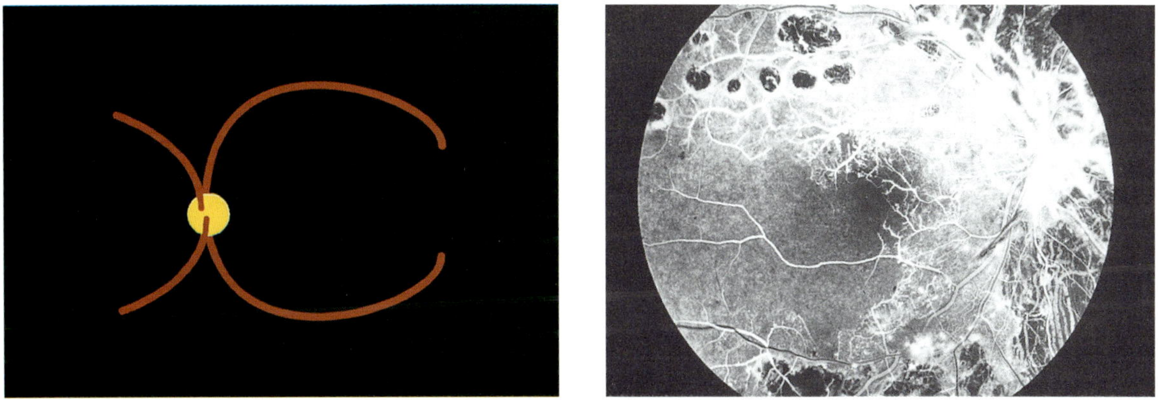

(a) (b)

Figure 1.12
(a) Diagram of retina as seen ophthalmoscopically. Extensive capillary non-perfusion–featureless macula. (b) Fluorescein angiogram of ischaemic maculopathy. Extensive capillary non-perfusion–dark areas.

microaneurysms may be identified on fluorescein angiography as are ophthalmoscopically visible, because intraretinal oedema may obscure deeper microaneurysms.

Exudates

Intraretinal exudate, visible as creamy yellow plaques, flecks or dots, reflects the deposition of lipoprotein at the junction between thickened

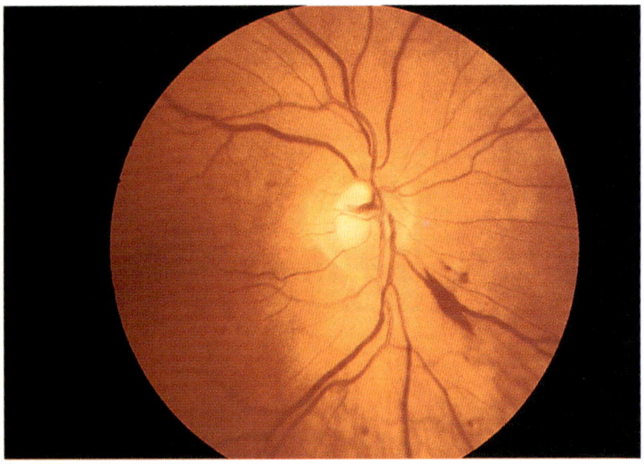

Figure 1.13
Nerve fibre layer haemorrhage.

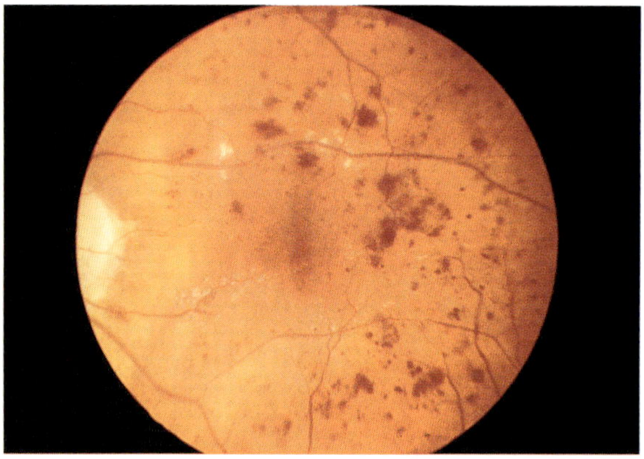

Figure 1.14
Cluster haemorrhages.

retina adjacent to areas of microvascular leakage, and surrounding non-thickened retina (*Fig. 1.9b*). Extensive posterior pole exudation may indicate renal failure. The presence of exudate is not associated with increased risk of progression to proliferative retinopathy,[1] and their main relevance is in relation to macular oedema. It is important to note, however, that a speckled appearance similar to intraretinal exudate may be produced by large areas of capillary non-perfusion following the resolution of cloudy swelling, and this may be of prognostic significance in regard to the development of proliferative retinopathy. Fluorescein angiography may be required to differentiate the two entities.

Intraretinal haemorrhages

In non-proliferative retinopathy, a variety of forms of intraretinal haemorrhage may be seen throughout the fundus. Flame-shaped haemorrhages occur within the retinal nerve fibre layer, the long axis of the haemorrhage aligned with the nerve fibres (*Fig. 1.13*). Deeper in the retina, punctate dot haemorrhage or larger blot haemorrhages with irregular margins may occur. Cluster haemorrhages are large dark and lie between the superficial and deep retinal capillary plexi (*Fig. 1.14*). It is important to note that haemorrhage which overlies retinal blood vessels is by definition preretinal, not intraretinal, and implies the presence of proliferative retinopathy (*Fig. 1.5b,c*). On fluorescein angiography all haemorrhages mask choroidal fluorescence to some degree; cluster haemorrhages typically demarcate areas of capillary non-perfusion and may represent haemorrhagic retinal infarcts. With increasingly widespread intraretinal haemorrhages and/or microaneurysms the risk of progression to proliferative diabetic retinopathy within 1 year is increased fourfold.[1]

Cotton wool spots

Cotton wool spots appear as localized whitish elevations of the retinal nerve fibre layer, the striations of which may be visible within the lesion. With large areas of microvascular infarction the retina takes on a diffusely grey appearance termed 'cloudy swelling', which may be difficult to distinguish from retinal oedema. As these lesions resolve, a process that may take many months, a punctate appearance similar to intraretinal exudate may develop. Fluorescein angiography demonstrates a variable area of capillary closure, corresponding to the infarct, often with surrounding capillary dilatation and leakage. A single cotton wool spot may arise from a small area of capillary non-perfusion, and thus has little predictive power for the subsequent development of proliferative retinopathy.[5] Large cotton wool spots or areas of cloudy swelling may, however, represent axoplasmic hold-up adjacent to arteriolar occlusion, with correspondingly greater prognostic significance. With increasing severity of cotton wool spots, there is a doubling of the risk of progression to proliferative disease within 1 year,[1] and the presence of five or more cotton wool spots is associated with a significantly increased risk of progression.[6] Note also that multiple cotton wool spots, particularly in a peripapillary distribution, may be associated with accelerated hypertension.

Intraretinal microvascular abnormalities (IRMAs)

Intraretinal microvascular abnormalities consist of vascular elements within the retina which branch with a frequency, number and angulation unlike that of normal retinal vessels. However, unlike retinal new vessels, which may also show abnormal branching patterns, IRMAs lie within the retina and therefore do not overlie retinal vessels or give rise to preretinal or vitreous haemorrhage. They may be located some distance to the side of veins, in contrast to retinal new vessels, which frequently arise directly from veins. In addition, the density of the inner retinal matrix through which they proliferate often gives rise to a more bizarre pattern than extraretinal new vessels. On fluorescein angiography IRMAs are seen at the edge of larger areas of capillary non-perfusion, branching into multiple hairpin-like loops. The tips of these loops are directed towards the centre of the non-perfused area, and stain with fluorescein, but do not leak like extraretinal new vessels. With increasingly widespread IRMAs, and thus capillary non-perfusion, the risk of developing proliferative retinopathy within a year increases fourfold.[1] In up to two-thirds of eyes in which IRMAs are identified, extraretinal neovascularization has already occurred.

Venous abnormalities

Beading is a term used to describe veins in which there is an irregular increase in calibre. It should be distinguished from the generalized vasodilatation of early retinopathy. As beading becomes more severe, the vein may take on the appearance of a string of sausages (venous segmentation) (*Fig. 1.2d,e*). Fluorescein angiography demonstrates the presence of extensive capillary non-perfusion in the area of beading, commonly extending up to the wall of the vein, which may stain or leak dye. Segmentation occurs in those parts of the vein's course in which confluent capillary non-perfusion extends up to the vein wall; as the vein passes into relatively better perfused regions, the wall takes on a more normal appearance. The extent of venous abnormality is an indicator of the proportion of the fundus in which capillary non-perfusion is present. With increasing severity of venous beading the risk of progression to proliferative retinopathy within 1 year is increased more than fourfold, and the presence of venous beading is a more powerful predictor of subsequent development of proliferative diabetic retinopathy than the presence of any other single abnormality.[1] Proliferative retinopathy may already be present in more than 50% of eyes affected by venous beading.

With localized occlusion of retinal veins, the blocked segment may be bypassed initially by multiple dilated capillary channels and later by single or duplicate larger collateral vessels (venous reduplication or venous loops). Such loops generally form at the margin of areas of non-perfused retina. Venous loops may also arise from traction associated with extraretinal fibrovascular proliferation on either the concavity or convexity of the loop, and may thus indicate that proliferative retinopathy is already present. In one study, venous looping or reduplication was invariably associated with the presence of proliferative retinopathy.

Other signs of capillary non-perfusion

Retinal ischaemia may be associated with retinal thinning, loss of the nerve fibre layer, and pigment epithelial disturbance. Vessels crossing such areas frequently become whitened. Fluorescein angiography, in addition to showing hypofluorescence in areas of capillary non-perfusion, may demonstrate hyperfluorescence from the margins of these areas. In addition, dye may leak from vessels passing through such areas, and stain the vessel wall. These signs may be of value if media opacity prevents angiographic resolution of capillary detail.

PROLIFERATIVE RETINOPATHY

Retinal neovascularization/new vessels elsewhere (NVE)

Retinal new vessels typically take the spider-like form of multiple radial loops arising from a central feeding vessel derived from a vein (*Fig. 1.3c*). They differ from IRMAs in that they overlie normal retinal vessels and may be associated with retrohyaloid or intragel haemorrhage. Signs of local ischaemia such as cluster haemorrhages, white vessels, venous beading, venous loops and IRMAs may also be present. They commonly arise posterior to the equator at the margins of areas of peripheral capillary non-perfusion. In eyes that have undergone vitrectomy or posterior vitreous detachment, they may appear as raspberry-like structures, usually in the area temporal to the macula, within the retinal arcades and often overlying venules or arterioles. Fluorescein angiography shows retinal new vessels as foci of increasing fluorescence, with dye leakage occurring most prominently at the growing tips of the vessels. Between 20 and 30% of eyes with neovascularization limited to retinal vessels will progress to optic disc neovascularization within a year. Without photocoagulation, the 2 year incidence of severe visual loss, defined as visual acuity ≤ 5/200, is approximately 7% in eyes with retinal new vessels and no retrohyaloid or intragel haemorrhage or mild retinal new vessels and haemorrhage. Eyes with moderate to severe retinal neovascularization associated with preretinal or vitreous haemorrhage, however, have a 30% incidence of severe visual loss over 2 years; this can be halved by panretinal photocoagulation.[7] Such eyes are said to possess Diabetic Retinopathy Study High Risk Characteristics (DRS-HRC).

Indications for panretinal photocoagulation in proliferative diabetic retinopathy: Diabetic Retinopathy Study High Risk Characteristics.[7]

- Optic disc neovascularization (NVD) of moderate to severe degree
- Optic disc neovascularization (NVD) of any degree if associated with vitreous or preretinal haemorrhage
- Retinal neovascularization (NVE) if associated with vitreous or preretinal haemorrhage

Optic disc neovascularization/new vessels disc (NVD)

Optic disc neovascularization appears as an abnormally branching vascular network arising from the optic disc. Preretinal and vitreous haemorrhage may be present, and signs of severe retinal ischaemia such as cluster haemorrhages, white vessels, venous beading, venous loops and IRMAs are commonly widespread. Progressively increasing hyperfluorescence of the neovascular complex, leakage of dye into the surrounding preretinal space, and widespread retinal capillary non-perfusion is demonstrable on fluorescein angiography. Approximately 50% of eyes with mild neovascularization of the optic disc progress to moderate or severe neovascularization within 1 year. The 2-year incidence of severe visual loss in eyes with optic disc neovascularization associated with vitreous or preretinal haemorrhage, and in eyes with moderate to severe optic disc neovascularization not associated with vitreous or preretinal haemorrhage, is between 26 and 37%.[7] Scatter photocoagulation approximately halves the incidence of severe visual loss in these eyes are which are also said to possess DRS-HRC.

Fibrous proliferation optic disc/elsewhere

Neovascular tissue has a fibrous component that tends to increase with time, and is visible as whitish, often longitudinally striated tissue with a tendency to contraction which may be apparent in the distortion or displacement of surrounding structures. It may occur around the optic disc (fibrous proliferation on the optic disc, FPD), along the vascular arcades (fibrous proliferation elsewhere, FPE), on the surface of the retina, or between the retina and the posterior hyaloid face. In some cases fibrous proliferation occurs without adverse effect and spontaneously arrests after an interval, but in others the contraction of fibrous bands between vitreous and retina may produce traction retinal detachment and other features of advanced diabetic eye disease.

ADVANCED DIABETIC EYE DISEASE

Preretinal haemorrhage

Preretinal haemorrhage (*Fig. 1.5b*) lies between the retina and the incompletely detached posterior hyaloid face, and may form a fluid level, giving a characteristic boat-shaped or flat-topped appearance. Although the associated new vessels may be obscured by blood, preretinal haemorrhage strongly suggests the occurrence of proliferative retinopathy, and the need for panretinal photocoagulation. Dense premacular haemorrhage is associated with a high risk of early macular traction detachment and is an indication for vitrectomy or Nd:YAG membranotomy.

Vitreous haemorrhage

Vitreous haemorrhage (*Fig. 1.5c*) usually arises from preretinal new vessels, and as such lies in front of the retina and may obscure the majority of fundus detail. B-scan ultrasound may be necessary to exclude associated retinal detachment. In eyes with localized or sparse vitreous haemorrhage, however, it may be possible to identify the neovascular complex from which the blood was derived. In most eyes with vitreous haemorrhage, panretinal photocoagulation is indicated, but if haemorrhage persistently precludes this, vitrectomy may be required, particularly in the insulin-dependent diabetic. It is important to note, however, that vitreous haemorrhage may also result from retinal vascular avulsion, vitreous contraction in the presence of inactive new vessels, or retinal tears.

Retinal detachment

Traction retinal detachment appears as a greyish, concave elevation of the retina, from the apex of which fibrous bands may be seen to connect to the posterior hyaloid face (*Fig. 1.6b*). Peripheral traction detachments may remain relatively localized with minimal impact on vision. If the macula is involved, however, marked central visual loss occurs, and if macular function is acceptable, vitrectomy may be undertaken to reattach the retina. Should tractional forces cause a retinal tear (*Fig. 1.6c*), any resulting combined traction-rhegmatogenous detachment may be recognized by a change in the configuration of the detached retina from concave to convex, but if media opacity is present, B-scan ultrasound may be required for diagnosis. Vitrectomy is appropriate in eyes with the prospect of acceptable postoperative visual function.

Neovascular glaucoma

Iris neovascularization (rubeosis iridis) may result from severe widespread retinal ischaemia or extensive traction retinal detachment. As a rule it spreads peripherally from the pupil margin, arborizes over iris stroma, and then encroaches on the anterior chamber drainage angle, obstructing the trabecular meshwork, and producing a rise in acute intraocular pressure, corneal decompensation pain and visual loss. It is important to recognize, however, that the drainage angle appears to be involved first in around 10% cases.

MACULOPATHY

Macular exudate

Certain patterns of macular exudate deposition are recognizable. In focal maculopathy, exudates are typically arranged in a complete or incomplete circle around the leaking microvascular abnormality (*Fig. 1.9b*) (circinate maculopathy). Exudate is less prominent in more diffuse forms of maculopathy and may be most marked at the periphery of the diffusely oedematous macula. Large plaques of exudate centred on the fovea may be seen in long-standing macular oedema and cause marked visual loss, and a combination of peripheral and central plaques may occur. Exudate may be particularly prominent in renal failure.

Indications for macular laser treatment: Early Treatment Diabetic Retinopathy Study Clinically Significant Macular Oedema.[8]

- Thickening of the retina at or within 500 μm of the centre of the macula
- Hard exudates at or within 500 μm of the centre of the macula, if associated with thickening of the adjacent retina
- A zone or zones of retinal thickening one disc area or larger any part of which is within one disc diameter of the centre of the macula

Retinal thickening

Intraretinal oedema is manifest as thickening of the retina. Macular thickening correlates well with visual loss, is the principal feature of clinically significant macular oedema, and as such represents the principal indication for laser treatment. However, its identification may be difficult, requiring high-magnification stereoscopic evaluation either of the retina or of high-quality retinal photographs, and therefore clear ocular media, appropriate equipment and optimal examination conditions. It is hoped that newer methods of retinal evaluation such as optical coherence tomography and retinal thickness analysis will alleviate this problem. In relation to treatment, the key signs of diabetic maculopathy are those relating to microvascular leakage from microaneurysms and/or dilated capillaries, which are well visualized on fluorescein angiography, but it is important to recognize that hyperfluorescence is not invariably associated with retinal thickening. The incidence of significant visual loss in patients with clinically significant macular oedema is approximately halved by appropriate laser treatment.[8]

RETINOPATHY VARIANTS

Renal disease

A characteristic pattern of retinopathy may be seen in renal failure, dominated by massive posterior pole exudation. Profound visual loss as a result of deposition of a lipid plaque at the fovea is a common sequel, and the response to macular laser is typically poor. In addition, significant capillary non-perfusion may arise from acute arteriolar occlusion in association with renovascular hypertension, and consequent proliferative retinopathy may also prove refractory to laser. Renal transplantation, and to a lesser extent dialysis may produce a marked improvement in retinopathy, but visual recovery may be poor in eyes with macular pigment epithelial scarring secondary to plaque exudate.

Pregnancy

Pregnancy is associated with significant progression of retinopathy,[9] most commonly after the 16th week of pregnancy. Progression to proliferative retinopathy is commoner if at the onset of pregnancy retinopathy is more severe or glycaemic control poor, or if marked improvement in glycaemic control occurs in the first trimester.[3] Regular review and prompt treatment of sight-threatening retinopathy is essential, and improvement in glycaemic control should ideally occur prior to the onset of pregnancy.

Hypertension

The UK Prospective Diabetes Study recently documented[10] that in type II diabetics, tight control of blood pressure (below 150/85) reduced by 37% the risk of microvascular complications (especially the need for photocoagulation), and reduced by 47% the risk of doubling of the visual angle over a 9-year period. These findings make the recognition of fundus signs of hypertension of paramount importance in the diabetic. These include signs of acute hypertension such as peripapillary cotton wool spots, optic disc swelling, retinal arteriolar occlusion, and choroidal signs such as Elschnig spots, Siegrist streaks and serous retinal elevation, and more chronic signs, such as arteriolar attenuation, microaneurysms, haemorrhages, arteriovenous crossing changes, and alterations in retinal arteriolar reflex.

REFERENCES

1. Early Treatment Diabetic Retinopathy Study Research Group, Fundus photographic risk factors for progression of diabetic retinopathy. ETDRS Report no. 12, *Ophthalmology* (1991) **98**:823–33.
2. Early Treatment Diabetic Retinopathy Study Research Group, Grading diabetic retinopathy from stereoscopic color fundus photographs–an extension of the modified Airlie House classification. ETDRS Report no. 10, *Ophthalmology* (1991) **98**:786–806.
3. Chew EY, Mills JL, Metzger BE et al, Metabolic control and progression of retinopathy. The Diabetes in Early Pregnancy Study. National Institute of Child Health and Human Development Diabetes in Early Pregnancy Study, *Diabetes Care* 1995; **18**:631–7.
4. Kohner EM, Sleightholm M, Does microaneurysm count reflect severity of early diabetic retinopathy? *Ophthalmology* (1986) **93**:586–9.
5. Roy MS, Rick ME, Higgins KE, McCulloch JC, Retinal cotton-wool spots: an early finding in diabetic retinopathy? *Arch Ophthalmol* (1986) **70**:772–8.
6. Kohner EM, The natural history of diabetic

retinopathy, *J R Coll Physicians Lond* (1972) **6**:259–70.

7. Diabetic Retinopathy Study Research Group, Photocoagulation treatment of proliferative diabetic retinopathy: the second report of diabetic retinopathy study findings, *Ophthalmology* (1978) **85**:82–106.
8. Early Treatment Diabetic Retinopathy Study Research Group, Photocoagulation for diabetic macular edema, ETDRS Report no. 4, *Int Ophthalmol Clin* (1987) **27**:265–72.
9. Klein BE, Moss SE, Klein R, Effect of pregnancy on progression of diabetic retinopathy, *Diabetes Care* (1990) **13**:34–40.
10. Turner R, Holman R, Stratton S et al, Tight blood pressure control and the risk of macrovascular and microvascular complications in type 2 diabetes: UKPDS 38, *Br Med J* (1998) **317**:703–13.

2 Diabetic maculopathy

Louis MT Collum and David E Wallace

INTRODUCTION

Diabetic maculopathy can be defined as oedema of the retina, with or without associated hard exudates, involving the macular area. This may be compounded by the presesnce of ischaemia, making the condition difficult to treat. It is the commonest cause of visual loss in the diabetic population, including both insulin- and non-insulin-dependent patients.[1,2] Early treatment of maculopathy by laser photocoagulation is essential and has been shown to reduce the incidence of visual loss significantly.[3]

EPIDEMIOLOGY

The incidence of macular oedema is important in determining the health care needs of a population, as it is a significant risk factor for the development of visual loss.[4] In a large population-based study, macular oedema located within one disc diameter of the centre of the macula occurred in 9% of the diabetic population. Forty per cent of these had central macular involvement. For those patients who had been diabetics for more than 20 years, the prevalence of macular oedema increased to approximately 25%.[5]

A number of risk factors for the development of macular oedema have been identified. Older age at diagnosis, male sex and poorer control of blood sugar (higher $HgbA_{1c}$ levels than average) have been associated with an increased risk of clinically significant macular oedema in patients with type I diabetes.[6] In both younger- and older-onset diabetics the presence of a higher $HgbA_{1c}$, longer duration of diabetes and more severe retinopathy at baseline examination were associated with an increased incidence of the condition.[7]

The prevalence of macular oedema is strongly associated with the severity of retinopathy, occurring in 3% of eyes with non-proliferative retinopathy, in 38% of eyes with moderate to severe non-proliferative retinopathy and in 71% of eyes with proliferative diabetic retinopathy.[8] These studies underline the importance of glycaemic control in the prevention of clinically significant macular oedema. Population-based studies,[7] in contrast to clinic-based studies,[1] suggest that the incidence of macular oedema is greater in younger- than in older-onset diabetics. However, patients encountered in the clinic with macular oedema are most likely to be older-onset diabetics, due to their greater frequency in the population. This group of maturity-onset diabetics represents the majority of patients with diabetes and they are more likely to have significantly impaired vision with macular oedema. Fifty per cent of older-onset patients with macular oedema had vision worse than 20/40, compared with 20% of younger onset diabetic patients.[2] They are also more likely to have coexisting pathology, such as cataract, macular degeneration and glaucoma, when compared to younger-onset diabetics. In contrast to cataract and glaucoma, there is no definitive association between diabetes and age-related maculopathy.[9]

Therefore, diabetic macular oedema is an important cause of legal blindness[10] and also of partial visual impairment. This can result in occupational difficulties for patients, which are not represented in blindness statistics.

PATHOGENESIS

The exact cause of diabetic microvascular disease is unknown. The two characteristic features are focal intraretinal capillary closure and increased retinal vascular permeability. Capillary occlusion may include the perifoveolar capillaries, resulting in the development of an ischaemic maculopathy. Diabetic maculopathy may present as focal or diffuse retinal thickening or oedema, with or without the presence of hard exudates.[11]

Starling's law is the general principle which describes the passage of fluid between intravascular and interstitial components in tissue.[12] The five main pathways for oedema formation in the body are:

1. High capillary pressure.
2. Increased capillary permeability.
3. High negative tissue oncotic pressure.
4. Low blood oncotic pressure (protein loss).
5. Lymphatic blockage.

Lymphatic blockage is not applicable to the retina as the eye is devoid of lymphatic circulation. Therefore, the retina is more vulnerable to oedema than other tissues. Kristinsson proposed that these pathways for oedema formation be applied to the eye, to further our understanding of the pathogenesis of macular oedema.[13]

Histologically, macular oedema is the presence of extracellular fluid within the retina. Defects in the retinal capillary endothelium are associated with a breakdown of the inner blood–retinal barrier in the sensory retina. This allows the passage of macromolecules and ions from retinal capillaries into the retina, resulting in macular oedema.[14] However, it is suggested that not all the intraretinal oedema comes from retinal vessels, but that abnormalities in the retinal pigmented epithelium, the outer blood–retinal barrier, may also contribute by leakage through retinal pigmented epithelial cells.[15] Bresnick[8] and Patel[16] have both proposed a role for hyperperfusion in the pathogenesis of macular oedema. Retinal vasodilation leads to increased capillary pressure, resulting in retinal oedema or hard exudate formation. Hypertension is associated with diabetic maculopathy in epidemiological studies.[17] Increased systemic blood pressure combined with impaired autoregulatory mechanisms may result in increased capillary pressure. The treatment of hypertension medically can be associated with a decrease in macular oedema.[8]

Increased permeability as a result of blood–retinal barrier breakdown is a major factor in the pathogenesis of macular oedema. The degree of permeability has been shown to be related to progression of diabetic retinopathy.[18]

The accumulation of osmotically active substances in the extracellular space, such as hard exudates, occurs in diabetic maculopathy. Ferris and Patz[14] postulate that these substances could cause a negative oncotic pressure, causing an additional influx of fluid into the extravascular space, resulting in retinal oedema. However, in eyes with diffuse oedema, hard exudates are much less prominent. Therefore, the exact role of negative oncotic pressure in the pathogenesis of macular oedema is unknown.

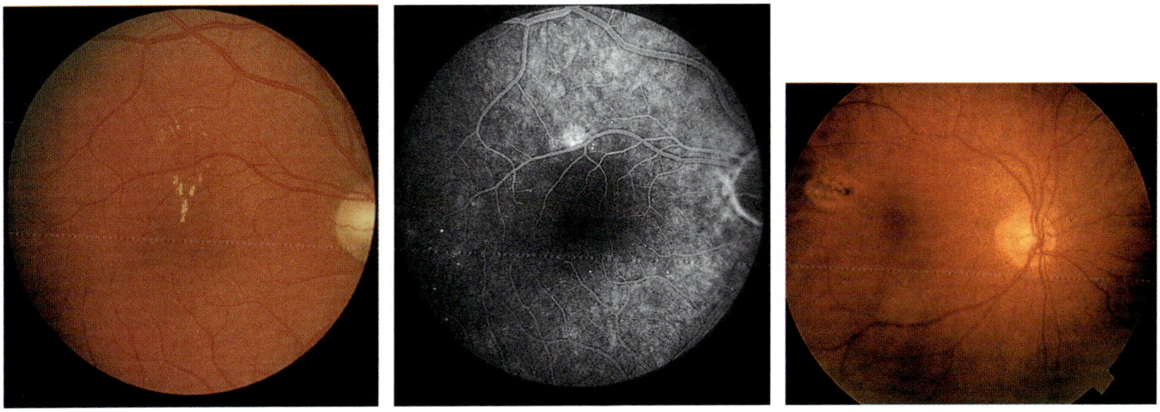

(a) (b) (c)

Figure 2.1
Focal maculopathy. A 27-year-old insulin-dependent diabetic presented for examination with a visual acuity of 6/6 unaided in the right eye. Fundal examination revealed clinically significant macular oedema with hard exudate encroaching on the centre of the macula (a). Fluorescein angiography confirmed the area of leakage (b). Photocoagulation was performed which resulted in resolution of the exudate (c).

Low blood oncotic pressure occurs in the nephrotic syndrome, which is seen in diabetes. Hypoproteinaemia results in decreased oncotic pressure of blood and may contribute to the pathophysiology of macular oedema.

CLASSIFICATION

Diabetic maculopathy can be divided into several subgroups, reflecting the underlying pathological process.

1. Focal maculopathy.
2. Diffuse maculopathy.
3. Ischaemic maculopathy.
4. Mixed maculopathy.

Each subgroup has specific clinical features. The pattern of each disease will also differ and thus require individual treatment approaches.

Focal maculopathy consists of clusters of microaneurysms or dilated retinal capillaries, located within areas of focal retinal oedema. These are often surrounded by rings of hard exudate. Leaking microaneurysms are well defined by fluorescein angiography. They may be located in the deep or superficial capillary networks of the retina. Leakage results in a flow of fluid towards normal capillaries, where resorption occurs. At these distal sites lipoproteins are deposited, which are seen as hard exudates (*Fig. 2.1a–c*).

Diffuse macular oedema results from a generalized breakdown of the blood–retinal barrier. The extent of oedema varies between patients. It may occur centrally or involve the whole of the posterior pole. Cystoid macular oedema is often seen with diffuse maculopathy (*Fig. 2.2a,b*). On fluorescein angiography, the capillary bed is diffusely dilated, with many widened intercapillary spaces. Hard exudate is usually absent and retinal microaneurysms are few in number. Diffuse macular

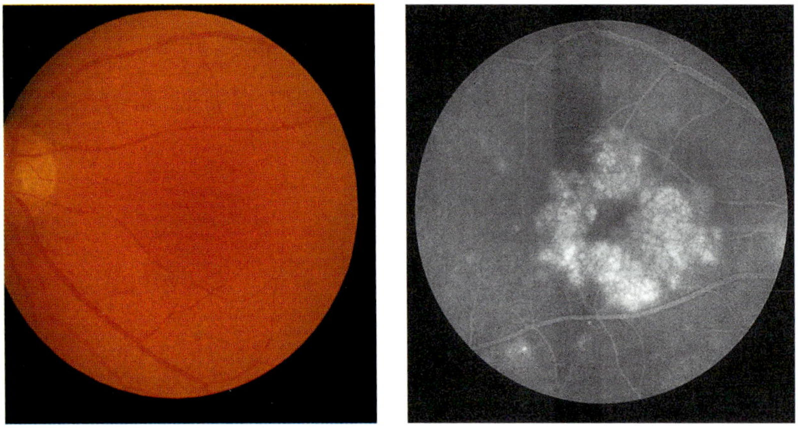

(a) (b)

Figure 2.2
Cystoid macular oedema. Diffuse maculopathy may have a cystoid appearance (a) as seen in this example of the right eye of a 69-year-old insulin-dependent diabetic, with vision reduced to 6/18. Fluorescein angiography confirmed the polycystic pattern of dye leakage (b).

oedema is more common in maturity-onset diabetics and may be associated with systemic factors, such as hypertension or severe fluid retention.

Macular ischaemia occurs where capillary closure involves the macular region. On close inspection, features of capillary non-perfusion may be evident on clinical examination. These include the presence of small white capillaries in the foveal region, deep haemorrhages and the presence of cotton wool spots at the posterior pole. Evidence of widespread ischaemia, such as the presence of neovascularization, can indicate that the ischaemic process can also involve the macula (*Fig. 2.3a–c*). Fluorescein angiography shows capillary closure, with widening of the central foveal avascular zone. It occurs more commonly in non-insulin-dependent diabetic patients. Unfortunately, macular ischaemia is often a complicating factor in diabetic maculopathy, leading to a poor visual prognosis.

Although it is possible to subdivide diabetic maculopathy into the above groups, many eyes show a combination of these features.[8] The pattern of involvement may not be evident until fluorescein angiography is performed (*Fig. 2.4a,b*).

DIAGNOSIS

The early detection of macular oedema is important so that referral and appropriate treatment may be given to prevent visual loss. Clinically significant macular oedema, as defined in the Early Treatment Diabetic Retinopathy Study (ETDRS),[3] is best detected using slit lamp biomicroscopy. A 78- or 90-dioptre lens is commonly used, but in borderline cases the use of a contact lens is more effective.

Kinyoun et al[19] examined the interobserver agreement in the assessment of macular oedema between retinal specialists, using ophthalmoloscopy and contact lens biomicroscrepy, and photographic graders, using 30° stereoscopic colour fundus photographs. In detecting hard exudate, the two methods were comparable. For eyes with questionable or no retinal thickening contact lens fundus biomicroscopy was superior to photographic grading or assessment with a non-contact lens.

Fluorescein angiography allows accurate and reproducible classification of diabetic retinopathy and identifies sources of leakage in diabetic

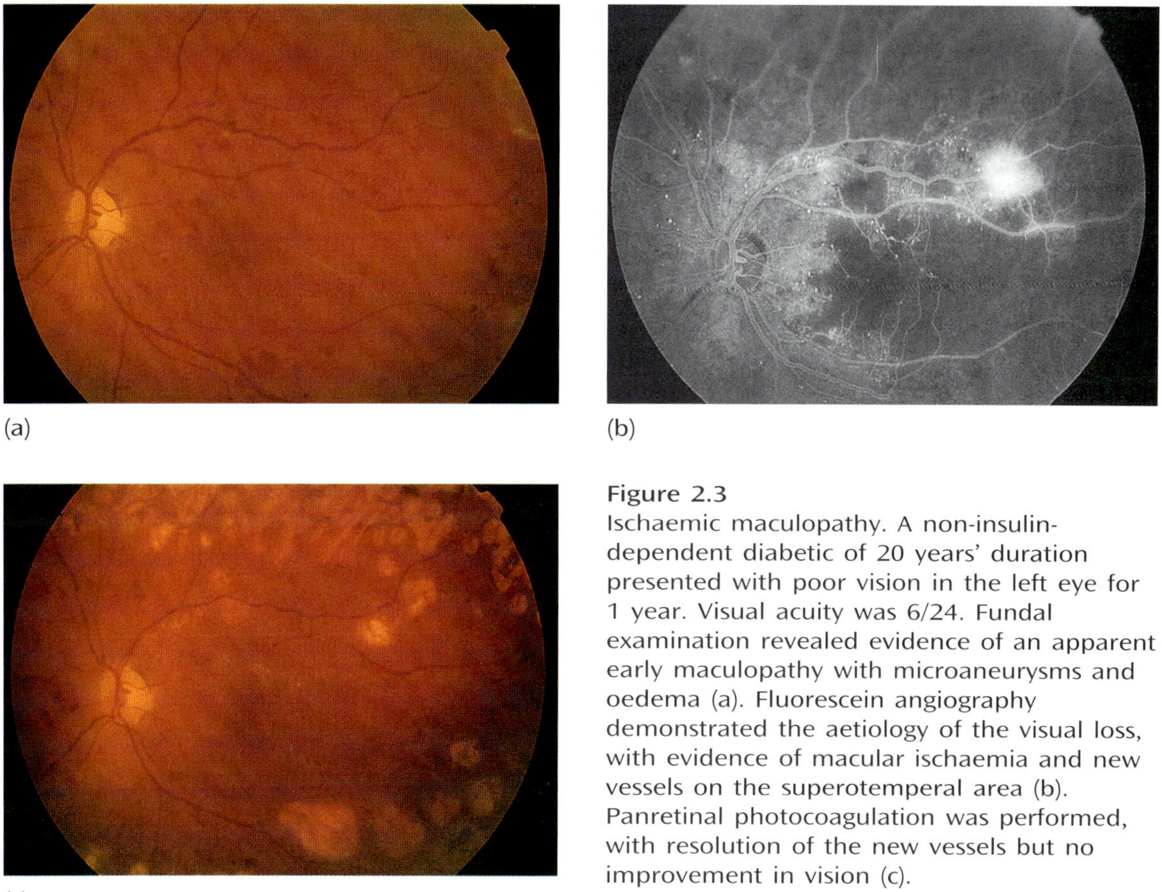

(a) (b) (c)

Figure 2.3
Ischaemic maculopathy. A non-insulin-dependent diabetic of 20 years' duration presented with poor vision in the left eye for 1 year. Visual acuity was 6/24. Fundal examination revealed evidence of an apparent early maculopathy with microaneurysms and oedema (a). Fluorescein angiography demonstrated the aetiology of the visual loss, with evidence of macular ischaemia and new vessels on the superotemporal area (b). Panretinal photocoagulation was performed, with resolution of the new vessels but no improvement in vision (c).

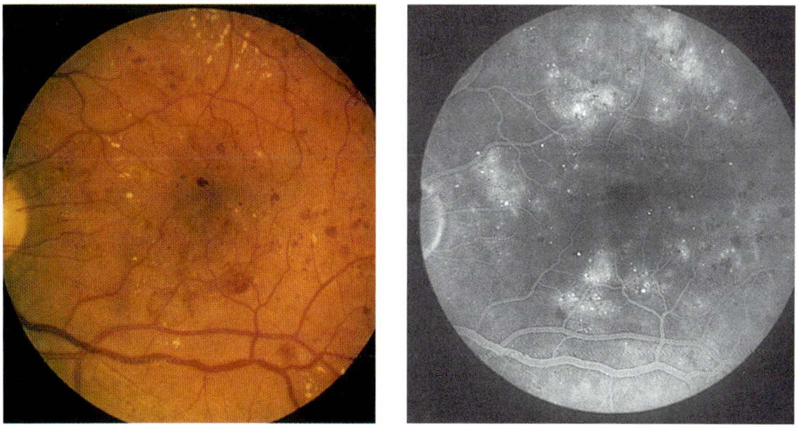

(a) (b)

Figure 2.4
Mixed maculopathy. A non-insulin-dependent diabetic, of 9 years' duration, presented with gradual loss of vision in his left eye to 6/36. Fundal examination revealed a small amount of exudate in the macular area (a). Fluorescein angiography outlined the responsible microaneurysms but also demonstrated an ischaemic component, with enlargement of the foveal avascular zone (b), accounting for the visual loss.

maculopathy.[20] In most studies, fluorescein angiography was performed before and after treatment in the management of diabetic maculopathy.[21,22] Routine fluorescein angiograms are not required in all cases of diabetic maculopathy, as a diagnosis of clinically signficant macular oedema can be made on clinical examination.

In a study where laser photocoagulation was directed at clinically identifiable leaking microvascular lesions, posttreatment fluorescein angiograms suggested that there was satisfactory control of the disease.[23] However, in the cases of mixed maculopathy, fluorescein angiography can play an important role in defining areas requiring treatment and demonstrating areas of ischaemia. Moreover, if leaking persists after photocoagulation, in the absence of a readily identifiable source or focus of leakage, angiography can play a role in identifyng a refractory area. Also in patients with nuclear sclerosis where visualization of the fundus can be difficult, angiography has a role to play in detecting the areas of leakage.

MANAGEMENT

In determining the clinical guidelines for the treatment of diabetic maculopathy, there are a number of issues to be addressed:

1. What treatment is beneficial?
2. Who should be treated?
3. When should they be treated?

Laser photocoagulation treatment for diabetic maculopathy has been reported to have varying success rates using different treatment and wavelength modalities.[22,24–26] However, the majority of these reports have not provided definitive evidence of treatment success, owing to an accumulation of factors, such as small numbers in studies, lack of randomization and different stages of the disease at initiation of therapy. The ETDRS is a multicentre, randomized clinical trial which was designed to evaluate the benefits of photocoagulation and aspirin treatment in the management of patients with non-proliferative or early proliferative diabetic retinopathy.[3,21] It specifically addressed the question of the effectiveness of photocoagulation in the treatment of diabetic macular oedema. The study showed that after 3 years of follow-up, 12% of eyes which had been assigned to treatment of macular oedema had experienced significant visual loss, as opposed to 24% of eyes that had not received treatment. Significant visual loss was defined as a loss of three or more lines on the ETDRS visual acuity chart, equivalent to a doubling of the visual angle. Therefore, the prompt photocoagulation of clinically significant macular oedema reduces the visual loss by half in a subgroup of eyes with mild to moderate non-proliferative diabetic retinopathy (NPDR) and macular oedema.

Clinically significant macular oedema

The ETDRS defines clinically significant macular oedema as:

1. Thickening of the retina at or within 500 μm of the centre of the macula.
2. Hard exudate at or within 500 μm of the centre of the macula, associated with thickening of the adjacent retina.
3. A zone or zones of retinal thickening one disc area or larger, any part of which is within one disc diameter of the centre of the macula.

Eyes with clinically significant macular oedema showed a positive significant treatment effect after 8 months and the effect of treatment continued to remain significant thereafter. Eyes with less severe oedema at baseline did not show a significant treatment effect for at least 3 years. Therefore, the presence or absence of clinically significant macular oedema is the most important factor in deciding whom to treat. It is recommended that laser treatment for eyes with clinically significant macular oedema be undertaken without delay owing to the proven effectiveness of this treatment.[21]

The timing of treatment should coincide with the onset of clinically significant macular oedema. Prior to this development, the risk of visual loss is low. If there are early signs of diabetic macular oedema, but no clinically significant macular oedema, a period of close observation is preferable, as to date no evidence of increased benefit of early treatment is proven. This is especially relevant if the centre of the macula is involved, with increased risk of damage from direct treatment close to the macula or migration from treatment scars.[27] It is advised that patients with early macular oedema should be reviewed at 4–6 month intervals.

Treatment has been shown to be beneficial, regardless of the level of visual acuity at baseline. It is also easier to preserve visual acuity than to regain losses in visual acuity. This underlies the importance of screening, so that beneficial treatment can be applied at the onset of clinically significant macular oedema, thus preventing visual loss.

As previously discussed, the different subgroups of diabetic maculopathy have specific features and different rates of progress. Hence the treatment requirements of each subtype differ. Treatment may be applied as:

- direct focal treatment to leaking microaneurysms
- modified grid treatment for larger areas of leakage
- grid photocoagulation for diffuse macular oedema.

The ETDRS has provided a clinically proven basis for the treatment of diabetic macular oedema and it has been widely adopted.

Preparation for laser treatment

Before undergoing laser therapy patients must be fully informed regarding the treatment. This information should include details of anaesthesia, the use of contact lenses during treatment, the sensation experienced during treatment and possible side effects of treatment. Proper informed consent can thus be obtained.

The best corrected visual acuity must be recorded prior to treatment. The patient's pupil may be dilated with a combination of tropicamide 1% and phenylephrine 2.5% eye drops. Most procedures can be performed with topical anaesthesia and the application of a contact lens. If pain is significant, retrobulbar or peribulbar anaesthesia may be required. This has the added advantage of providing akinesia as well as anaesthesia, which is of benefit in applying laser treatment close to the fovea.

The fundus contact lens permits visualization of the posterior pole and is the lens of choice for treating macular lesions. The central aperture of the Goldmann three–mirror contact lens may also be used for treating lesions at the posterior pole. Non-contact lenses including the 78- and 90-dioptre lenses may also be used, although the fundus contact lens is preferable in terms of clarity and the orientation of the image. Laser treatment can result in complications, often due to lack of experience and loss of orientation (*Figs 2.5 and 2.6*).

Treatment of focal maculopathy

In focal maculopathy there are well-defined areas of leakage which may be located at or away from the fovea. If located at the fovea the amount of visual disturbance is related to the degree of retinal thickening and the amount of exudate

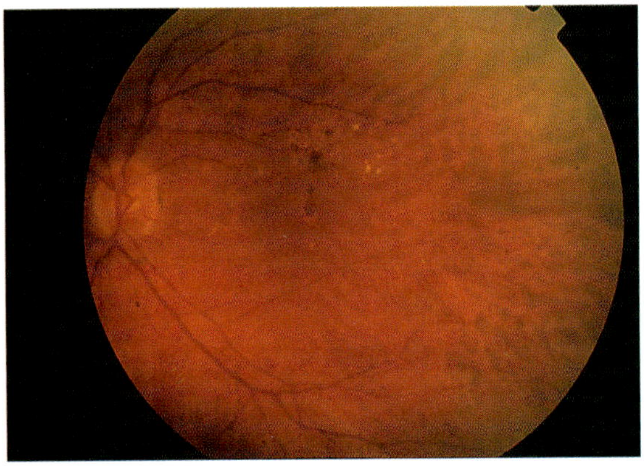

Figure 2.5
Foveal burn. Inadvertent foveal burn during treatment of focal maculopathy in a 71-year-old non-insulin-dependent diabetic, with vision reduced from 6/6 to 6/36.

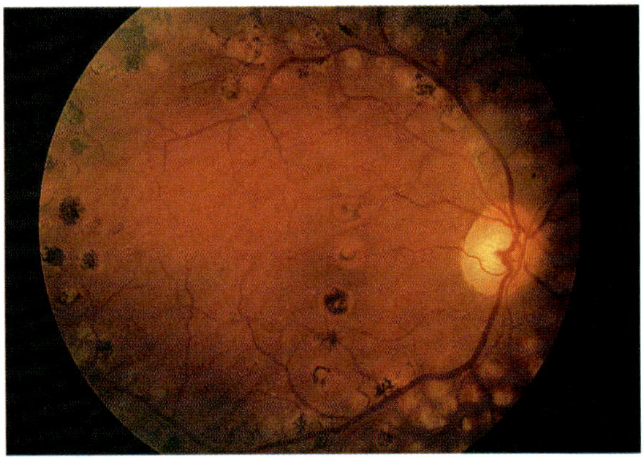

Figure 2.6
Loss of orientation during panretinal photocoagulation in an insulin-dependent diabetic with proliferative retinopathy. Fortunately, visual acuity was unaffected.

present. If the fovea is not involved, central vision may be normal, the patient may be asymptomatic or there may be fluctuations in visual acuity.

The aim of treatment in focal maculopathy is to prevent leakage from microvascular lesions.[21] This allows resorption of hard exudate and fluid. In most cases lesions are well defined and angiography is not required. However, if treatment is to be applied close to the fovea, fluorescein angiography is recommended.

Treatment requirements for focal maculopathy are:

- argon green
- spot size–50–100 μm
- length of exposure–0.1 seconds
- power–sufficient to produce a minimal reaction (blanching of the retinal pigmented epithelium (RPE) or microaneurysm).

In treating focal maculopathy, microaneurysms are treated directly. The aim is to produce a darkening or blanching of the lesion. Treatment is applied to lesions up to two disc diameters from the centre of the fovea and treatment closer than 500 μm is not required initially. Treatment of microaneurysms greater then two disc diameters from the centre of the macula may be required, if associated with hard exudates or retinal thickening extending into the treatment zone (*Fig. 2.7a–c*).

If there are large circinate rings present, it is beneficial to apply a modified grid treatment using a larger spot size. Treatment requirements are:

- argon green
- spot size–200 μm
- length of exposure–0.1 seconds
- power–sufficient to produce a minimal reaction (blanching of the RPE).

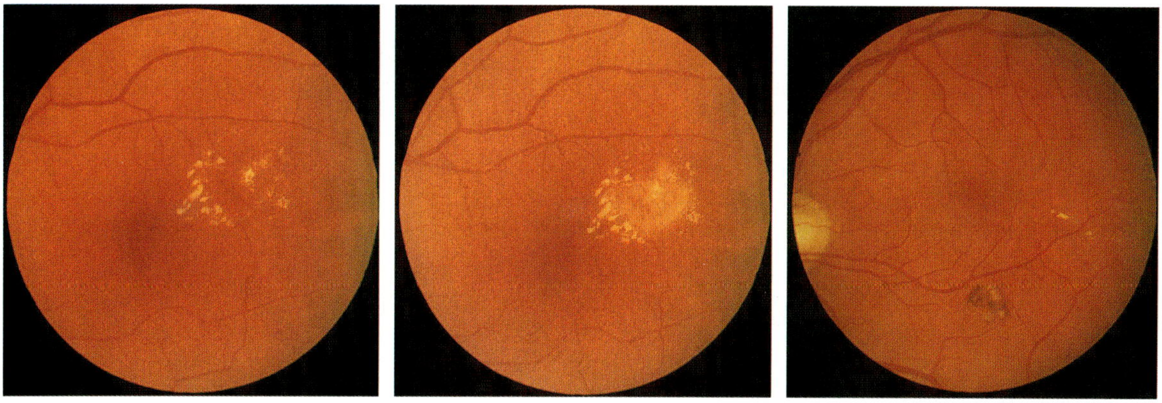

(a) (b) (c)

Figure 2.7
Focal maculopathy. A 69-year-old non-insulin-dependent diabetic presented for annual examination with vision of 6/6 in the right eye. She was noted to have a ring of exudate in the macular area (a). Photocoagulation was performed (b) (immediately posttreatment). Resolution of exudate occurred in 6 months (c).

Therefore, in the presence of a combination of the above features, a combination of focal and modified grid treatment may be required. A patient whose fovea is not involved has the best prognosis. Unfortunately, if long-standing foveal involvement is present with oedema or hard exudate, laser treatment may result in resolution of the maculopathy, but the vision is likely to remain poor due to irreversible damage.

Patients should be re-evaluated 1 month after treatment, when any additional leakage should be treated. It is important to note that the amount of exudate may appear to increase initially due to the resorption of retinal oedema and that resorption of exudate may take up to 1 year to be complete.

Treatment of diffuse maculopathy

Diffuse oedema occurs secondary to diffuse leakage from capillaries. In these patients hard exudate and retinal microaneurysms are not a significant feature. Patients typically present complaining of a recent decrease in vision, which is usually bilateral. Visual acuity is commonly 20/80 or less and diffuse oedema is more common in maturity onset diabetics and may occur secondary to panretinal photocoagulation. The extent and degree of oedema is variable.

Treatment of diffuse oedema is by a grid pattern of laser application.[21,28] A burn of mild to moderate intensity is applied to the oedematous area, while avoiding the fovea. Burns can be placed on the papillomacular bundle, but not closer than 500 μm to the centre of the macula. It is best to leave a space of one burn width between each application. However, if there is less intensive leakage the treatment can be spread over a wider area. Treatment is extended in all directions up to two disc diameters from the centre of the macula or to the border of existing panretinal photocoagulation treatment. One eye should be treated at a time.

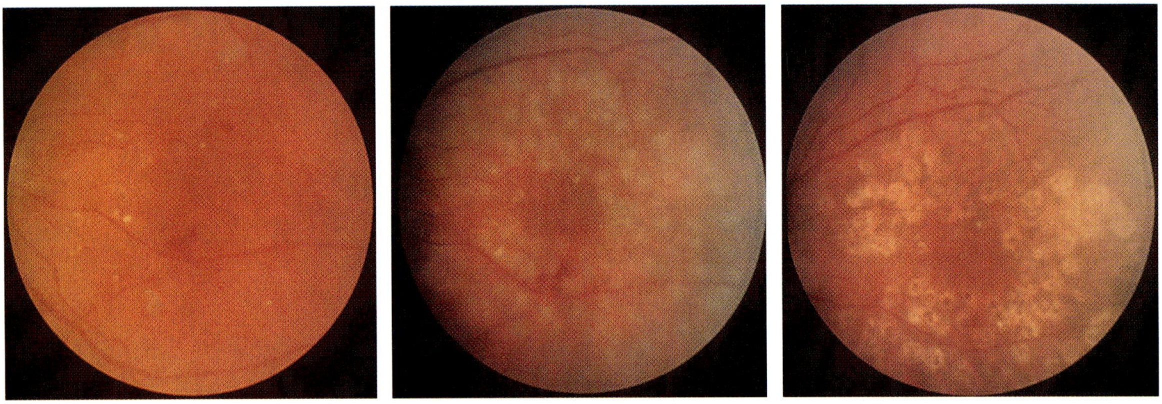

(a) (b) (c)

Figure 2.8
Diffuse maculopathy. A 63-year-old non-insulin-dependent diabetic presented with visual acuity reduced to 6/18 in the left eye. There was marked diffuse maculopathy (a), (b) and the patient underwent grid laser therapy (c), with stabilization of vision.

Treatment requirements for diffuse maculopathy are:

- argon green (alternative: krypton)
- spot size–50–200 μm
- length of exposure–0.1 seconds
- power–sufficient to produce a minimal reaction (blanching of the RPE).

Grid therapy for diffuse macular oedema has a variable response. The oedema may resolve, but if irreversible damage has occurred prior to laser application, visual acuity may be unchanged. Another reason for poor vision after treatment can be the persistence of a central area of oedema (*Fig. 2.8a–c* and *Fig. 2.9a–c*).

A side effect of this treatment is the development of paracentral scotomas and the patient may notice a haze over the treated eye. Most of these subjective complaints disappear with time but can be demonstrated to persist on visual field testing.[28] The importance of using argon green instead of shorter wavelengths is to reduce the danger of inner retinal damage due to absorption by the macular pigment, xanthophyll. Krypton red may be more effective than argon green in the treatment of diffuse macular oedema by grid photocoagulation.[29]

Treatment of ischaemic diabetic maculopathy

Ischaemic diabetic maculopathy occurs secondary to non-perfusion of macular capillaries. It may be accompanied by oedema, if there is associated incompetence of residual capillaries. Unfortunately, no effective treatment for this condition has been developed.

Treatment of mixed maculopathy

Mixed maculopathy is not uncommon and exhibits features of all three groups. Visual acuity on presentation of these patients is usually poor. The different components of maculopathy are best assessed with fluorescein angiography (*Fig. 2.10a,b*). Despite a combination of focal and grid treatment, the prognosis in these patients is invariably poor.

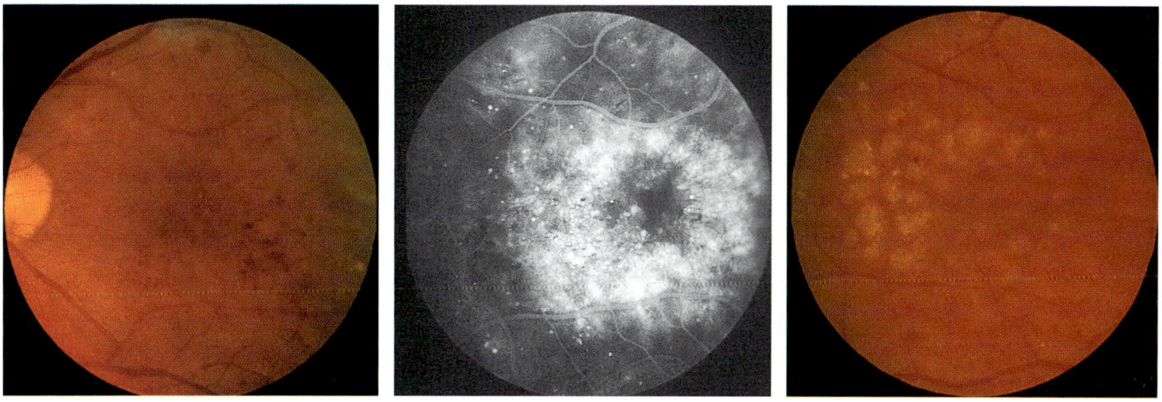

(a) (b) (c)

Figure 2.9
Diffuse maculopathy. A 57-year-old non-insulin-dependent diabetic presented with reduced visual acuity in the right eye. Fundal examination revealed a diffuse maculopathy (a), which was confirmed on fluorescein angiography (b), showing many areas of leakage. Despite adequate grid treatment (c) and resolution of oedema, the vision did not improve.

FOLLOW-UP

Appropriate follow-up of patients with diabetic maculopathy is essential. Patients are reviewed at 4 weeks and no treatment is added at this stage unless obvious treatable lesions have been missed. The next assessment is performed at 4 months and if clinically significant macular oedema is present, re-treatment is advised at this stage.

SPECIAL CONSIDERATIONS

Pregnancy

Pregnancy has been shown to influence the natural history of diabetic retinopathy, leading to worsening of this condition.[30–32] In the absence of any baseline retinopathy at the start of pregnancy, the risk of development of background retinopathy is approximately 25% of patients,[32,33] with small risk of visual loss.

Background diabetic retinopathy present at the start of pregnancy often worsens during the second trimester.[34] This can be associated with the development of macular oedema, especially in pregnant women with proteinurea and hypertension.[35] Macular oedema has a significant ischaemic component in these patients and may be associated with the development of proliferative retinopathy. Panretinal photocoagulation for proliferative retinopathy may also worsen the maculopathy.[35]

Therefore, an ophthalmological examination should be performed in young diabetic women who are considering pregnancy. If necessary, appropriate treatment can be applied for retinopathy and additional factors, such as hypertension, controlled before conception. If minimal retinopathy is present at the start of pregnancy, fundal examination every 3 months is sufficient unless visual symptoms occur.

If background retinopathy is present, baseline fundal photography is of benefit so that progres-

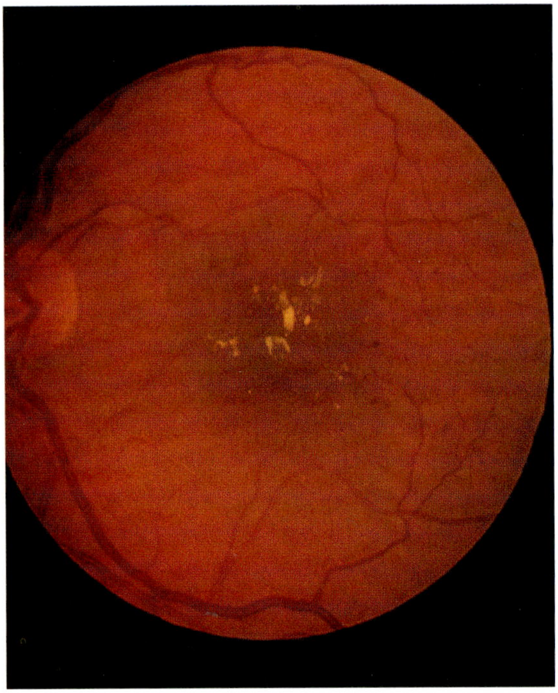

(a)

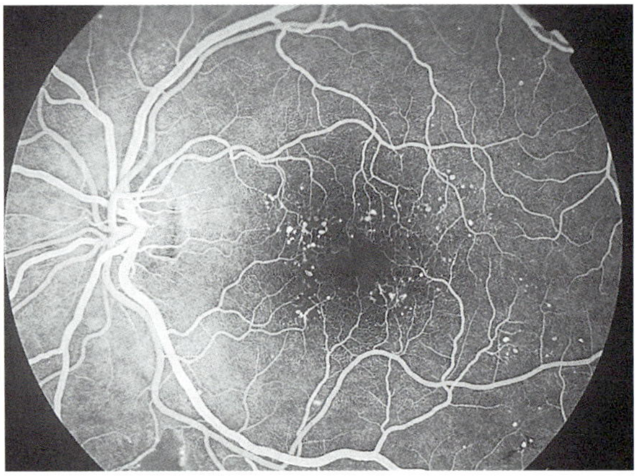

(b)

Figure 2.10
Mixed maculopathy. Fundal photography shows microaneurysms and haemorrhages, with small amounts of hard exudate involving the macular region (a). Fluorescein angiography demonstrates multiple areas of leakage with evidence of ischaemia (enlargement of the foveal avascular zone) (b).

sion can be detected. Ocular examination should be performed in the first and second timesters, with monthly examinations in the third. If progression is detected, examination at 2-weekly intervals may be required. Fluorescein angiography may be of value in the management of maculopathy in pregnant diabetic patients, where vision is threatened. It allows accurate assessment of capillary non-perfusion and the detection of early neovascularization. Though there is no evidence of this procedure having any detrimental effect on the developing fetus,[36] it should be avoided in pregnancy unless there is significant visual compromise.

Cataract surgery

Diabetics are at an increased risk of developing cataracts compared to non-diabetics. Cataracts are the leading cause of legal blindness in older-onset diabetics and are second only to proliferative diabetic retinopathy in the younger-onset group.[2] Cataract surgery in diabetics is associated with an increased incidence of postoperative complications, including postoperative progression of retinopathy, macular oedema and iris neovascularization.[37]

In a meta-analysis of visual acuity following cataract surgery, Dowler et al found that maculopathy prior to surgery was six times more likely to be associated with a postoperative visual acuity of less than 6/12.[38] The poorer outcome of diabetics compared to non-diabetics may be related to the difficulty of recognition and treatment of maculopathy prior to surgery owing to the presence of cataract and/or the exacerbation of pre-existing maculopathy after surgery. The exact mechanisms responsible for the worsening of maculopathies are unknown, but may be related to increased permeability of the abnormal retinal vasculature which is present in diabetics.

Therefore, diabetic patients who are scheduled for cataract surgery should have a comprehensive medical and ophthalmic examination. Patients with clinically significant macular oedema should have treatment prior to surgery. However, this may not prevent recurrence of clinically significant macular oedema postoperatively.[39] After surgery patients should have a detailed retinal examination within 3 months, with appropriate treatment as required.

Panretinal photocoagulation

Decreased visual acuity following panretinal photocoagulation has been recognized since the introduction of this treatment in the managment of proliferative diabetic retinopathy.[40] MacDonald and Schatz reviewed the pre- and postoperative fluorescein angiograms of 175 eyes with proliferative diabetic retinopathy treated by panretinal photocoagulation. In this series, 43% of patients developed macular oedema between 6 and 10 weeks following laser treatment. Macular oedema persisted in 27% of these patients and visual loss of two more lines occurred in 8%.[41]

The management of a patient with both clinically significant macular oedema and retinopathy that is approaching the high-risk stage (very severe non-proliferative retinopathy or moderate proliferative retinopathy) may be difficult. The ETDRS recommends the combination of early mild scatter and focal photocoagulation for the macular oedema.[42] Delaying scatter photocoagulation until focal photocoagulation is completed is unlikely to be associated with an increased risk of severe visual loss, provided that the retinopathy is not progressing in the meantime. In view of these findings it is suggested that pre-existing macular oedema should be treated in combination with, or prior to panretinal photocoagulation, so as to reduce the incidence of this complication.

PREVENTION

As previously described, maculopathy is associated with a higher level of glycosylated haemoglobin than average and more severe retinopathy at baseline examination, in diabetic patients. The results of the Diabetes Control and Complications Trial support the recommendation that with insulin-dependent diabetes the aim should be to achieve blood glucose levels as close to the non-diabetic range as is safely possible, thereby reducing the incidence and progression of the retinopathy.[43,44]

SCREENING

The maximum benefit in the treatment of diabetic maculopathy is obtained if the patients are treated at the onset of clinically significant macular oedema before any loss of vision has occurred.[21] Therefore, the identification of diabetics who are at risk of losing vision is of the uppermost importance, so that they can benefit from current treatment recommendations. The current methods of screening for retinopathy include full fundal examination or photography with visual acuity recordings. However, there is a high rate of underestimation of serious retinopathy. There is poor sensitivity with these methods, but they have good specificity, being able to establish whether retinopathy is present or not.[38] This is especially true in the detection of maculopathy, as macular oedema may be difficult to determine in the absence of hard exudate formation and before the onset of visual deterioration. Therefore, any screening methods or fundal examination must pay particular attention to any retinopathy within the macular region, particularly within one disc diameter of the fovea. The monitoring of patients' visual acuity must be incorporated in the screening programmes, as a decrease in visual acuity may be the first evidence of the onset of diabetic maculopathy.

The screening of diabetic retinopathy is required on a regular basis. The intervals between screening are determined by the severity of retinopathy on examination, the type and duration of diabetes and the age of the patient. Also, as discussed previously, special consideration must be taken following cataract surgery and during pregnancy.

Diabetic retinopathy is uncommon before the age of 14 years. Therefore, diabetic children should be screened from this age onwards, on an annual basis. If mild non-proliferative diabetic retinopathy develops, they should be examined every 6 months because clinically significant macular oedema may develop.

In maturity-onset diabetics, screening should commence with the diagnosis of the disease, as it will not be clear when these patients have become diabetic and retinopathy may already be present. In the absence of retinopathy a yearly examination is satisfactory. In the presence of mild non-proliferative diabetic retinopathy 6 monthly examinations, with special regard to diabetic macular oedema, should be carried out.

In the presence of more severe retinopathy, regardless of age of onset, follow-up examinations should be performed every 2–3 months, with appropriate treatment as required.[45]

ACKNOWLEDGEMENT

We would like to acknowledge the assistance of the Fundal Diagnostic and Photographic Department of the Royal Victoria Eye & Ear Hospital.

REFERENCES

1. Aiello LM, Rand LI, Briones JC et al, Diabetic retinopathy in Joslin Clinic patients with adult-onset diabetes, *Ophthalmology* (1981) **88**:619–23.
2. Klein R, Klein BEK, Moss SE, Visual impairment in diabetes, *Ophthalmology* (1984) **91**:1–8.
3. Early Treatment Diabetic Retinopathy Study Research Group, Photocoagulation for diabetic macular edema. ETDRS Report no. 1, *Ophthalmology* (1985) **103**:1796–806.
4. Moss S, Klein R, Klein B, The incidence of visual loss in a diabetic population, *Ophthalmology* (1988) **95**:1340–8.
5. Klein R, Klein BEK, Moss SE et al, The Wisconsin Epidemiologic Study of Diabetic Retinopathy. IV. Diabetic macular oedema, *Ophthalmology* (1984) **91**:1464–74.
6. Vitale S, Maguire MG, Murphy RP et al, Clinically significant macular edema in type I diabetes, *Ophthalmology* (1995) **102**:1170–6.
7. Klein R, Klein BEK, Moss SE et al, The Wisconsin Epidemiologic Study of Diabetic Retinopathy. XI. The incidence of diabetic macular edema, *Ophthalmology* (1989) **96**:1501–10.
8. Bresnick GH, Diabetic macular edema. A review, *Ophthalmology* (1986) **93**:989–97.
9. Klein R, Klein BEK, Moss SE, Diabetes, hyperglycaemia, and age-related maculopathy, *Ophthalmology* (1992) **99**:1527–34.
10. Clark JB, Gray RHB, Lim KKT, Burns-Cox CJ, Loss of vision before ophthalmic referral in blind and partially sighted diabetics in Bristol, *Br J Ophthalmology* (1994) **78**:741–4.
11. Garner A, Histopathology of diabetic retinopathy in man, *Eye* (1993) **7**:250–3.
12. Guyton AC, *Textbook of Medical Physiology*. 9th edn (WB Saunders: Philadelphia, 1996) 358–9, 368–70.
13. Kristinsson JK, Diabetic retinopathy. Screening and prevention of blindness, *Acta Ophthalmol Scand* (1997) **75**(223 Suppl):52–60.
14. Ferris F, Patz A, Macular edema. A complication of diabetic retinopathy, *Surv Ophthalmol* (1984) **28**(Suppl): 452–61.

15. Weinberger D, Fink-Cohen S, Gaton DD et al, Non-retinovascular leakage in diabetic maculopathy, *Br J Ophthalmology* (1995) **79**:728–31.
16. Patel V, Rassom S, Newson R et al, Retinal blood flow in diabetic retinopathy, *BMJ* (1992) **305**:678–83.
17. Dobson PM, Gibson JM, Longterm follow-up of medical conditions in patients with diabetic exudative maculopathy, *Eye* (1991) **5**:699–703.
18. Engler C, Krogsa B, Lund-Anderson H, Blood–retinal barrier permeability and its relation to progression of diabetic retinopathy in type 1 diabetics. An 8–year follow-up study. *Graefes Arch Clin Exp Ophthalmol* (1991) **229**:442–6.
19. Kinyoun J, Barton F, Fisher M et al, Detection of diabetic macular edema. Ophthalmoscopy versus photography. ETDRS Report no. 5, *Ophthalmology* (1989) **96**:746–51.
20. Early treatment of diabetic retinopathy study group; classification of diabetic retinopathy from fluorescein angiograms. BTDRS report no. 11, *Ophthalmology* (1991) **98**:807–22.
21. Early Treatment Diabetic Retinopathy Study Research Group, Treatment techniques and clinical guidelines for photocoagulation of diabetic macular edema. ETDRS Report no. 2, *Ophthalmology* (1987) **94**:761–74.
22. Blankenship GW, Diabetic macular edema and laser photocoagulation, *Ophthalmology* (1979) **86**:69–75.
23. Abu El-Azrar A, Morse PH, Laser photocoagulation control of diabetic macular oedema without fluorescein angiography, *Br J Ophthalmology* (1991) **75**:97–9.
24. British Multicentre Study Group, Photocoagulation for diabetic maculopathy; a randomised controlled clinical trial using xenon arc, *Diabetes* (1983) **32**:1010–16.
25. Merrin S, Yanko L, Ivry N, Treatment of diabetic maculopathy by argon laser, *Br J Ophthalmol* (1974) **58**:85–91.
26. Patz R, Schatz H, Berkaw JW et al, Macular edema: an overlooked complication of diabetic retinopathy, *Ophthalmology* (1973) **77**:34–42.
27. Early Treatment Diabetic Retinopathy Study Research Group, Focal photocoagulation treatment of diabetic macular edema. Relationship of treatment effect to fluorscein angiographic and other retinal characteristics at baseline. ETDRS Report no. 19, *Arch Ophthalmol* (1995) **113**: 1144–55.
28. Olk RJ, Modified grid argon (blue-green) laser photocoagulation for diffuse diabetic macular edema, *Ophthalmology* (1986) **93**: 938–50.
29. Olk JR, Argon-green (514 nm) vs krypton-red (647 nm) modified grid laser photocoagulation for diffuse diabetic macular edema, *Ophthalmology* (1990) **97**:1101–13.
30. Moloney JB, Drury MI, The effect of pregnancy on the natural course of diabetic retinopathy, *Am J Ophthalmol* (1982) **93**:745–56.
31. Best RM, Chakravarthy U, Diabetic retinopathy in pregnancy, *Br J Ophthalmol* (1997) **81**:249–51.
32. Klien BE, Moss SE, Klein R, Effect of pregnancy on progression of diabetic retinopathy, *Diabetes Care* (1990) **13**:34–40.
33. Axer-Siegel R, Hod M, Fink-Cohen S et al, Diabetic retinopathy during pregnancy, *Ophthalmology* (1996) **103**:1815–19.
34. Phelps Rl, Sakol L, Metzger BE et al, Changes in diabetic retinopathy during pregnancy. Correlations with regulation of hyperglycemia, *Arch Ophthalmol* (1986) **104**:1806–10.
35. Sinclair SH, Nesler C, Foxman R et al, Macular oedema and pregnancy in insulin-dependent diabetes, *Am J Ophthalmol* (1984) **97**:154–67.
36. Halperin LS, Olk RJ, Soubrane G, Coscas G. Safety of fluorescein angiography during pregnancy, *Am J Ophthalmol* (1990) **109**:563–6.
37. Benson WE, Brown GC, Tasman W et al, Extracapsular cataract extraction with placement of posterior chamber lens in patients with diabetic retinopathy, *Ophthalmology* (1983) **100**:730–8.
38. Dowler JGF, Hykin PG, Lydman SL et al, Visual acuity following extracapsular cataract extraction in diabetes: a meta-analysis, *Eye* (1995) **9**. 313–17.
39. Jaffe GJ, Burton TC, Progression of non-proliferative diabetic retinopathy following cataract extraction, *Arch Ophthalmol* (1988) **106**: 745–9.

40. Meuyers SM, Macular oedema after scatter laser photocoagulation for proliferative diabetic retinopathy, *Am J Ophthalmol* (1980) **90**:210–16.
41. MacDonald HP, Schatz H, Macular edema following pan-retinal photocoagulation, *Retina* (1985) **5**:5–10.
42. Early Treatment Diabetic Retinopathy Study Research Group, Early photocoagulation for diabetic retinopathy. ETDRS Report no. 9, *Ophthalmology* (1991) **98(Suppl)**:757–65.
43. The Diabetes Control and Complications Trial Research Group, The effect of intensive treatment of diabetics on the development and progression of long-term complications in insulin-dependent diabetes mellitus, *N Engl J Med* (1993) **329**: 977–86.
44. The Diabetes Control and Complications Trial Research Group, The effect of intensive diabetes treatment on the progression of diabetic retinopathy in insulin-dependent diabetes mellitus. The diabetes control and complications trial, *Arch Ophthalmol* (1995) **113**:36–51.
45. Buxton MJ, Sculpher MJ, Ferguson DA et al, Screening for treatable diabetic retinopathy; A comparison of different methods, *Diabet Med* (1991) **8**:371–7.

3 Differential diagnosis of diabetic retinopathy

Gabriel Coscas, Isabelle Meunier and Gisèle Soubrane

Different conditions such as retinal vein occlusion, hypertensive retinopathy, ocular ischaemic syndrome, radiation retinopathy, retinal telangiectasia, Coats' disease and sickle cell retinopathy can mimic diabetic retinopathy at different stages of the disease. These conditions should be particularly considered in cases of undiagnosed or recently diagnosed diabetes mellitus or in cases of asymmetric or atypical retinopathy.

The diagnostic approach should be based on the analysis of systemic data and of the clinical pattern (especially venous abnormalities) and of the location and extent of retinal ischaemia. In addition, some of these diseases can be associated with diabetic retinopathy, especially retinal vein occlusion and hypertensive retinopathy.

HYPERTENSIVE RETINOPATHY

Hypertensive retinopathy includes all the changes in the retinal vessels related to hypertension, including both essential hypertension (95% of cases) and hypertensive disease (5%). The vascular changes have been graded according to their prognostic value and to distinguish the changes related to arteriolosclerosis with those related to hypertension.

Arteriolosclerosis is not specific but only a compensatory reaction to increased vascular stress in patients with hypertension and to the height of diastolic pressure. Generalized retinal arteriolosclerosis is graded I–IV, based on the severity of the thickening of the vessel wall and the extent of compression of the underlying venules at arteriolovenular crossings.

Hypertensive retinopathy can mimic any stage of diabetic retinopathy with similar retinal changes, for example, microaneurysms and hard exudates. However, certain vascular changes are directly correlated with hypertension and help to distinguish these retinopathies especially in patients with both systemic diseases. There is a definite relationship between the narrowing of the arterioles and the diastolic pressure, and the haemorrhages and hard exudates have a characteristic pattern in hypertensive retinopathy that is not seen as often in diabetic retinopathy, i.e. macular scar with peripapillary haemorrhages and papillary oedema. In addition, the duration of the systemic disease should be considered: diabetic retinopathy is unusual before diabetes has existed for 10 years. The most striking feature of hypertensive retinopathy is diffuse arteriolar narrowing which is correlated more with the diastolic pressure than the systolic. The reduction of calibre of arterioles related to the calibre of veins can be graded I–IV.

One may also see focal constriction, a localized, symmetric, waist-like narrowing of the arterioles. The degree of the constriction is directly related to the acuteness of development or exacerbation of the hypertension and to the height of the diastolic pressure.

Arteriovenous crossing changes are characteristic of chronic hypertensive disease, even though they can sometimes occur in normotensive patients (after 50 years of age).

In cases of prolonged or advanced hypertension, one may see other lesions as well. There may be haemorrhages, located in the nerve fibre layer, with a flame-shaped appearance. Deeper haemorrhages suggest more severe hypertension. Cotton wool spots, typically observed around the optic disc, are usually few in number and small in size. They usually disappear within a few weeks. Hard exudates vary in size from a dot to a disc diameter or more and may produce the appearance of a macular star. In hypertension, residues usually appear grey or silver as compared with the waxy exudates of diabetes. Microaneurysms are particularly located around cotton wool spots. Vessel sheathing is an increase in the optical density of the vessel wall caused by lateral thickening. When the entire vessel is opaque this may appear to be an occluded vessel, but the patency of such vessels has been demonstrated by fluorescein angiography.

Classifications of hypertension and arteriolosclerosis

The attempt to relate ophthalmoscopic findings to the severity of hypertensive disease has brought about many classifications. The early classification of Keith–Wagener–Barker[1] correlates the retinal findings with the hypertensive disease state. The Wagener–Clay–Gipner classification[2] combines both the acute and the chronic aspects of hypertensive disease. The Scheie classification[3] grades separately the retinal changes of hypertension and of arteriolosclerosis. The classification of Leishman[4] underlines the fact that hypertensive retinopathy depends on the degree of elevation of the blood pressure and also on the age of the patient.

More recently, fluorescein angiography (FA) has shown more details of early and late changes in the retinal capillary bed, the degree of its perfusion and the development of intraretinal channels. FA has also allowed analysis of the permeability of the capillaries by showing leakage and oedema. In diabetic retinopathy, the changes in the capillary bed usually increase very steadily. In hypertensive retinopathy, these changes, combined with retinal and papillar oedema, are mainly observed in malignant hypertension and in young patients.

In treated hypertension, most of these symptoms regress rapidly leaving only disorganization of the architecture of the capillary bed. Elschnig's spots, which are retrospective markers of choroidal involvement in resolved hypertension, are irregular spots of pigmented epithelium atrophy.

RETINAL VEIN OCCLUSION

This retinopathy can reproduce many lesions similar to those of diabetic retinopathy. The visual defects and retinal damage caused by venous occlusion depend on the degree of vein occlusion and capillary perfusion and on the development of collateral pathways for venous outflow in this endarterial vascular system. The degree and severity of retinal venous occlusion can range from minimal changes with normal visual acuity to ischaemic proliferative retinopathy with maculopathy and severe decrease of vision.

Background

Arterial hypertension and arteriosclerosis represent the main systemic risk factors for central retinal vein occlusion. Hypertension is reported in approximately 60% of patients (twice that in an age-matched population). Carotid artery disease and diabetes mellitus have been reported in association with central retinal vein occlusion, particularly the ischaemic form. Open-angle glaucoma appears to be related to central retinal vein occlusion. Glaucoma could lead to worsening of the prognosis of central vein occlusion by its haemodynamic effects of a decrease in blood flow. To date many studies are focusing on the role of hyperviscosity in retinal venous occlusion (abnormalities of erythrocytes and/or platelet aggregation). Smoking appears not to be a factor in the occurrence of central retinal vein occlusion.

Classification

Central retinal vein occlusion was separated into two categories, haemorrhagic and venous stasis retinopathy by Hayreh. But fluorescein angiography now allows us to distinguish more precisely between the ischaemic, non-perfused type and the oedematous, well-perfused type, as well as to recognize mixed and intermediate forms.[5] It can be difficult to determine with accuracy the ischaemic or non-ischaemic type on initial evaluation owing to the not infrequent increase of the degree of capillary non-perfusion which occurs during follow-up. In such a case, the patient must be re-evaluated by fluorescein angiography after haemorrhages have been absorbed.

Clinical features

Oedematous (non-ischaemic) central retinal vein occlusion

Oedematous (well-perfused) central retinal vein occlusion is the most frequent, and a much milder and more variable disease in appearance, symptoms, and course than is ischaemic central retinal vein occlusion. Patients with well-perfused vein occlusion are on average of 5 years younger (mean age 63 years) than those with ischaemic vein occlusion. The majority of patients have an initial visual acuity of 20/50 or better. The features of non-ischaemic central retinal vein occlusion are varied. Engorgement of the venous tree is prominent, with characteristic dilation and increased tortuosity; there are often associated cotton wool spots. Disc oedema is a marker of the acute phase. Retinal haemorrhages vary markedly: they may appear only peripherally in the four quadrants, or they may be rather prominent in the posterior pole. The decrease in vision is due to macular oedema or macular haemorrhages. Fluorescein angiography demonstrates a prolonged venous transit time, dilation of the retinal venous circulation, mild staining of the walls of veins, and disc and macular oedema (including cystoid macular oedema) (*Fig. 3.1*). The intraocular pressure is frequently lower in the eye with occlusion.

Many patients (40–50%) have a final visual acuity less than 20/40 due to persistent cystoid macular oedema, macular cystic changes, pigmentary changes, or residual microvascular abnormalities that could lead to permanent visual loss. Disc collateral channels, which sometimes develop in late retinal vein occlusion, can be very useful to differentiate this condition from other retinal vasculopathies and diabetic retinopathy. Some eyes with an oedematous vein occlusion (5–22%, depending on the duration of follow-up) will progress towards a more severe ischaemic form. This evolution is due to progression of the vein occlusion with resultant retinal capillary non-perfusion.

Ischaemic central retinal vein occlusion

Patients with an ischaemic pattern of vein occlusion usually complain of a sudden painless decrease in visual acuity. Visual acuity ranges from 20/40 to seeing hand movements. Confluent deep haemorrhages infarcting the retinal outer layers are the most frequent fundus. Preretinal haemorrhage or vitreous haemorrhage sometimes occurs as a result of bleeding through the internal limiting membrane. The entire venous tree is tortuous, dilated, and dark. Cotton wool

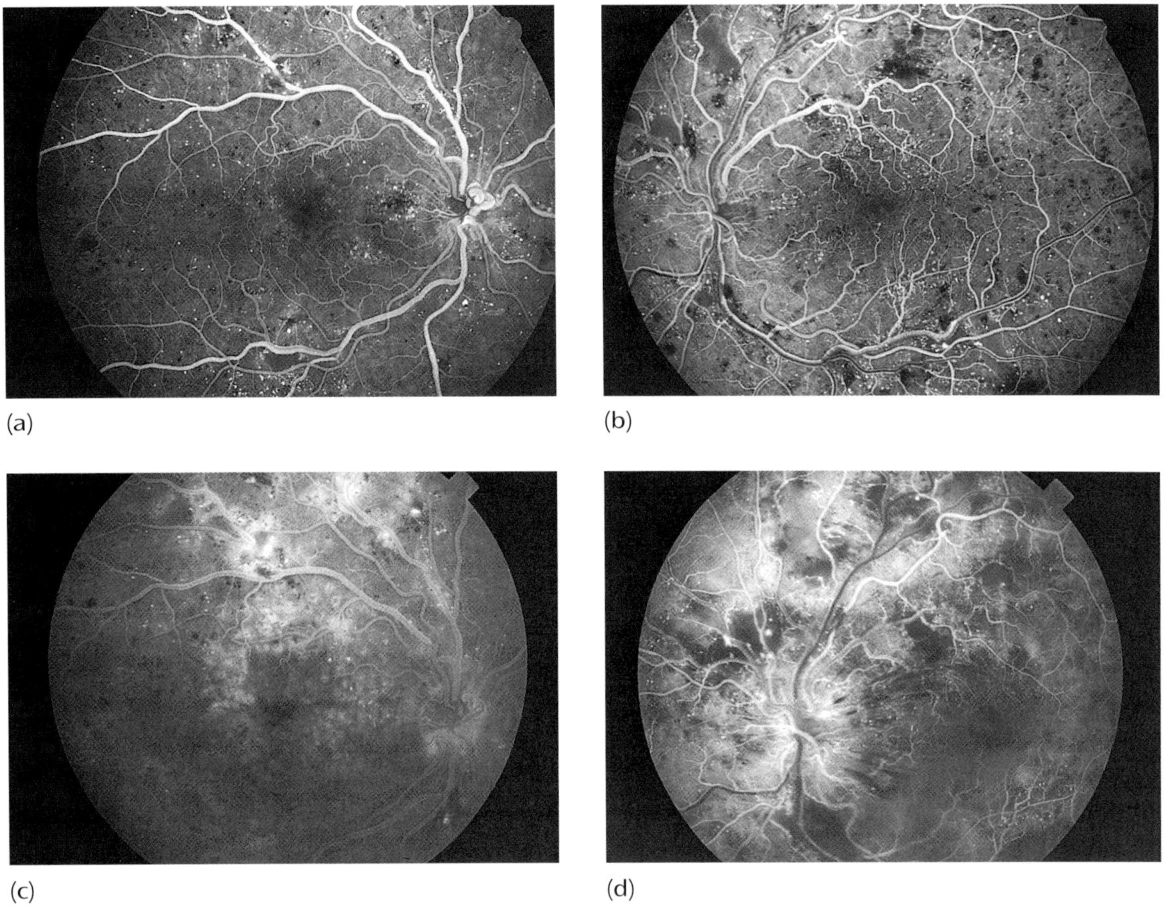

Figure 3.1
Central retinal vein occlusion combined with proliferative diabetic retinopathy in a 48-year-old diabetic patient. (a), (b) Initial fluorescein angiography. (a) Right eye: Microaneurysms are widespread at the posterior pole with moderate dye leakage and macular oedema. Capillary non-perfusion is noted along the temporal vessels. The inferotemporal vein has an irregular diameter along the ischaemic area with staining of its walls (venous beading). The patient has collateral channels of the optic disc. (b) Left eye: There is evidence of more extensive capillary non-perfusion in the midperipheral fundi. (c), (d) Fluorescein angiography 10 months later for a severe deterioration of vision in left eye. (c) Right eye: Fluorescein angiography demonstrates more extensive non-perfusion areas, particularly in superotemporal zone, and aggravation of macular oedema. (d) Left eye: A central retinal venous occlusion is now present. Retinal haemorrhages are more numerous and noted in all the four quadrants. The retinal circulation time is prolonged. There is papillary oedema, and severe dropout of the retinal capillary bed.

spots are present in proportion to the severity. The venous pulse is absent. The arterioles are frequently narrowed. Fluorescein angiography discloses precisely the extent and severity of capillary non-perfusion, even in the presence of widespread confluent haemorrhages. The foveal avascular zone is enlarged with large non-perfused areas, and peripheral views may show very extensive areas of non-perfusion. Microaneurysms may not be noted at the time of initial occlusion but become manifest shortly thereafter. Late staining along the large retinal veins is a characteristic feature in moderate and severe forms of central retinal vein occlusion. Patients can have a bilateral non-simultaneous central retinal vein occlusion (6–17%) and late cases can mimic diabetic retinopathy.

The prognosis for ischaemic central retinal vein occlusion (CRVO) is poor because of macular capillary non-perfusion and neovascularization. After resolution of the retinal haemorrhages, varying degrees of permanent capillary non-perfusion or dropout usually remain in the macular zone. In contrast to the case in diabetic retinopathy, retinal and disc neovascularization are relatively infrequent. In severe ischaemic CRVO, the most serious complication is anterior segment neovascularization with rubeosis and neovascular glaucoma (NVG). This NVG occurs in 8–25% of all central retinal vein occlusions. The incidence increases dramatically where there is approximately 50% capillary non-perfusion in the fundus. Neovascular glaucoma may occur as early as 2 weeks after CRVO. The average time of onset is approximately 3 months following occlusion and the natural course is more rapid and severe than in proliferative diabetic retinopathy.

Panretinal photocoagulation is the method of treatment of ischaemic CRVO. Clinical trials (CRVO study) show that it does not affect the final visual acuity outcome but is effective in regression of neovascularization. In our experience, eyes with greater than 50% capillary non-perfusion as seen on fluorescein angiography should benefit from prophylactic treatment.

RADIATION RETINOPATHY

Radiation retinopathy appears to be more frequent as new ocular radiotherapy techniques and indications come into use, not only for melanomas but also for angiomas and possibly for some types of ill-defined choroidal neovascularization in age-related macular degeneration.

Background

After local or external beam irradiation, patients may develop retinopathy or optic neuropathy 6 months to 3 years after treatment (average of 18 months). The risk increases with the dose and is influenced by the radiation technique. Doses of 25–35 Gy are required to induce radiation retinopathy. External radiation produces more severe retinopathy. Diabetes mellitus and chemotherapy are additive risk factors.

Clinical features

Several lesions that mimic diabetic retinopathy can be noted, including intraretinal haemorrhages, hard exudates, cotton wool spots, microaneurysms, telangiectatic vessels, and sheathed vessels. Visual impairment ranges from mild to severe, and is secondary to macular ischaemia or macular oedema. The most severe change is the progressive development of non-perfusion areas not only in the periphery but also in the posterior pole. This retinopathy, as well as diabetic retinopathy, combines lesions due to capillary non-perfusion with lesions due to capillary hyperpermeability. Microaneurysms are less frequent in radiation retinopathy than in diabetic retinopathy. In the proliferative form of radiation retinopathy, ischaemia is usually located in the area that received a high level of radiation, rather than with a preferentially nasal location as in diabetic retinopathy.

Radiation optic neuropathy also occurs with doses similar to those inducing radiation retinopathy. In the acute phase, the optic disc is swollen, surrounded by intraretinal haemorrhages, hard exudates and subretinal fluid. Progressively, over several weeks or months, the optic disc becomes pale and atrophic with variable visual acuity.

To date, there is no prevention for radiation retinopathy except to fractionate the doses and decrease the total cumulative dose. Preventive panretinal photocoagulation of peripheral non-perfusion areas could be considered before the occurrence of neovascularization, vitreous haemorrhage, and neovascular glaucoma.

OCULAR ISCHAEMIC SYNDROME

Carotid artery disease includes ocular symptoms from amaurosis fugax to the ocular ischaemic syndrome. The ocular manifestations can be the first manifestation of carotid artery disease. This ocular ischaemic syndrome can mimic diabetic retinopathy except for the history of amaurosis fugax , the presence of widely scattered blot and dot retinal haemorrhages, and in some severe forms, the presence of panuveitis, neovascular glaucoma, and rapidly progressing cataract.

Background

Classically, transient obstruction of either or both of the ipsilateral carotid and ophthalmic arteries can lead to transient loss of vision in one eye (amaurosis fugax). One-third of untreated patients will have a stroke, a rate approximately four times greater than that in an age-matched population.

Clinical features

When there is chronic rather than transient ocular ischaemia one often finds a unilateral retinopathy (ipsilateral to the carotid artery lesion), which includes cotton wool spots and dilated arterioles and veins. The vision is not affected. This retinopathy was first recognized as a sign of carotid artery disease by Hollenhorst in 1958.[6] In some cases, the clinical presentation may be reduced to enlargement of retinal arterioles on the side of the pathological carotid artery.

Another type of chronic ophthalmic artery obstruction, characterized by venous tortuosity and by deep haemorrhages and microaneurysms in the midperiphery and periphery, is produced by hypoperfusion (venous stasis retinopathy, Kearns and Hollenhorst[7]). Fluorescein angiography discloses areas of capillary non-perfusion and microaneurysms. The entire periphery of the eye is usually affected, although there may be more haemorrhages in one quadrant than another.

The third type of chronic arterial occlusion is the ocular ischaemic syndrome. This syndrome is usually associated with bilateral and severe stenosis, but usually affects only one eye. This is characterized posteriorly by hypoperfusion retinopathy (*Fig. 3.2*) and choroidal perfusion defects. In some cases, neovascularization of either the disc (NVD) or the retina elsewhere (NVE) is associated. There may be episcleral dilatation and signs of anterior segment ischaemia (corneal oedema, anterior chamber cells, neovascular glaucoma). The most striking feature in the most severe form is the presence of severe orbital pain (ocular angina).

In severe forms of ocular ischaemic syndrome both carotid endarterectomy and carotid artery bypass surgery have been shown to be effective in increasing perfusion to the eye. After surgery, the signs of anterior ischaemia and pain may decrease. In addition, the ocular ischaemic syndrome may require panretinal photocoagulation or combined

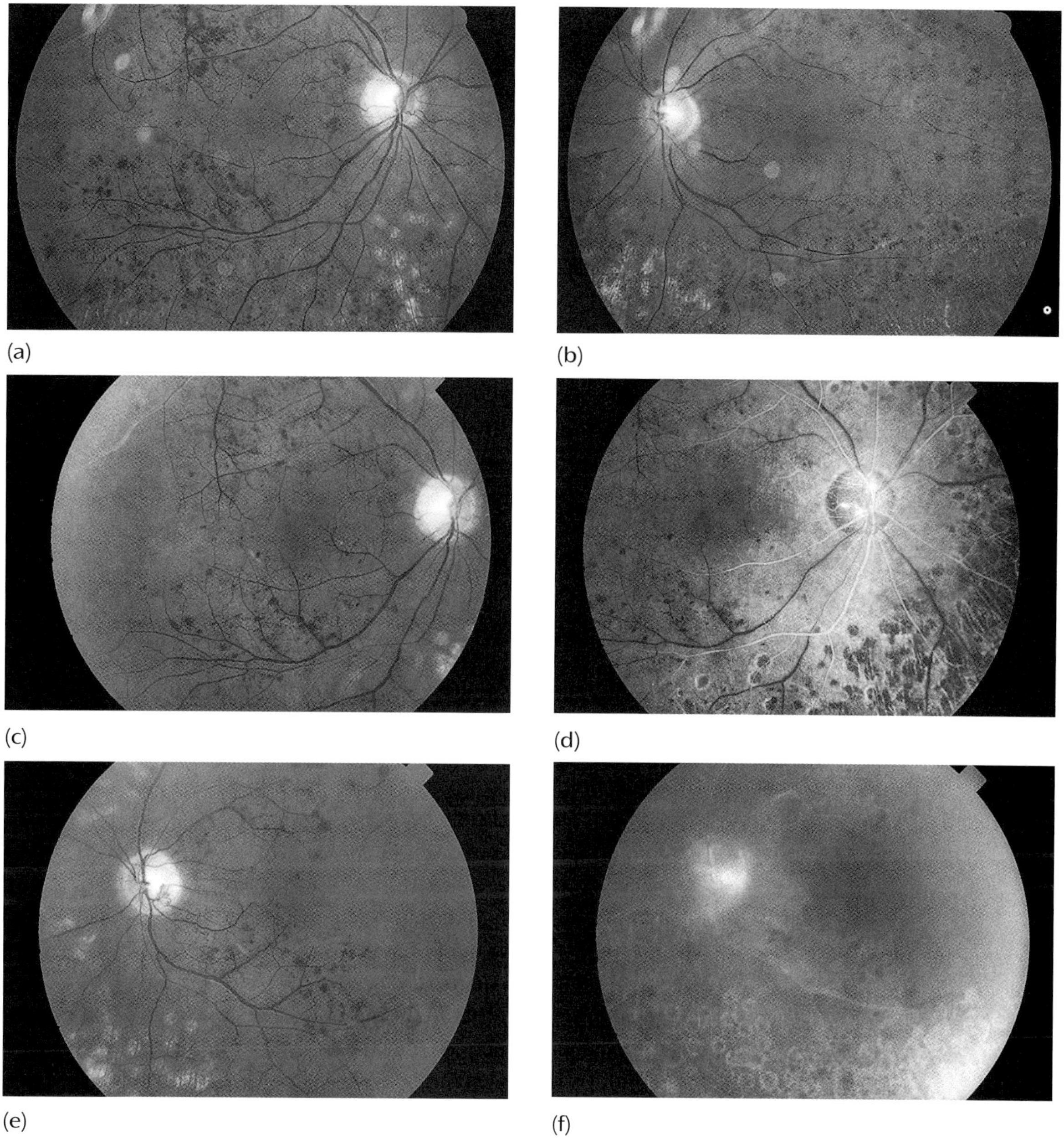

Figure 3.2
Ocular ischaemic syndrome in a 45-year-old man with severe carotid artery obstruction. The patient was referred for neovascular glaucoma of the right eye and rubeosis of the left eye. (a), (b) Red-free photographs. Scattered blot and dot haemorrhages are noted, combined with large areas of capillary non-perfusion, some degree of venous and arteriolar occlusion, and ischaemic optic neuropathy. (c)–(f) Fluorescein angiography performed 4 months later. There has been progression of capillary non-perfusion, particularly in the macular area. The perifoveal capillary network is completly destroyed in both eyes.

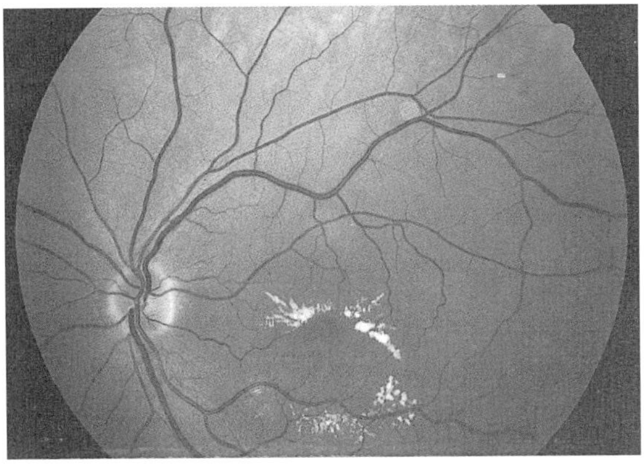

(a)

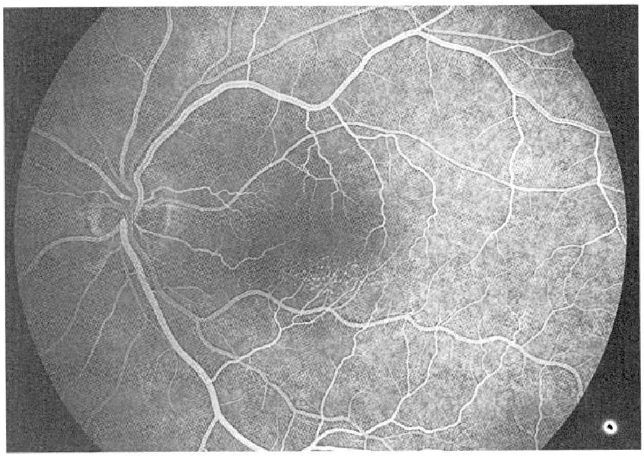

(b)

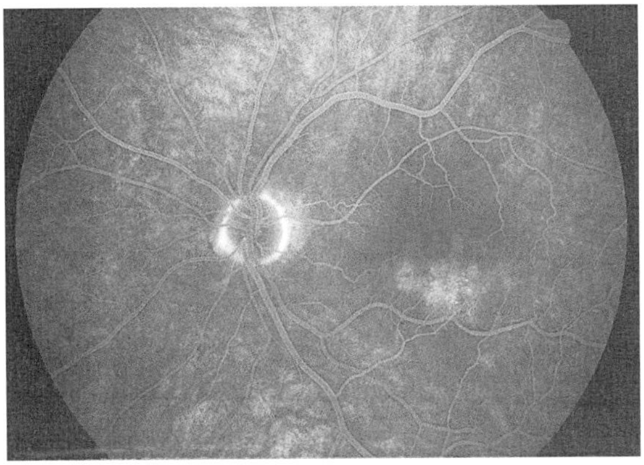

(c)

Figure 3.3
Retinal telangiectasis with severe exudation misdiagnosed as background retinopathy. (a) Red-free photograph. Circinate exudates are noted, involving the fovea (b). Fluorescein angiography showing irregular widening of the capillary-free zone, aneurysmal dilation of abnormal vessels with evidence of dye leakage, and (c) macular oedema in late phase.

panretinal photocoagulation and cyclocryotherapy to manage retinal neovascularization or neovascular glaucoma.

RETINAL TELANGIECTASIS

Juxtafoveal retinal telangiectasia can be independent of diabetic retinopathy, but has recently been recognized sometimes as an atypical presentation of background diabetic retinopathy that can occur either unilaterally or bilaterally. Telangiectasis can be part of Coats' disease as well.

The unilateral form is more common in young to middle-aged men (group 1). The lesions are small perifoveal and parafoveal telangiectatic capillaries with tortuosity, dilation, and irregular calibre. Lipid exudation and microaneurysms can be noted. These abnormalities can be localized to an area of 1–5 mm in diameter or scattered throughout the macula. In group 1A, the congenital form, macular oedema is the main complication and laser photocoagulation can be of benefit (*Fig. 3.3*). In group 1B, unilateral idiopathic parafoveolar telangiectasis, laser treatment is not beneficial. Visual prognosis is fair and laser treatement could lead to iatrogenic choroidal neovascularization.

Bilateral juxtafoveal retinal telangiectasis (group II) is a separate entity. Ocular symptoms occur later. The telangiectasis tends to be symmetric, located in the temporal area of the macula. Retinal oedema and hard exudates are less severe. Abnormal venules ('right angle' venules) can drain the telangiectatic areas. Retinal pigmented epithelial alterations and pseudovitelliform lesions can be noted. Choroidal neovascularization is the main complication than can develop, and causes severe loss of vision.

All patients with presumed telangiectasis should have a glucose tolerance test to rule out latent diabetes.

The term 'Coats' disease' should be reserved for patients with congenital retinal telangiectasis associated with massive hard exudation. The extent and the degree of retinal capillary alterations and exudation are variable and the clinical pattern can range from minimal macular exudation to massive yellow exudative detachment.

Background

Congenital telangiectasis is usually unilateral (80%), affecting mostly young males in their first or second decade of life, but up to one-third of patients are more than 30 years of age before the onset of symptoms.

Clinical features

This idiopathic retinal vascular disorder is characterized by irregular dilatation and incompetence of the retinal vessels. Abnormal dilatations may occur anywhere in the fundus on both arteries and veins. Vascular loops and beading neovascularization have been reported as well. Fluorescein angiography helps to visualize these telangiectasies and to localize precisely the degree and severity of leakage (cystoid macular oedema, circinate maculopathy, macular exudation detachment). Portions of the capillary bed may show non-perfusion, and this pattern is frequently observed in the peripheral fundus combined with large aneurysmal vascular abnomalies. The clinical course is variable, and total exudative retinal detachment with rubeosis iridis, glaucoma, and phthisis bulbi can occur in severe cases.

Photocoagulation or cryotherapy may induce the absorption of exudative lesions. However, close follow-up is required because new telangiectasis can develop in areas of retina that were previously uninvolved.

SICKLE CELL RETINOPATHY

Sickle cell retinopathy includes all the retinopathies caused by the sickling gene including sickle cell disease (SS), SC disease and sickle cell thalassemia (SThal). These retinopathies can mimic diabetic retinopathy except for three characteristic features: the preferential midperipheral location and progression of ischaemia; the peripheral arteriolar-venular anastomoses and emergence of new vessels in a sea fan pattern at the junction between perfused and non-perfused retina; and the peripheral salmon patch haemorrhages. Sickle cell retinopathy and Eales disease are not distinguishable except for the abnormal haemoglobin.

Background

The SS combination results in the worst systemic symptomatology. Other sickle haemoglobinopathies lead to milder and less severe systemic symptoms, but ocular complications are more likely to occur especially in SC and SThal diseases. Ocular changes do not occur in patients with sickle cell trait unless they have additional systemic and/or retinal disease.

Sickle cell haèmoglobin is most prevalent in black persons in North America, who show the following prevalences: AS haemoglobin 8–9%, SS disease 0.4%, SC disease 0.1–0.3% and SThal 0.5–1.0%. Caucasians are rarely affected by sickle haemoglobinopathies.

Clinical features

Like other retinopathies, sickle cell retinopathy may be separated into a non-proliferative and a proliferative form. Significant ischaemic retinopathy has been noted as early as the second decade of life, with both sexes equally at risk. A classification according to vascular abnormalities and the extent of peripheral ischaemia has been established and reflects the progression and severity of the retinopathy. The different stages are: stage I, peripheral arteriolar occlusion; stage II, peripheral arteriovenous anastomosis; stage III, peripheral neovascularization; stage IV, vitreous haemorrhage; stage V, retinal detachment.

Some patients also show occlusion of one or more paracentral arterioles and angiography should be performed to reveal these areas of capillary closure. Alternatively, peripheral ischaemia can extend towards the posterior pole, especially in the temporal zone of the macula. Besides the development of circumferential arteriovenous communications and sea fan neovascularization, the clinical pattern can include residual lesions after salmon patch haemorrhages have cleared, such as iridescent patches of haemosiderin, black patches of proliferated retinal pigment epithelium (RPE) (sunburn spots) or non-specific hyperpigmented scars (SThal, 20%; SS, 33%). Another common sign observed in these haemoglobinopathies, and not so often in cases of diabetic retinopathy, is venous tortuosity (SS, 47%; SC, 32%).

Vitreous haemorrhage (stage IV) is a frequent complication of retinal neovascularization in sickle cell retinopathy: it was found in 23% of patients with SC disease but in only 3% of patients with SS disease. Vitreous haemorrhage is infrequent in AS hemoglobinopathy, due to the rarity of retinal neovascularization in this disorder.

Occlusion of the central retinal vein or artery is a rare complication of sickle cell retinopathy (SS haemoglobinopathies). Angioid streaks have been described in some patients with sickle haemoglobinopathies, especially SS disease.

EALES DISEASE

Despite controversy about its definition and specific identity, Eales disease is actually classified as an idiopathic retinal vasculitis (primary retinal vasculitis). Vascular sheathing and focal occlusion involve the small peripheral retinal vessels. The most striking feature of Eales disease is the occurrence of retinal neovascularization at the junction of the perfused and non-perfused retina. Thus, this disease is frequently revealed by recurrent vitreal haemorrhages.

To date Eales disease appears as a characteristic clinical and angiographic syndrome that represents the clinical manifestation of different diseases such as sarcoidosis, systemic lupus erythematosus, diabetes mellitus, sickle cell disease, and collagen vascular disease.

Background

Eales disease is uncommon in Western countries but reported as a major cause of visual loss in India, Pakistan, and Afghanistan. It typically affects healthy young men between the ages of 20 and 30. Patients may mention symptoms of vitreal haemorrhage, such as floaters or decreased vision. This idiopathic vasculitis is most frequently bilateral, although often asymmetric. An equal prevalence among both men and women is actually suggested.

Clinical features

Signs of ocular inflammation may be noted in Eales disease, especially early in its natural course. Thin white lines to thick heavy exudative

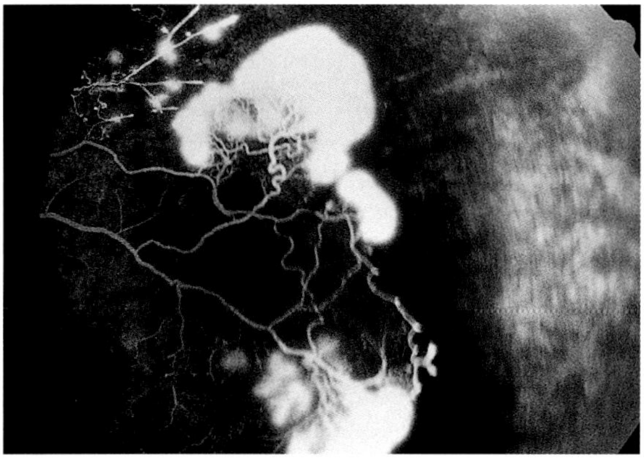

Figure 3.4
Classic peripheral neovascularization in a case of Eales disease (primary retinal perivasculitis). Peripheral proliferative retinopathy at the junction of perfused and non-perfused retina. Note the staining of the neovascular sea fan.

sheathing may be observed, associated with cystoid macular oedema, vitreal cells, keratic precipitates and cells in the anterior chamber in the acute phase. Nevertheless, in most patients there is no evidence of inflammation at the time of examination.

Microaneurysms, arteriovenous shunts, and venous beading are associated and localized at the junction between the perfused and non-perfused retina.

Fluorescein angiography makes it possible to determine and quantify the area of peripheral vascular non-perfusion and proliferation. This pattern is strictly identical to that in sickle cell disease. The temporal retina is most commonly affected. In addition, fluorescein angiography discloses in a few patients macular non-perfusion and/or telangiectasis that can mimic background retinopathy.

As a result of the retinal non-perfusion, new vessels can form either on the disc (NVD) or elsewhere in the retina (NVE) (*Fig. 3.4*). The NVEs present a sea fan appearance.

Patients with Eales disease retain good acuity. Some patients will have permanent visual loss owing to cystoid macular oedema, macular holes, retinal telangiectasis, or epiretinal membrane.

No treatment is known to prevent or reverse non-perfusion or capillary dropout.

RETINAL VASCULITIS

Any lesion found in diabetic retinopathy can also be observed in cases of retinal vasculitis, which may result from uveal inflammation, as part of systemic disease, or as a primary disorder of the retinal vasculature.

Background

Retinal vasculitis is observed in a variety of systemic or ocular diseases such as systemic lupus erythematosus (SLE), polyarteritis nodosa, Behçet's disease, and idiopathic retinal vasculitis, pars planitis, Vogt–Koyanagi–Harada syndrome, and sarcoidosis. The major histocompatibility complex plays an important role in differentiating some of these types of vasculitis. Specific human leukocyte antigen (HLA) types have been linked to retinal vasculitis (DR4), birdshot retinochoroidopathy (A29), Behçet's disease (B5, Bw51), multiple sclerosis (A3, B7, B18, Dw2, DRw3), and Wegener's granulomatosis (B8).

Phlebitis and periphlebitis are characteristic inflammatory changes and occur more frequently than arteriolar changes. Periphlebitis appears as irregular whitish cuffs of exudate that can line the vein anywhere from the optic nerve head to the peripheral retina. These inflammatory lesions are not linked with venous branchings or arteriovenous crossings.

Fluorescein angiography enhances the visualization of venous and arteriolar inflammation, especially at the early stages. It also shows precisely the extent of location of retinovascular changes and of subsequent capillary non-perfusion and/or neovascularization. In the late stages, ghost vessels can be noted which appear as white cords and have permanently closed lumens. Deposition of immune complex in precapillary arterioles may be reflected by the formation of cotton wool spots, which represent microinfarcts.

Kyrieleis arteriolitis is a peculiar form of segmental arteritis with occurence of yellowish plaques but no angiographic abnormalities of the vessels. These arterial changes are most typically associated with toxoplasmosis but have been seen in syphilis, tuberculosis, and herpes zoster retinopathy. The location of vascular inflammation (central vs peripheral), the predominant vessels involved (artery vs vein), and other specific ocular features (e.g. necrotic retinitis, granulomatous uveitis, vitreal snowballs) may suggest a specific diagnosis. Physical examination is required to diagnose certain systemic diseases such as Behcet's disease and connective tissue disorders definitively.

Immunological studies, such as testing for the presence of autoantibodies (antinuclear and anticardiolipin antibodies), enzyme linked immunosorbent assays (ELISA), Venereal Disease Research Laboratory (VDRL) and fluorescent treponemal antibody absorption tests, and HLA typing are useful in distinguishing between collagen vascular disease, toxoplasmosis, toxocariasis, syphilis, and Behcet's disease. Hyperreactive responses to skin testing are helpful in the diagnosis of tuberculosis and Behcet's syndrome, while cutaneous anergy suggests sarcoidosis, herpes zoster, or peripheral uveitis. Viral and fungal cultures are essential in the evaluation of immunosuppressed patients. Testing for agglutinins has been useful in rickettsial infections. Radiological studies aid in the diagnosis of sarcoidosis and tuberculosis. Computed tomographic scanning and magnetic resonance imaging may detect cerebral vascular lesions in multiple sclerosis, neurosarcoidosis and neurolupus. Vitreous analysis has been used to rule out bacterial and fungal infections, Whipple's disease, and reticulum cell sarcoma.

SARCOIDOSIS

Sarcoidosis is a systemic granulomatous disease of undetermined aetiology and pathogenesis with a high incidence of pulmonary involvement. The diagnosis can be made from combined systemic and ophthalmological features including pulmonary and lymph node involvement, uveitis, laboratory data, and biopsy confirmation of non-caseating granuloma. Sarcoidosis should be considered in the differential diagnosis of any form of ocular inflammation. About 40% of cases have ocular involvement as the first sign of the disease.

Sarcoidosis retinopathy can mimic diabetic retinopathy with macular oedema and diffuse macular capillary hyperpermeability or with peripheral ischaemia whether or not combined with preretinal or prepapillary neovascularization. In contrast with diabetic retinopathy, however, sarcoidosis presents with combined anterior and posterior inflammation and does not cause macular ischaemia. The anterior ocular inflammation in sarcoidosis may involve almost any part or the globe and ocular tissues. The anterior uveitis may be granulomatous or non-granulomatous, acute or chronic, localized or diffuse. While large or mutton-fat keratic precipitates are not specific for sarcoidosis, iris nodules on the pupillary border (Koeppe nodules) or in the midstroma (Busacca nodules) are characteristic. Chronic anterior uveitis in sarcoidosis is frequently associated with cystoid macular oedema.

The vitreous cellular reaction in sarcoidosis can range from minimal (with just a few vitreous cells) to vitreous snowballs. Retinal periphlebitis typically occurs in the midperiphery of the retina associated with small exudates ('candle wax drippings'). Choroidal granulomas can be multiple or small, widespread at the posterior pole or single and very large resembling a choroidal tumour. The optic nerve may be involved with disc neovascularization, disc oedema or a granuloma. Combined fluorescein angiography and Indocyanine Green (ICG) angiography are particularly useful to localize retinal and choroidal involvement. Fluorescein angiography shows the degree and extent of retinal vascular involvement, while ICG is useful to show the degree of choroidal involvement with granulomas. Granulomas are most widepread at the posterior pole and in midperipheral retina. They are hypofluorescent during ICG angiography and may not be visible at all on fluorescein angiography. In some cases, branch vein or central retinal vein occlusion can cause a complication of periphlebitis or of a large papillary granuloma that compromises venous return. In addition, some cases of choroidal neovascularization have been reported, a complication that is particularly rare in diabetic retinopathy.

Laboratory tests provide confirmation of the diagnosis of sarcoidosis, although biopsy findings of non-caseating granuloma are not definitive.

Elevation of angiotensin-converting enzyme (ACE) and serum lysozyme may be noted in sarcoidosis. The elevation of lysozyme is more specific but not pathognomonic. Serum thermolysin-like metalloendopeptidase is elevated in chronic sarcoidosis even during corticosteroid therapy. Hypercalcaemia is another frequent marker. Cutaneous anergy is a characteristic but inconstant sign of chronic sarcoidosis.

CHRONIC MYELOGENOUS LEUKAEMIA

The frequency of ocular involvement in leukaemia ranges from 31 to 80%. The eye is more frequently involved in acute leukaemia than in chronic leukaemia and the retinopathy is more striking. It includes dilation, tortuosity and beading of retinal veins, retinal vascular sheathing with a string-of-sausage appearance, cotton wool spots, exudates, and all types of retinal haemorrhages. White-centred haemorrhages are frequently associated with leukaemic retinopathy.

Patients with chronic myelogenous leukaemia are more likely to show retinal peripheral microaneurysms, retinal vascular closures, and retinal neovascularization that mimic diabetic retinopathy. These changes are directly correlated with increased blood viscosity and reduced blood flow. Hard exudates may be noted in a circular, or circinate, pattern surrounding microaneurysms or a point of leakage. Neovascularization occurs most often in the peripheral retina in chronic leukaemia, and at the optic nerve head in acute leukaemia.

REFERENCES

1. Keith NM, Wagener HP, Barker NW. Some different types of essential hypertension: their course and prognosis. *Am J Med Sci* (1939) **197**:332.
2. Wagener HP, Clay GE, Gipner JF, Classification of retinal lesions in the presence of vascular hypertension, *Trans Am Ophthalmol Soc* (1947) **45**:57.
3. Scheie HG, Evaluation of ophthalmoscopic changes of hypertension and arteriolar sclerosis, *Arch Ophthalmol* (1953) **49**:117.
4. Leishman R, The eye in the general vascular disease: hypertension and arteriosclerosis, *Br J Ophthalmol* (1957) **41**:641.
5. Coscas G, Dhermy P, *Occlusions veineuses rétiniennes* (Masson: Paris, 1987).
6. Hollenhorst RW, The neuro-ophthalmology of strokes, *Neuro-ophthalmology* (1965) **2**:109.
7. Kearns TP, Hollenhorst RW, Venour-stasis retinopathy of occlusive disease of the carotid artery, *Mayo Clin Proc* (1963) **38**:304.

4 Extraretinal ocular pathology in diabetes

O Paul van Bijsterveld and Nynke Klaassen-Broekema

CORNEA

In patients with type I and II diabetes nonspecific corneal epithelial lesions[1] are present in more than one-half of all patients[2,3] and these are the results of basement membrane abnormalities.[4,5] Tsubota et al[6] observed no apparent changes in the epithelial cells themselves on biomicroscopic examination, whereas using a wide-field specular microscope they did find minor irregularities in the epithelium. In most patients the epithelial lesions tend to be transient and only few patients mention discomfort. However, recurrent erosion syndromes can occur, for example following photocoagulation, as well as delayed healing after surgical trauma.[7]

In addition to the epithelial cells of the cornea, the diabetic endothelium also shows morphological[8] and functional[9] disturbances. In type I and II diabetes there are significant differences in size (polymegathism) and shape (pleomorphism) of endothelial cells as compared to age-matched nondiabetic persons.[8] Cell density was found to be significantly decreased in only type I diabetes in the fourth and fifth decades. Other studies, however, did not find any differences in endothelial cell densities.[10,11]

The etiology of polymegathism and pleomorphism of corneal endothelial cells in diabetes is unknown. It is hypothesized, though, that aldose reductase–the enzyme which reduces glucose to sorbitol–is responsible for endothelial cell damage,[12,13] since this enzyme is known to be implicated in the pathogenesis of a number of other diabetic complications.[12] In addition, Meyer et al[14] have shown in a rat model that topically applied aldose reductase inhibitors can inhibit and partially reverse the diabetes-induced endothelial cell changes.

As a regular hexagonal pattern of endothelial cells provides the most stable covering of the membrane of Descemet, an irregular pattern will most probably result in a vulnerable monolayer that might be associated with abnormal endothelial cell function. Lass et al[9] did find an increased endothelial permeability in type I diabetes that, remarkably enough, was sufficiently compensated by an increased pump rate. On the basis of their fluorophotometric studies the authors speculate that the latter might be the result of an increase in pump site density. Also, histochemical studies[15] indicate the presence of adaptivity of reserve pump capacity within the human corneal endothelium in response to various stressors such as metabolic changes, age and dystrophic corneal disease.

Since adaptive reserve pump capacity is able to compensate for increased endothelial cell layer permeability, corneal thickness in diabetics is expected to be normal and the results of several studies seem to demonstrate this.[8,9] Busted et al[16] and Olsen and Busted,[17] on the contrary, did find increased corneal thickness. They even found small folds in Descemet's membrane which they considered to be the result of an increased hydration of the cornea. The different findings in the latter study might be explained by the presence of moderate to severe retinopathy in the patients studied, whereas in the study of Lass[9] only patients with mild background retinopathy without proliferative disease were included.

Corneal sensitivity is reduced in patients with diabetes,[18] especially in those patients with retinopathy.[19] Corneal sensitivity is also reduced in patients on oral antidiabetic medication, but insulin-dependent patients seem to have corneal sensitivity. Ishida et al[20] found alterations in the thickness of the basal lamina of Schwann cells, axonal degeneration, and irregular distribution of nerve beading in the corneas of rats with streptozin-induced diabetes. The tear fluid production is normal in patients with diabetes mellitus.[21]

In spite of the observed changes in threshold values–testing corneal sensitivity–the majority of patients are still adequately able to detect corneal foreign bodies. On the other hand, in patients with serious diabetic complications such as tractional retinal detachment and/or vitreous hemorrhage with a reduced corneal sensitivity, neurotrophic ulcers can occur.[22] Also, the pathological changes in corneal innervation are likely to be responsible, at least partially, for delayed epithelial healing following surgery or photocoagulation.

TRANSIENT CHANGES IN REFRACTION IN DIABETES

Development and metabolism of the lens

The lens is formed by an invagination originating from the surface ectoderm and subsequent separation of the lens vesicle. As soon as the lens vesicle is detached from the surface ectoderm an elastic capsule is secreted around the lens. Growth occurs during life by division of a single layer of cells situated immediately under the anterior lens capsule. These epithelial cells then develop into fiber cells; the oldest fibers are situated in the center, the younger fibers are positioned in the periphery. The fiber cells are densely packed, leaving little room for the extracellular space, which is estimated to amount to not more then 10% of the lens substance.

As the lens is not vascularized, nutrients are supplied and waste products are removed by the circulating aqueous humor. The lens capsule permits diffusion of small molecules such as glucose, amino acids, salts, and vitamins to supply energy and maintain ionic balance and protein synthesis. The epithelial cells actively transport amino acids through the lens capsule against a concentration gradient which is of importance to maintain ionic balance and protein synthesis. The epithelial cells through the action of adenosine triphosphatase (ATPase) also operate to create an increase in the ratio of potassium and sodium over that in the aqueous, to maintain ionic balance.

There are essentially three ways in which glucose can be metabolized by the lens, namely glycolysis, the aerobic glucose metabolism, and by means of the aldose reductase pathway. Glucose is the essential source of energy for the lens. The concentration of glucose in the aqueous humor is approximately that of the blood. The concentration in the lens is about one-tenth of this. Glucose enters the lens by diffusion, permeates the extracellular space and is transported to the lens fibers. The rate of entry of glucose into the lens fibers is approximately the same as the utilization of the sugar, so that there is little sugar demonstrable in the lens fibers.

The oxygen tension of the aqueous humor is that of the venous blood, therefore the lens is relatively anoxic and under normal conditions glycolysis is by far the most important pathway. This anaerobic breakdown of glucose to lactic acid appears to be sufficient to satisfy the metabolic needs of the lens. Glucose is first phosphorylated in the presence of ATP by the enzyme hexokinase, forming glucose 6-phosphate and ADP. Glucose 6-phosphate is then transformed to fructose and finally to lactic acid. The limiting factor for glycolysis under normal circumstances is the phosphorylation of glucose by the enzyme hexokinase.

It is estimated that about 2.5% of the glucose is broken down by oxidation, but the aerobic pathway supplies about one-third of the energy derived from glucose, as much ATP is formed. Oxidation of glucose produces an increased concentration of CO_2, because the pentose phosphate pathway is also used. Pentose is formed and also nicotinamide adenine dinucleotide phosphate ($NADPH_2$) for synthetic processes.

The lens contains the enzyme aldose reductase, which in the presence of the reduced coenzyme $NADPH_2$ produces sorbitol from glucose and the oxidized coenzyme. Sorbitol is further broken down by another enzyme, polyol dehydrogenase, in the presence of the coenzyme nictotinamide adenine dinucleotide (NAD), forming fructose and $NADH_2$. Fructose can be reduced further to lactic acid. As the affinity of hexokinase for glucose is about two hundred times greater then the affinity of aldose reductase, under normal circumstances only a fraction of the glucose will be used for the aldose reductase pathway.

If the blood sugar rises and the concentration of glucose increases in the aqueous humor, and also, through diffusion, the lens, the rate of glycolysis will not increase, as the limiting factor is the phosphorylation of glucose by the enzyme hexokinase, which is already proceeding at the maximum possible rate. Under these conditions glucose is also broken down by the aldose reductase pathway. As the enzyme is located in the epithelial cells immediately under the capsule and in the anterior cortex, sorbitol and other metabolites will accumulate there.

Passing visual symptoms

Transient changes in refraction in patients with diabetes mellitus have been known for quite some time. The concept of Duke-Elder has long been accepted. He felt that in acute diabetes there is a loss of salts and electrolytes due to polyuria and polydipsia with subsequent dehydration of the body. The composition of the aqueous humor is similar to that of the blood. It becomes hypotonic in comparison to the osmotic value of the lens as the lens retains its composition longer because substances diffuse only slowly from the lens because of the lens capsule. This results in osmotic swelling of the lens with a subsequent shift towards myopia.

If diabetes is treated, the composition of the blood and aqueous humor return to normal values and as the lens only slowly becomes isotonic it releases the extra fluid over a period of time, causing a shift towards hyperopia. Later, when the lens metabolism became better understood, the swelling of the lens was attributed to the osmotic swelling as a result of accumulation of sorbitol in the anterior cortex, but the association of more or less acute diabetes with myopia and the normalization of diabetes with hyperopia remained essentially unchallenged until relatively recently.

However, there is now overwhelming evidence of an association between moderate hyperglycemia and hyperopia[23–27] and little or no evidence of any association between moderate hyperglycemia and myopia.[26] Moreover, Planten et al,[28] with the aid of ultrasonic A-scans, failed to reveal any difference in the optic parameters or the position of the lens during or after changes in blood glucose content, which demonstrates that only changes in the refractive indices between cortex and nucleus of the lens were responsible for the shift towards hyperopia, rather than changes in the radius of curvature of the lens or its position. Relatively small changes in the refractive index of the lens can be responsible for marked refractive changes.[29]

Eva and associates[26] argued very convincingly that an elevated glucose level in the aqueous at the onset of diabetes counterbalances the osmotic pressure caused by sorbitol and other polyol metabolites that might have formed in the lens through the aldose reductase pathway. Osmotic swelling cannot be expected in the lens as long as the glucose levels in the aqueous are high. Only long-standing and moderately severe cases of diabetes, in which the glucose level of the aqueous increases relatively little and diffuses into the lens and activates the aldose reductase pathway, will cause a sufficient accumulation of metabolites to cause osmotic swelling with a shift towards hyperopia.

It would seem, then, that the nature of the refractive changes is dependent on the relative strength of the osmotic forces in the lens and the aqueous humor. If the lenticular osmotic forces are more pronounced a shift towards hyperopia can be expected. On the other hand, if the osmotic forces of the aqueous are stronger, one can expect myopia to develop. This would explain the development of myopia in severe acute onset diabetes. The very rapid rise in glucose in the aqueous before sufficient metabolites have accumulated in the lens to balance the osmotic forces inside and outside the lens. This change does not last long; once metabolites have accumulated in the lens and the sugar concentration in the aqueous is decreased, hyperopia sets in. Vigorous treatment of diabetes will temporarily move the osmotic force in the lens, with subsequent hydration and development of hyperopia.[30]

CATARACT AND DIABETES

It is common knowledge that high blood sugar can cause opacities in the lens. Two types of cataract have been identified in diabetic patients and their association with hyperglycemia has been well established. One type occurs at a relatively young age, often referred to as 'juvenile cataracts'. Their appearance is somewhat arbitrarily set at under 40 years of age. These cataracts are considered 'typical' for diabetes, yet biomicroscopically they share many characteristics with other metabolic cataracts. They mature relatively rapidly and are usually bilateral. Their development is related to the severity of diabetes and can be expected if diabetic control is poor (*Fig. 4.1*). An association with the duration of diabetes is less clear.

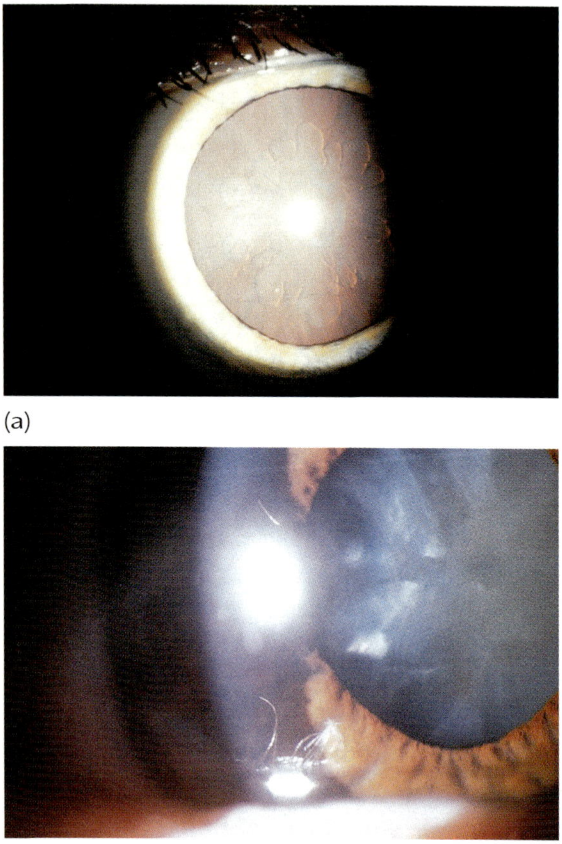

(a)

(b)

Figure 4.1
A rapidly developing dense cataract in a patient with ketoacidosis and a very high blood sugar concentration. (Courtesy of Peter Hamilton.)

The other form is indistinguishable from presenile and senile cataracts, except that they tend to occur at a younger age and have a more rapid progression, particularly in women. From a biochemical standpoint the pathological process underlying both types of cataracts is believed to be identical, namely osmotic stress which results in interference with metabolic processes. What is ultimately responsible for the morphological differences between the juvenile and the adult diabetic cataracts is the age of the lens capsule and the lens material at the time of diabetes.

Diabetic juvenile cataract

On biomicroscopic examination juvenile diabetic cataracts show some characteristic features that have been well documented. In the anterior and somewhat later in the posterior cortex, located just beneath the capsule, one can observe a layer of dot-like or flake-like opacities somewhat reminiscent of a 'snow storm'.[31] These opacities are not pathognomonic for juvenile diabetes, as similar morphologic opacities are found in other metabolic diseases. Gradually, the opacities progress into the middle and deeper parts of the cortex. At this point the posterior cortex usually becomes involved and later on the nucleus of the lens becomes hazy.

Perhaps the only pathognomonic feature of the juvenile diabetic cataract is the 'diabetic needles'.[32] Although it is not always present, it is very characteristic. In retroillumination one can observe in these cases peculiar, spoke-like structures in the periphery of the lens that have an equal diameter over their entire length and can thus be differentiated from ordinary spokes if these presenile changes happen to be present also (*Fig. 4.2*).

As the cataract progresses a dense subcapsular central disciform opacity can sometimes develop. From the disk, opacities usually radiate for a short distance towards the periphery. These polar opacities impede the vision to a marked degree (*Fig. 4.3*). Histopathologically, these opacities represent excessive thickening of the anterior polar capsule.[33] Juvenile cataracts are rare.

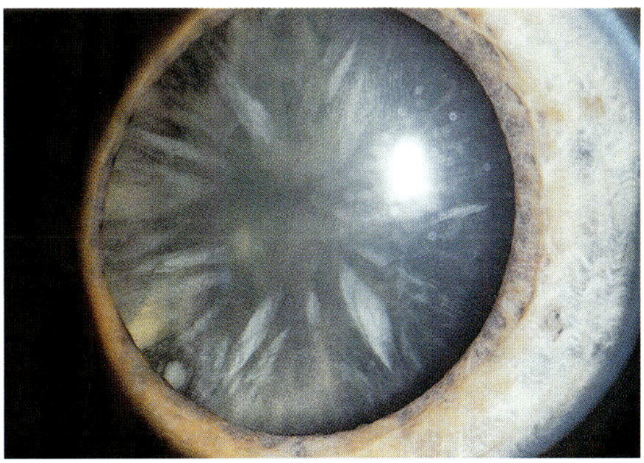

Figure 4.2
Probably the only truly pathognomonic feature of juventile diabetic cataract is the 'diabetic needle'. (Courtesy of Peter Hamilton.)

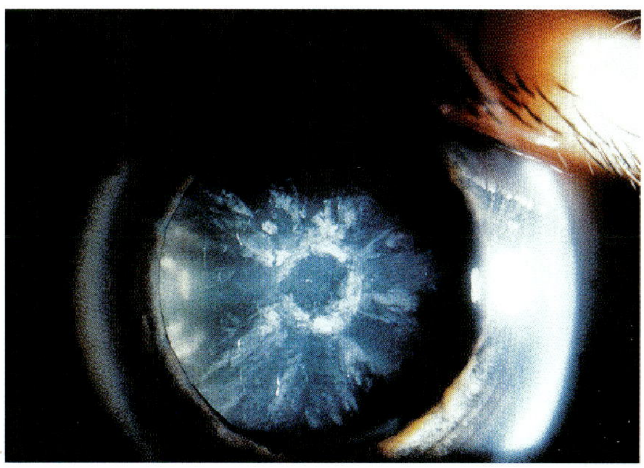

Figure 4.3
Anterior lens opacity in the polar region in a diabetic patient. Note the dot lens opacities in the subcapsular region of the anterior cortex of the lens. (Courtesy of Peter Hamilton.)

The adult diabetic cataract

Any lens undergoes certain chemical and physical changes as it ages. The older central fibers are getting increasingly compressed by the relentless growth of the outer cortical fibers and the lens becomes relatively flatter. At the end of the fifth decade the progressive sclerosing process of the lens, and more particularly of the nucleus of the lens, becomes clinically manifest as loss of accommodation that is a decrease in molding ability of the lens as a result of the gradual loss of elasticity of the capsule. There is also thickening of the lens capsule. Furthermore, there is gradual dehydration with loss of water-binding capacity.

The lens metabolism decreases and waste material accumulates which in the end leads to opacification of the lens. In both senile and adult diabetic cataracts, the changes may involve primarily the cortex, the nucleus, or subcapsular regions and be classified further according to their development. Early and frequent changes usually involve the cortex of the lens. These changes in the ageing lens are 'water clefts', lamellary separation of the lens fibers and cuneiform opacities. The nucleus may become hazy and may even display yellowish, reddish, and brownish colors.

The lens in diabetics may show opacification that follows certain definite morphological patterns indistinguishable from presenile and senile changes. Yet chemically, the diabetic cataract differs significantly from the senile cataracts in that in the adult diabetic cataracts there is an increase in the concentration of glucose, sorbitol, and fructose in comparison to the normal population. Adult diabetic cataracts are common; in fact they have been shown to occur more often in the diabetic population than in a normal population[34] and they usually tend to occur at an earlier age and progress more rapidly, particularly in women.[35,36]

Tight control of diabetes mellitus at all times is difficult to achieve. Episodes of hyperglycemia result in increased concentrations of glucose in the aqueous, with correspondingly increased glucose levels in the lens. This overtaxes the hexokinase pathway, which in turn leads to the activation of the aldose reductase pathway, with the accumulation of sorbitol in the epithelium and the anterior portion of the cortex of the lens. Thus an osmotic gradient is created, causing hydration of the lens and a change in the refractive index of the cortical area that will result in a shift towards hyperopia. Many diabetics experience such transient changes in refraction.

Kinoshita[37] demonstrated that the aldose reductase-initiated extracellular accumulation of sorbitol leads to an osmotic force in the lens that can provoke cataract formation. Sorbitol accumulates because its production is faster than its conversion to fructose. Diffusion of sorbitol out of the lens is slow because the polar character of this alcohol sugar makes easy penetration through membranes difficult. The accumulation of sorbitol increases the intralenticular osmotic force with subsequent hydration of the lens in order to neutralize the osmotic gradient between the aqueous and the lens.

Increased lens hydration leads to altered lens membrane permeability and subsequent biochemical changes that will ultimately result in cataract formation. As the lens membrane permeability changes, sodium will enter the lens by diffusion and the high potassium:sodium ratio in the lens will decrease. The concentration of glutathione, myoinositol, ATP, and free amino acids in the lens also decreases.

Because of these biochemical changes, degeneration of the epithelial cells in the axial regions shows as vacuolation.[40] The superficial cortical fibers swell, disintegrate, and show vacuoles. Protein synthesis decreases as a result of the increase of intralenticular concentration of sodium and is finally abolished. Cortical opacities proceed to nuclear cataracts with complete loss of osmotic integrity. There is considerable support for this osmotic hypothesis of cataract formation.[38–41]

On the other hand, Bron et al[36] have pointed out that as aldose reductase is much more concentrated in the epithelial cells than the rest of the lens, sorbitol will primarily accumulate in the epithelial cells and the anterior section of the cortex, and there appears to be a marginal expectation that sufficient sorbitol accumulates in the cortex to explain the lens swelling and cataract formation on an osmotic basis alone. They feel that the very low levels of sorbitol in adult diabetic lenses make an osmotic mechanism for the increased risk of cataract less likely. They suggest that other mechanisms such as glycation and oxidative stress may play an important role.

INTRAOCULAR PRESSURE AND DIABETES

Primary chronic ocular hypertension and glaucoma

The relationship between diabetes mellitus and significant deviations from the average intraocular pressure in the population, increased intraocular pressure, and glaucoma has often been and still is contested. Small wonder, as diabetes mellitus is a complex metabolic disease that will affect at one time or another those factors that are responsible for the changing of the intraocular pressure.

Hyperglycemia, for example, can lead either to a fall in intraocular pressure as the result of an osmotic mechanism or to an increase in intraocular pressure. Hypoglycemia can also lead to a fall in intraocular pressure[42] due to the release of adrenalin. A drop in intraocular pressure can also be expected in those cases with insulin-dependent diabetes during acute hypocalcemia.[43]

From the data available, it would seem that on the average the intraocular pressure in diabetics with autonomic neuropathy is not different from that in persons without diabetes.[44] While some clinicians have claimed the intraocular pressure in diabetics to be higher than in patients without diabetes,[45–47] Armaly and Baloglou[48] claimed the intraocular pressures in diabetics to be lower than in the general population.

Recently, the dispute on the association between diabetes mellitus and glaucoma has flared up again. Quite a number of clinicians have reported the two diseases to be associated. Dielemans et al[49] concluded that newly diagnosed patients with diabetes mellitus and high levels of blood glucose are associated with elevated intraocular pressure and high-tension glaucoma. Klein et al[50] found the presence of open-angle glaucoma to be increased in people with older-onset diabetes.

Mitchell et al[51] found a significant and consistent association between diabetes and glaucoma that was independent of the effect of diabetes on the intraocular pressure, which suggests that there is a real association between these diseases. Clark and Mapstone[52] found in patients with closed-angle glaucoma and in patients with ocular hypertension a significantly increased prevalence of familial type (non-insulin-dependent) diabetes mellitus.

Redmond[53] however, pointed out that the link between diabetes and glaucoma is disputed and Thielsch et al[54] found no evidence from their population-based investigation to support an association between diabetes and primary open-angle glaucoma. It must be remembered that demonstrating a positive association between two diseases that are relatively frequent in middle age is difficult.

Many clinicians have assumed that an increased intraocular pressure conferred some protection for the eye against the development of retinopathy.[55] Jain[56] studied the intraocular pressure as a function of the level of the retinopathy and found that the mean value of the intraocular pressure was significantly lower in patients with retinopathy than in diabetics without retinopathy, which seemed to support the clinical impression that increased intraocular pressure protected against retinopathy.

Becker[45] found that in patients with diabetes who had high basic pressures, the water-drinking test was in a high proportion of cases positive, and that provocation with topical corticosteroids produced a significant increase in intraocular pressure in 80% of patients without retinopathy or with simple background retinopathy and in only 30% of those patients with malignant retinopathy. One of the conclusions of the author is that the high intraocular pressure seems to confer some protection against the development of malignant retinopathy.

In the study of Valone et al[57] it was demonstrated that patients with unilateral increased intraocular pressure had less severe manifestations of diabetic retinopathy on the side that had increased intraocular pressure.

Unchallenged and of important clinical significance are the findings that in diabetics with glaucoma there is a more rapid functional deterioration as shown in more rapid visual field loss and more rapid increase in cup to disk ratio. Also, in relatively slightly increased intraocular pressure, visual field defects can be expected early.[45] An interesting observation was made by Zeiter and Shin,[58] who found that patients with primary open-angle glaucoma and predominantly inferior field defects in one or both eyes are more likely to have diabetes.

Secondary ocular hypertension and glaucoma

When diabetic retinal disease reaches the phase of proliferative retinopathy, or sometimes even earlier, neovascularization of the iris can be expected (*Fig. 4.4*). It is assumed to be induced by hypoxia of the iris or indirectly by diffusion of a vasoproliferative factor from the hypoxic retina. This neovascularization of the iris, coined 'rubeosis iridis' by Salus, is by no means pathognomonic for diabetes.[59] Newly formed vessels start appearing, usually in both eyes, at any point on the anterior surface of the iris; however, the area of the pupillary margin and the periphery of the iris are predilection sites. The detection of early neovascularization of the iris is greatly facilitated by fluorescein angiography. One can sometimes see the newly formed vessels originating from what seems to be a normal iris vessel.[59]

These newly formed vessels consist of tubes of simple endothelial lining with little supportive tissue. If tufts of these newly formed vessels are growing towards the chamber angle, and start covering or even invading the corneoscleral meshwork, extensive peripheral anterior synechiae can be the result. Corneal endothelial cells may grow posteriorly over the angle and the

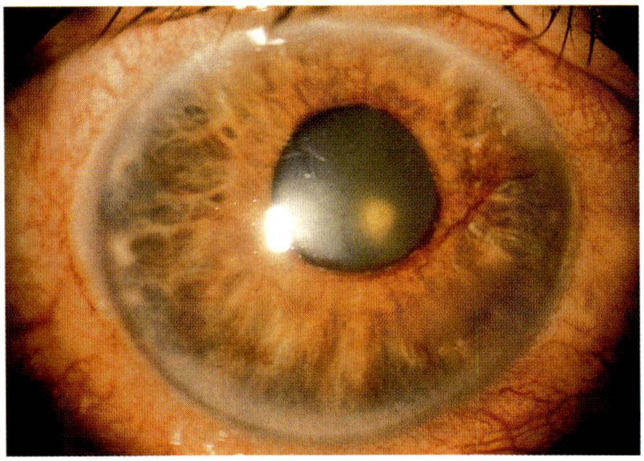

Figure 4.4
Rubeosis iridis diabetica. New vessels are visible on the anterior surface of the iris. (Courtesy of Peter Hamilton.)

peripheral iris surface,[60] increasing the resistance to outflow of the aqueous and causing a rise in intraocular pressure.

Increased intraocular pressure can also originate from an increased outflow resistance as a consequence of repeated bleeding from the newly formed vessels or leakage of protein and cells from these vessels.[61] Posterior synechiae may form as the pupillary margin and anterior surface of the lens adhere because of neovascularization or inflammatory exudate, which presents as threads of egg white, as there is invariably a chronic inflammatory response and atrophy of the iris which can lead to ectropion uveae.

Neovascularization can on occasion disappear spontaneously, after panretinal coagulation,[62–65] often with a decrease in intraocular pressure, or after hypophysectomy. Matsushima et al[66] described an interesting case in which 3 months after a cataract extraction neovascular glaucoma developed in a patient with diabetes mellitus and severe anemia as a result of gastrointestinal hemorrhage due to advanced stomach cancer. After the anemia improved the neovascularization of the iris disappeared. Here the severe anemia is believed to have accelerated the development of the neovascular glaucoma.

If neovascularization of the iris is complicated by glaucoma the prognosis is poor, as the situation develops as a rule into a painful, intractable hemorrhagic glaucoma. The treatment is very difficult. Because of the tendency of the newly formed vessels to bleed, intraocular filtration procedures are not indicated. Cyclodiathermy is the operation of choice, but the pressure-lowering effect is only temporary. Because of the pain and poor vision, enucleation is tempting, but one has to be cautious as the condition is bilateral.

Ocular hypotony and diabetes

In severe diabetic ketosis the eye becomes hypotonic. The eyeball becomes so soft that it has been likened to a 'poached egg'. Complications are rare. As soon as the ketosis responds to treatment the intraocular pressure returns to normal values. The mechanism of the hypotonia in diabetic ketosis is unkown. It is likely that it is a consequence of the combination of salt depletion and water dehydration, metabolic acidosis, and hyperosmolarity with hyperglycemia.

Any one of these factors alone cannot be responsible for the marked hypotonia, as it is not observed in severe dehydration alone such as occurs in cholera, nor is it observed in acidosis alone such as occurs in both uremic and respiratory acidosis. Hyperosmolarity in hyperglycemia in diabetic ketosis alone can also not be responsible for the ocular hypotony, since in nonketotic hyperosmolar diabetic coma there is no ocular hypotonia.

DISORDERS OF THE OPTIC NERVE IN DIABETES

Apart from a genetically determined autosomal recessive or sporadic hereditary progressive optic atrophy, with many neurologic and systemic abnormalities,[67] there are two well-recognized disease entities of the optic nerve associated with diabetes: optic disk edema and optic neuropathy. There is considerable doubt if there exists a specific diabetic optic neuritis. Optic or retrobulbar neuritis can occur in the course of diabetes,[68,69] but the incidence of this acute painless and often bilateral loss of vision with central or pericentral scotoma is probably not higher than in an age-matched nondiabetic population.[70]

Edema of the optic disk

Acute swelling of the optic disk in juvenile diabetics[71–73] is a well-recognized syndrome. The swelling of the optic disk may be unilateral or bilateral and in the beginning there is no pallor. Edema of the optic disk has to be differentiated from papilledema due to increased intracranial pressure and psuedopapilledema with or without drusen; from papillitis; and from adult ischemic optic atrophy with severely affected visual acuity that has no tendency to return to normal values and that ends with optic atrophy.

Patients with edema of the optic disk are almost always younger than 30 years of age and have long-standing juvenile diabetes which is usually well controlled (*Fig. 4.5*). There is no relationship between the degree of the edema of the optic disk and the level of diabetic retinopathy. In half of the cases an illness preceeds the onset of the swelling of the disk. Visual loss is usually moderate and is not related to the degree of swelling of the disk and has the tendency to return to normal or near normal within 6 months. In mild cases no hemorrhages are present on the swollen disks, but in severe cases capillary telangiectasia and hemorrhages in the nerve fiber layer and fluorescein-leaking capillaries can be expected. Occasionally, cystoid macular edema and exudative macular star figures can develop.

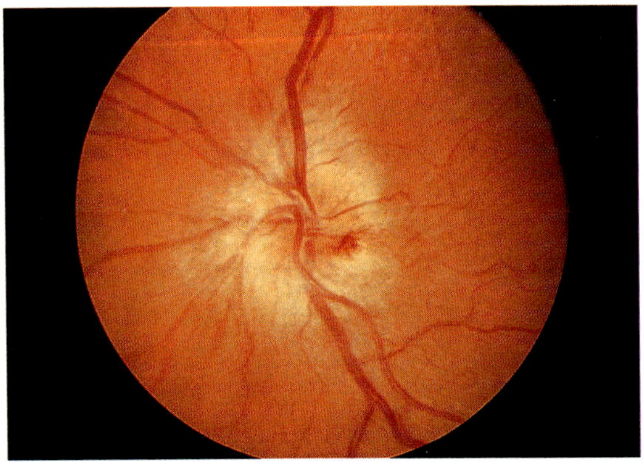

Figure 4.5
Non-neurologic optic disk oedema in juvenile-onset diabetes. The oedematous disc shows superficially located and somewhat dilated capillaries. (Courtesy of Peter Hamilton.)

Visual field defects can occur and are of an arcuate nature that may or may not persist. Occasionally, an enlarged blind spot or altitudinal defects are found. In those cases, in which the visual field defects appear to be permanent, a certain pallor of the optic disk will develop. Since the swelling of the optic disk occurs abruptly in many patients, this disease is thought to have a vascular origin.

Optic neuropathy

Optic neuropathy is a condition that evolves rather slowly in the course of diabetes. In the beginning there is a decrease in nerve function without any clinically visible changes in either the nerve fiber layer or the optic nerve. Later clinically visible damage to the nerve fiber layer can be observed and later still damage of the optic nerve becomes apparent. There is some merit in dividing the evolution of optic neuropathy into three stages as championed by Chihara.[74]

In stage 1 only electrophysiologic abnormalities are found. At this time there is no visible retinopathy. In the second stage, clinically visible defects in the nerve fiber layer can be detected (*Fig. 4.6*), and in the third stage a manifest atrophy of the optic nerve with or without cupping of the optic disk is present. In the last two stages diabetic retinopathy is clinically visible, and there is a general relation between the degree of retinopathy and the severity of the nerve fiber layer defects. In the initial stage no nerve fiber loss can be detected clinically.

However, there is a wide range of electrophysiologic abnormalities such as reduction of oscillatory potentials on the electroretinogram,[75] reduction in dark adaptation,[76] reduction in the visual evoked response,[77] abnormal color sensation,[78] reduction in contrast sensitivity,[79] and

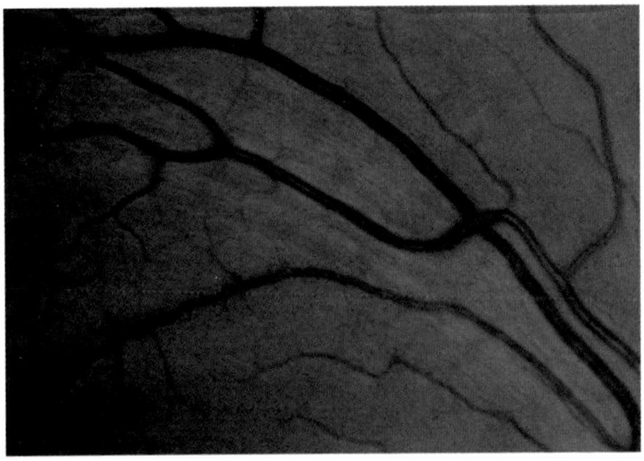

Figure 4.6
A red-free photograph of a retinal nerve fiber layer defect, visible as a dark band in connection with the optic nerve. (Courtesy of Peter Hamilton.)

reduction in conduction velocity in the optic nerve.[80]

The pathogenesis of these electrophysiologic abnormalities has not yet been elucidated with certainty, but nerve fiber damage as a consequence of metabolic rather than vascular abnormalities is believed to be more important. Particularly, problems in the metabolism of myoinositol have received much attention. It is known that myoinositol, a water-soluble 6-carbon cyclic hexanol, is an important substrate in maintaining nerve function. Myoinositol is metabolized to IP3 (inositol 1,4,5-triphosphate). This metabolite mediates the release of calcium from intracellular store sites. Associated with IP3 is diacylglycerol, an activator of protein kinase C. IP3 and diacyclglycerol play an important role in the intracellular metabolism. Hyperglycemia inhibits the uptake of myoinositol.

A depletion of myoinositol has been reported in the diabetic retina,[81] which in turn may cause a reduced protein kinase C which will lead to an impaired sodium–potassium ATPase function and so explain reduced electrophysiologic nerve function and reduced conduction velocity.[80–82,83] Also, the glycosylation of enzymes[84] and impaired polymerization of tubulin[85] may play a role in the reduction of conduction velocity.

The second stage is characterized by loss of nerve fibers. Clinically, optic nerve fiber loss can be visualized in red-free light with the ophthalmoscope. These nerve fiber layer defects can be seen as arcuate dark bands in the retina. In the early stages the optic disk may appear normal but there may be visual field defects present.[86] In about one-fifth of patients with diabetes of 10 years' duration or more these defects can be spotted even before any clinical sign of diabetic retinopathy is present. A general depression of retinal sensitivity[87] or relative scotomas[88] are usually present.

The pathogenesis of retinal nerve fiber layer remains uncertain and a number of pathological factors have been proposed. As the enzyme aldose reductase is present in neural tissue, it stands to reason that sorbitol accumulation as a primary cause of optic neuropathy has figured prominently, and in fact an increase in the level of endoneural sorbitol has been demonstrated,[89] but the increased osmolality is too small to cause the capillaries to collapse.[90] In fact in one clinical study no increase in the endoneural fluid pressure could be demonstrated.[91] Also, the inhibition of aldose reductase did not prevent optic atrophy.

In the period before major diabetic changes in the retina have taken place, the main pathogenic factors may have to be attributed to primary axonopathy. Continuous supply of axoplasmic enzymes and cytoskeletal proteins by way of axonal transport maintains nerve function. If this transport is disrupted in any way, nerve dysfunction or loss of retinal nerve fibers is the result.[92,93] At a later stage, parts of the capillary bed become obstructed and ischemic retinal changes set in, which are visible as areas of nonperfusion on fluorescein angiography. The local hypoxia may result in dysfunction and loss of the nerve fibers. The appearance of cotton-wool sports in the ischemic retinal areas is a clinically visible sign of stagnant axoplasmic transport.[94] Besides ischemic changes leading to damage of the nerve fiber layer, other factors possibly contributing to nerve fiber layer damage, such as excitotoxins, heat shock protein, and growth factor[85,95] to name but a few, may also be responsible for nerve fiber damage in diabetic patients.

DIABETIC OPHTHALMOPLEGIA

Isolated cranial nerve palsies occasionally develop in diabetes. The third,[96,97] sixth[97] and, rarely, the fourth[96] cranial nerves are the most likely to be involved. The etiology is unclear, although several clinicopathological studies on the oculomotor nerve palsy in diabetes[98,99] are strongly indicative of a focal ischemic lesion. It is assumed[98,99] that widespread damage to arterioles, as is the case in diabetes, might cause local secondary ischemic lesions that effect the vasa vasorum of the involved cranial nerve.

Both Asbury et al[98] and Weber et al[99] found the substrate of the ischemic lesion to be a circumscribed demyelinated lesion of the affected third nerve in either its intracavernous or its subarachnoid portion. It was obvious that the central part of the nerve was more affected than the peripheral parts, indicating that the peripheral nerve fibers are less vulnerable to ischemia than are the central fibers. As the pupillomotor fibers of the third nerve are mainly located in the peripheral nerve part,[100,101] it is not surprising that in diabetic ophthalmoplegia of the third nerve the pupil will be spared.

Risk factors for diabetic nerve palsies are age and duration of diabetes,[102,103] although in some patients the ophthalmoplegia is the first manifestation of diabetes. Patients with ophthalmoplegia are usually adult but it can occur in younger patients. Moderate to severe retinopathy and neuropathy are also known to be associated with the development of diabetic ophthalmoplegia.[102]

The development of isolated cranial nerve palsies is not restricted to diabetes mellitus. Other causes of an acquired isolated third nerve palsy can be neoplasm, trauma, aneurysm, miscellaneous diseases, and ischemia.[100,101] Diabetic ophthalmoplegia is part of the ischemia group and is, in fact, quite common.[102,103] It is estimated that in ophthalmoplegia of ischemic origin about 18% can be attributed to diabetes.[104]

The causes of a sixth nerve palsy are similar. However, an acquired isolated sixth nerve palsy is, in comparison to a third nerve palsy, much more likely to be caused by neoplasm or diseases such as leukemia, multiple sclerosis, and pseudomotor cerebri. Ischemia is the cause in about 10–15%[96,105] of which 26% can be attributed to diabetes.[104]

The clinical picture of an acquired third nerve palsy in diabetes is quite characteristic. It is almost always preceded by headache–usually, but not necessarily, located at the same side as the ophthalmoplegia–that lasts for a few days. Subsequently, there is ptosis and diplopia. As a rule the pupil is spared. Although there is almost always a complete paralysis of the external muscles, full recovery can be expected within 9 months. In contrast to a third nerve palsy, the sixth nerve palsy is very rarely preceded by headache. The course of the disease is, however, similar to a third nerve palsy with a rapid onset and a compete recovery in a few months.

MUCORMYCOSIS

The term 'mucormycosis' is well established in medical literature and should therefore continue to be used for mycoses of the order of Mucorales. The designation 'zygomycosis', derived from the class name Zygomycetes, should be abandoned, as the various members of the Zygomycetes do not cause the same type of diseases and it consequently does not convey useful information for the clinician.[106]

Mucormycosis can infect a number of different sites of the body and these distinct forms are referred to as rhinoorbitocerebral, gastrointestinal, pulmonary, and cutaneous infections. The most common variety is the rhinoorbitocerebral form and as it has ophthalmic implications, only this form is treated here.

Pathogens and epidemiology

The various members of the family of the Mucorales are ubiquitously distributed fungi that can be found on decaying fruits and vegetables and on moulding bread. These opportunistic fungi have a low virulence but they can infect debilitated persons, particularly diabetics in ketoacidosis. The most frequently isolated genera of the Mucoraceae associated with mucormycosis in diabetics are *Rhizopus*, *Rhizomucor* and *Absidia*, but other genera are occasionally involved.

All Mucorales are molds as they grow as hyphae. Differentiation of the most important genera of the Mucoraceae is based to an important extent on morphological characteristics such as the presence and location of rhizoids, the presence of apophyses, and the morphology of columnellae. The organisms grow within 1 week on most media, except on those which contain cyclohexamide, but curiously enough, the agents of mucormycosis are very difficult to culture from infected tissue.[107] Hyphae are relatively easily demonstrated in fixed-tissue biopsies stained with hematoxilin-eosin, Grocott–Gomori methenamine silver nitrate or periodic acid-Schiff stain or on touch slides taken from biopsy material after treatment with potassium hydroxide. The hyphae are broad, 10–20 μm in diameter, non- or sparsely septate, and branching at right angles.

The predilection of the hyphae of these molds for invading the blood vessels, particularly the arterioles, where they cause local thrombosis with the release of septic emboli, ischemia, and infarction,[108,109] combined with the ability of these fungi to produce enzymes capable of causing necrosis, makes infection with Mucoraceae a very dangerous and often fatal disease that has a survival rate of slightly over one-third of the patients.[110]

Pathogenesis

Why diabetics with ketoacidosis are at such risk of becoming infected with Mucorales is not entirely clear. The loss of the ability to prevent germination in macrophages, the failure to produce adequate quantities of toxic phagocytic agents and oxidative metabolites, and the decrease in anti-infective serum factors may play an important role.[96]

Rhinoorbitocerebral mucormycosis

Mucoraceae belong to the normal flora of the nose and pharynx. If the host defences are markedly decreased, infection therefore usually begins in the upper turbinate or paranasal sinuses, less frequently in the palate or pharynx.[111] The usual presenting signs and symptoms of the infection, therefore, can be expected there. Later, the eye and eventually the brain and meninges become involved.[113–119]

A thick blackish discharge tinged with blood becomes visible in the nose, and black eschars are situated around the nasal orifices. On inspection, reddish-black necrotic areas can be seen on the turbinates and the septum. Radiographic examination can reveal thickened mucosa if the sinuses are involved and there may be an air-fluid level present. If there is bone destruction this can be best visualized using a CT scan.

If the mold reaches the orbit, signs and symptoms of orbital cellulitis will develop, with orbital and facial pain, headache and loss of extraocular muscle function and proptosis. In this stage there is usually a marked conjunctival swelling. Vision is lost due to thrombosis of the central retinal artery and the retinal veins are swollen. Hyphae may be observed in the vitreous.

If the cranial nerves are involved, usually branches of the trigeminal and facial nerve, areas of anesthesia, ptosis, and a fixed and dilated pupil are present, as well as symptoms of facial nerve palsy. In the end cavernous sinus thrombosis and thrombosis of the internal carotid artery and the formation of a cerebral abscess can ensue with lethargy, delirium, coma, and death, which can be expected in 1–2 weeks after infection.

Treatment

First and foremost, as in all saprophytic infections as a result of debilitating diseases, the treatment has to be directed towards the underlying disease, such as diabetes with ketoacidosis. The best antifungal treatment for infection caused by Mucorales is amphotericin B.[108] The drug is nephrotoxic and kidney function should be carefully watched. Extensive surgical debridement should be carried out wherever possible.

REFERENCES

1. Ioli-Spade G, Ulteriore contributo allo studio della cherato distrofia epitheliale punctata diabetica, *Boll Ocul* (1964) **43**:775.
2. Schultz RO, Peters M, Sobocinski K et al, Diabetic corneal neuropathy, *Trans Am Ophthalmol Soc* (1983) **81**:107.
3. Schultz RO, Peters MA, Sobocinski K et al, Diabetic keratopathy as a manifestation of peripheral neuropathy, *Am J Ophthalmol* (1983) **96**:368.
4. Ishii Y, Lahav M, Mukai Y, Corneal changes in diabetic patients and streptozocin-diabetic rats. An ultrastructural correlation, ARVO abstracts, *Invest Ophthalmol Vis Sci* (1981) 154.
5. Kenyon KR, Wafai Z, Michels R et al, Corneal basement membrane abnormalities in diabetes mellitus, *Invest Ophthalmol Vis Sci* (1978) **17**:245.
6. Tsubota K, Chiba K, Shimazaki J, Corneal epithelium in diabetic patients, *Cornea* (1991) **10**:156–60.
7. Foulks G, Thoft R, Perry H, Tolentino F, Factors related to corneal epithelial complications after closed vitrectomy in diabetes, *Arch Ophthalmol* (1979) **97**:1076.
8. Schultz RO, Matsuda M, Yee RW et al, Corneal endothelial changes in type I and II diabetes mellitus, *Am J Ophthalmol* (1984) **98**:401–10.
9. Lass JH, Spurney RV, Dutt RM et al, A morphologic and fluorophotometric analysis of the corneal endothelium in type I diabetes mellitus and cystic fibrosis, *Am J Ophthalmol* (1985) **100**:783–8.
10. Busted N, Olsen T, Schmitz O, Clinical observations on the corneal thickness and the corneal endothelium in diabetes mellitus, *Br J Ophthalmol* (1981) **65**:687–90.
11. Pardos GJ, Krachmer JH, Comparison of endothelial cell density in diabetics and a control population, *Am J Ophthalmol* (1980) **98**:172.
12. Kador PF, Kinoshita JH, Role of aldose reductase in the development of diabetes-associated complications, *Am J Med* (1985) **79** (Suppl 5a):8.
13. Kinoshita JH, Aldose reductase in the diabetic eye: XLIII Edward Jackson Memorial Lecture, *Am J Ophthalmol* (1986) **102**:685.
14. Meyer LA, Ubels JL, Edelhauser HF, Corneal endothelial morphology in the rat, effects of aging, diabetes, and topical aldose reductase inhibitor treatment, *Invest Ophthalmol Vis Sci* (1988) **29**:940–8.

15. Geroski DH, Matsuda M, Yee RW, Edelhauser HF, Pump function of the human corneal endothelium. Effects of age and cornea guttata, *Ophthalmology* (1985) **92**:759.
16. Busted N, Olsen T, Schmitz O, Clinical observations on the corneal thickness and the corneal endothelium in diabetes mellitus, *Br J Ophthalmol* (1981) **65**:687–90.
17. Olsen T, Busted N, Corneal thickness in eyes with diabetic and nondiabetic neovascularisation, *Br J Ophthalmol* (1981) **65**:691–3.
18. Schwartz DE, Corneal sensitivity in diabetes, *Arch Ophthalmol* (1974) **91**:174–8.
19. Draeger J et al, *Corneal Sensitivity; Management and Clinical Importance* (Springer-Verlag: Vienna, 1984) 58–63.
20. Ishida N, Rao GN, del Cerro M, Aquavella JV, Corneal nerve alterations in diabetes mellitus, *Arch Ophthalmol* (1984) **102**:1380–4.
21. Anderson J, Baun O, Aamand HE, Tear secretion in juvenile diabetics with and without autonomic neuropathy, *Acta Ophthalmol* (1985) **63**:93–6.
22. Hyndiuk RA, Kazarian EL, Schultz RO, Seideman S, Neurotrophic corneal ulcers in diabetes mellitus, *Arch Ophthalmol* (1977) **95**:2193–6.
23. Rosen M, Diabetes mellitus with relative hyperopia, *Am J Ophthalmol* (1956) **41**:680–1.
24. Planten JTh, Physiologic optic approach of lens and cataract, *Ophthalmologica* (1975) **171**:249–53.
25. Feinblum SM, Clinical significance of refractive changes in diabetes, *Optom Weekly* (1972) **63**:199–206.
26. Eva PR, Pascoe PR, Vaughan DG, Refractive change in hyperglycaemia: hyperopia, not myopia, *Br J Ophthalmol* (1982) **66**:500–5.
27. Marmor MF, Transient accommodative paralysis and hyperopia in diabetes, *Arch Ophthalmol* (1973) **89**:419–21.
28. Planten JTh, Kooijman AC, de Vries B et al, Pathological-optic approach of cataract and lens, *Ophthalmologica* (1978) **176**:331–4.
29. Fledelius HC, Fuchs J, Reck A, Refraction in diabetes during metabolic dysregulation acute or chronic, *Acta Ophthalmol* (kbh) (1990) **68**:275–80.
30. Saito Y, Ohmi G, Kinoshita S et al, Transient hyperopia with lens swelling at initial therapy in diabetes, *Br J Ophthalmol* (1973) **77**:145–8.
31. O'Brien CS, Molsberry JM, Allen JH, Diabetic cataract, *JAMA* (1934) **103**:892.
32. Rosen E, Diabetic needles, *Br J Ophthalmol* (1945) **29**:645.
33. Paterson RA, Heath H, Chemical changes in human diabetic, cataractous and b,b/-iminodiproprionitrile treated rat lens capsules, *Exp Eye Res* (1967) **6**:233.
34. Klein BE, Klein R, Wang Q et al, Older-onset diabetes and lens opacities, *Ophthalmic Epidemiol* (1995) **2**:49–55.
35. Perkins ES, Cataract: refractive error, diabetes, and morphology, *Br J Ophthalmol* (1984) **68**:293–7.
36. Bron AJ, Sparrow J, Brown et al, The lens in diabetes, *Eye* (1993) **7**:260–75.
37. Kinoshita JH, Mechanism initiating cataract formation. Proctor Lecture, *Invest Ophthalmol* (1974) **13**:713–24.
38. Chylack LT Jr, Kinoshita JH, A biochemical evaluation of a cataract induced in high glucose medium, *Invest Ophthalmol* (1969) **8**:401–12.
39. Kador PF, Kinoshita JH, Diabetic and galactosaemic cataracts, *Ciba Found Symp* (1984) **106**:110–31.
40. Robison WG, Houlder N, Kinoshita JH, The role of lens epithelium in sugar cataract formation, *Exp Eye Res* (1990) **50**:641–6.
41. Kinoshita JH, Kador PF, Datiles MD, Aldose reductase in diabetic cataracts, *JAMA* (1981) **246**:257–61.
42. Frier BM, Hepburn DA, Fisher BM et al, Fall in intraocular pressure during acute hypoglycaemia in patients with insulin dependent diabetes, *BMJ Clin Res Ed* (1987) **294**:610–11.
43. Larkin DF, Eustache P, Fall in intraocular pressure during acute hypocalcemia in patients with insulin dependent diabetes, *BMJ Clin Res Ed* (1987) **294**:1353–4.
44. al-Sereiti MR, Turner P, Gale EA, Intraocular pressure and pupillary responses in patients with diabetes mellitus, *Postgrad Med J* (1991) **67**:250–1.

45. Becker B, Diabetes mellitus and primary open-angle glaucoma, *Am J Ophthalmol* (1971) **71**:1–13.
46. Klein BEK, Klein R, Moss SE, Intraocular pressure in diabetic persons, *Ophthalmology* (1984) **91**:1356–60.
47. Arora VK, Prasad VN, The intraocular pressure and diabetes—a correlative study, *Indian J Ophthalmol* (1989) **37**:10–12.
48. Armaly MF, Baloglou PJ, Diabetes mellitus and the eye. 2. Intraocular pressure and aqueous outflow facility, *Arch Ophthalmol* (1967) **77**:493.
49. Dielemans I, de Jong PT, Stolk R et al, Primary open-angle glaucoma, intraocular pressure and diabetes mellitus in the general elderly population. The Rotterdam Study, *Ophthalmology* (1996) **103**:1271–5.
50. Klein BEK, Klein R, Jensen SC, Open-angle glaucoma and older onset diabetes. The Beaver Dam Eye Study, *Ophthalmology* (1994) **101**:1173–7.
51. Mitchell P, Smith W, Chey T et al, Open-angle glaucoma and diabetes: the Blue Mountains eye study, Australia, *Ophthalmology* (1997) **104**:712–18.
52. Clark CV, Mapstone R, Progression of impaired glucose tolerance to diabetes mellitus in patients with primary glaucoma and hypertension, *Diabet Med* (1986) **3**:226–9.
53. Redmond R, Improving the detection of glaucoma. Link between glaucoma and diabetes is disputed, *BMJ* (1995) **310**:546–7.
54. Thielsch JM, Katz J, Quigley HA et al, Diabetes, intraocular pressure, and primary open angle glaucoma in the Baltimore Eye Survey, *Ophthalmology* (1995) **102**:48–53.
55. Mooney AJ, Diabetic retinopathy—a challenge, *Br J Ophthalmol* (1963) **47**:513–20.
56. Jain IS, Luthra CL, Diabetic retinopathy. Its relationship with intraocular pressure, *Arch Ophthalmol* (1967) **78**:198–200.
57. Valone JA, McMeel JW, Franks EP, Unilateral proliferative diabetic retinopathy I. Initial findings, *Arch Ophthalmol* (1981) **99**:1357–61.
58. Zeiter JH, Shin DH, Diabetes in primary open angle glaucoma patients with inferior visual field defects, *Graefes Arch Clin Exp Ophthalmol* (1994) **232**:205–10.
59. Schulze RR, Rubeosis iridis, *Am J Ophthalmol* (1967) **63**:487–95.
60. Gartner S, Henkind P, Neovascularisation of the iris (rubeosis iridis), *Surv Ophthalmol* (1978) **22**:291–312.
61. Zirm M, Protein glaucoma—overtaxing of flow mechanisms? Preliminary report, *Ophthalmologica* (1982) **184**:155–61.
62. Callahan MA, Hilton GF, Photocoagulation and rubeosis iridis, *Am J Ophthalmol* (1974) **78**:873–4.
63. Laatikainen L, Preliminary report on effect of retinal pancoagulation on rubeosis iridis and neovascular glaucoma, *Br J Ophthalmol* (1977) **61**:278–84.
64. Little HL, Rosenthal AR, Dellaporte A et al, The effect of panretinal photocoagulation on rubeosis iridis, *Am J Ophthalmol* (1976) **81**:804–9.
65. Pavan PR, Folk JC, Weingeist TA et al, Diabetic rubeosis and panretinal photocoagulation. A prospective controlled, masked trial using iris fluorescein angiography, *Arch Ophthalmol* (1983) **101**:882–4.
66. Matsushima S, Miura Y, Kojima H et al, A case of neovascular glaucoma associated with anemia and diabetes, *Folia Opthalmol Japon* (1996) **47**:340–4.
67. Lessel S, Rosman NP, Juvenile diabetes mellitus and optic atrophy, *Arch Neurol* (1977) **34**:759–65.
68. Topilow A, Bisland T, Diabetes mellitus as a cause of papillitis, *Am J Ophthalmol* (1952) **36**:855–8.
69. Skillern PG, Lockhart G, Optic neuritis and uncontrolled diabetes mellitus in 14 patients, *Ann Intern Med* (1959) **51**:468–75.
70. Walsh FB, Hoyt WF, *Clinical Neuro-ophthalmology* 3rd edn (Williams & Wilkins: Baltimore, 1969) 624, 1111.
71. Lubow M, Makley TA, Pseudopapilledema of juvenile diabetes mellitus, *Arch Ophthalmol* (1971) **85**:417–22.

72. Barr CC, Glaser JS, Blankenship G, Acute disc swelling in juvenile diabetes. Clinical profile and natural history of 12 cases, *Arch Ophthalmol* (1980) **98**:2185–92.
73. Pavan PR, Aiello LM, Wafai Z et al, Optic disc edema in juvenile-onset diabetes, *Arch Ophthalmol* (1980) **98**:2193–5.
74. Chihara E, Matsuoka T, Ogura Y et al, Retinal nerve fiber layer defect as an early manifestation of diabetic retinopathy, *Ophthalmology* (1993) **100**:1147–51.
75. Yonemura D, Aoki T, Tsuzuki K, Electroretinogram in diabetic retinopathy, *Arch Ophthalmol* (1962) **68**:19–24.
76. Ameniya T, Dark adaptation in diabetics, *Ophthalmologica* (1977) **174**:322–6.
77. Puvanendran K, Devathasan G, Wong PK, Visual evoked responses in diabetes, *J Neurol Neurosurg Psychiatry* (1983) **46**:643–7.
78. Bresnick GH, Condit RS, Palta M et al, Association of hue discrimination loss and diabetic retinopathy, *Arch Ophthalmol* (1985) **103**:1317–24.
79. Sokol S, Moskowitz A, Skarf B et al, Contrast sensitivity in diabetics with and without background retinopathy, *Arch Ophthalmol* (1985) **103**:51–4.
80. Parisi V, Uccioli L, Monticone G et al, Visual evoked potentials after photostress in early diagnosed insulin-dependent diabetes, *Graefes Arch Clin Exp Ophthalmol* (1995) **233**:601–4.
81. MacGregor LC, Rosecan LR, Laties Am et al, Microanalysis of total lipid, glucose, sorbitol and myo-inositol in individual retinal layers of normal and alloxan-diabetic rabbits, *Diabetes* (1984) **33**(Suppl 1):89A.
82. Kamijo M, Cherian PV, Sima AA, The preventive effect of aldose reductase inhibition on diabetic optic neuropathy in the BB/W rate, *Diabetologia* (1993) **36**:893–8.
83. Greene DA, DeJesus PV, Winegrad AI, Effects of insulin and dietary myo-inositol on impaired peripheral motor nerve conduction velocity in acute streptozocin diabetes, *J Clin Invest* (1975) **55**:1326–36.
84. Frank RN, On the pathogenesis of diabetic retinopathy. A 1990 update, *Ophthalmology* (1991) **98**:586–93.
85. Williams SK, Howarth NL, Devenny JJ et al, Structural and functional consequences of increased tubulin glycosylation in diabetes mellitus, *Proc Natl Acad Sci USA* (1992) **79**:6546–50.
86. Wisznia KI, Lieberman TW, Leopold IH, Visual field in diabetic retinopathy, *Br J Ophthalmol* (1971) **55**:183–8.
87. Szymanska K, The significance of static perimetry as a method of detection of early functional changes caused by diabetes, *Pediatr Adolesc Endocrinol* (1981) **9**:82–8.
88. Bell JA, Feldon SE, Retinal microangiopathy. Correlation of Octopus perimetry with fluorescein angiography, *Arch Ophthalmol* (1984) **102**:1294–8.
89. Stewart MA, Sherman WR, Jurien MM et al, Polyol accumulation in nerve tissue of rats with experimental diabetes and galactosemia, *J Neurochem* (1967) **14**:1057–66.
90. Low PA, Endoneurial fluid pressure and microenvironment of nerve. In: Dyck PJ et al, eds. *Peripheral Neuropathy* (WB Saunders: Philadelphia, 1984).
91. Bartz-Schmidt KU, Schmitz-Valckenberg P, Retinal nerve fiber layer photography and papillometry in juvenile diabetes mellitus, *Ophthalmologe* (1994) **91**:364–7.
92. Chihara E, Impairment of protein synthesis in the retinal tissue in diabetic rabbits: secondary reduction of fast axonal transport, *J Neurochem* (1981) **37**:247–50.
93. Chihara E, Sakugawa M, Entani S, Reduced protein synthesis in diabetic retina and secondary reduction of slow axonal transport, *Brain Res* (1982) **250**:363–6.
94. McLeod D, Marshall J, Kohner EM et al, The role of axoplasmic transport in the pathogenesis of retinal cotton wool spots, *Br J Ophthalmol* (1977) **61**:177–91.
95. Pfeiffer A, Schatz H, Diabetic microvascular complications and growth factors, *Exp Clin Endocrinol Diabetes* (1995) **103**:7–14.

96. Rush JA, Younge BR, Paralysis of cranial nerves III, IV and VI, *Am J Ophthalmol* (1981) **99**:76–9.
97. Moster ML, Savino PJ, Sergott RC et al, Isolated sixth-nerve palsies in younger adults, *Arch Ophthalmol* (1984) **102**:1328–30.
98. Asbury AK, Aldredge H, Hershberg R, Fisher CM, Oculomotor palsy in diabetes mellitus: a clinico-pathological study, *Brain* (1970) **93**:555–66.
99. Weber RB, Daroff RB, Mackey EA, Pathology of oculomotor nerve palsy in diabetics, *Neurology* (1970) **20**:835–8.
100. Sunderland S, Hughes ESR, The pupilloconstrictor pathway in the nerves to the ocular muscles in man, *Brain* (1946) **69**:301.
101. Dreyfus PM, Hakim S, Adams RD, Diabetic ophthalmoplegia, *Arch Neurol Psychiat* (1957) **77**:337.
102. Goldstein JE, Cogan DG, Diabetic ophthalmoplegia with special reference to the pupil, *A.M.A. Arch Ophthalmol* (1960) **64**:592–600.
103. Zorilla E, Kozak GP, Ophthalmoplegia in diabetes mellitus, *Ann Intern Med* (1967) **67**:968–.
104. Rucker CW, Paralysis of the third, fourth and sixth cranial nerves, *Am J Ophthalmol* (1958) **46**:787–.
105. Rucker CW, The causes of paralysis of the third, fourth and sixth cranial nerves, *Am J Ophthalmol* (1966) **61**:1293–8.
106. Sugar AM, Agents of mucormycosis and related species. In: Mandell GL, Bennett JE, Dolin R, eds. *Madell, Douglas and Bennett's Principle and Practice of Infectious Diseases*, 4th edn (Churchill Livingstone: New York 1995) 2311–20.
107. Rippon JW, *Medical Mycology*, 3rd edn (WB Saunders: Philadelphia, 1988).
108. Lehrer RI, et al, Mucormycosis, *Ann Intern Med* (1980) **93**:93.
109. Meyer RD, Armstrong D, Mucormycosis—changing status, *Crit Rev Clin Lab Sci* (1973) **4**:421–51.
110. Espinel-Ingroff A, Oakley LA, Kerkering TM, Opportunistic zygomycosis, *Mycopathologia* (1987) **97**:33–42.
111. Abidi E, Sismanis A, Choi K et al, Twenty-five years experience treating cerebro-rhino-orbital mucormycosis, *Laryngoscope* (1984) **94**:1060–2.
112. Bullock JD, Jampol JM, Fezza AJ, Two cases of orbital phycomycosis with recovery, *Am J Ophthalmol* (1974) **78**:811–5.
113. Lazzaro EC, Gloan B, Mucormycosis: case presentation and discussion, *Ann Ophthalmol* (1982) **14**:660–2.
114. Rasse M, Male O, Knosp E, Rhinocerebral mycoses caused by *Mucoraceae* species (mucormycosis). Case report and literature review, *Wien Klin Wochenschr* (1990) **102**:395–403.
115. Ammon A, Rumpf WK, Hommerich CP et al, Rhinocerebral mucormycosis during deferoxamine therapy, *Dtsch Med Wochenschr* (1992) **117**:1434–8.
116. Gonzalez A, del-Palacio A, Cuertara MS et al, Zygomycosis: review of 16 cases, *Enferm Infecc Microbiol Clin* (1996) **14**:233–9.
117. Oakley LA, Fisher JF, Dennison JH, Breadmold infection in diabetes. The life-threatening condition of rhinocerebral *zygomycosis*, *Postgrad Med* (1986) **80**:93–6.
118. Boelaert JR, Mucormycosis (*zygomycosis*): is there news for the clinician? *J Infect* (1994) **28** (Suppl 1):1–6.
119. Jones AC, Bentsen TY, Freedman PD, Mucormycosis of the oral cavity, *Oral Surg Oral Med Oral Pathol* (1993) **75**:455–60.

5 Medical treatment of diabetic retinopathy

Anselm Kampik and Arnd Gandorfer

INTRODUCTION

Because of the high and growing prevalence of diabetes mellitus worldwide, treatment, including medical treatment of diabetic retinopathy, is of major clinical and public health importance. Since the results of the multicentre clinical trials of the Diabetic Retinopathy Study Research Group (DRS) and the Early Treatment Diabetic Retinopathy Study Research Group (ETDRS), retinal photocoagulation has been proven to be the effective and even cost-effective therapy in well-defined stages of diabetic retinopathy.[1,2] If employed adequately this efficacy is proven not only for the prevention of severe visual loss in diabetic macular oedema and proliferative diabetic retinopathy, but also for the preservation and even improvement of visual acuity. In cases of persistent vitreous haemorrhage, traction-induced macular oedema, and tractional retinal detachment, the development of highly sophisticated vitreoretinal surgical techniques in combination with additional laser coagulation therapy is an indispensable tool to restore vision in such late stages of diabetic retinopathy, primarily not suitable for photocoagulation therapy.[3,4] In combination with good metabolic control of diabetes mellitus, these methods of treatment are able to avoid blindness from this disease.

Therefore, noone today would deny the advantages and efficacy of photocoagulation therapy in diabetic retinopathy. However, despite its undoubtedly proven benefit, photocoagulation is a thermal destructive treatment of the retina that impairs contrast sensitivity and night vision. In addition, laser photocoagulation of the retina is effective only in rather late stages of diabetic retinopathy when definite morphological and functional deficiencies of the patient's retina are already present (*Fig. 5.1*).

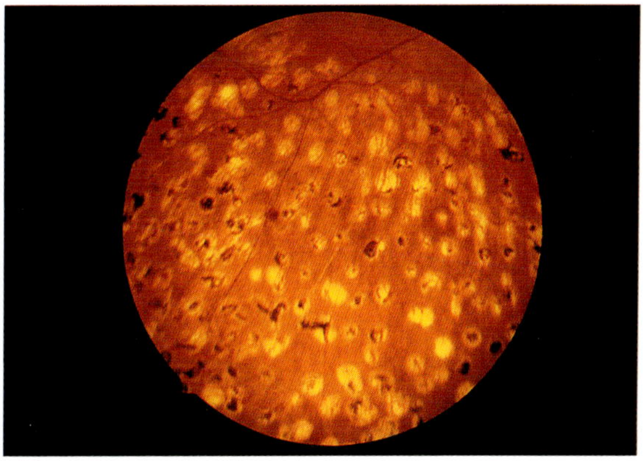

Figure 5.1
Despite its undoubtedly proven benefit, full scatter laser coagulation impairs contrast sensitivity and night vision.

Thus, a non-destructive, pharmacological therapy of diabetic retinopathy is a worthwhile aim. Ideally, medical treatment should interfere in a causative way with mechanisms leading to diabetic retinal changes at a very early stage of the disease

Table 5.1 Pharmacological substances and effect on diabetic retinopathy.

Pharmacological substance	*Therapeutic mechanism*	*Theoretical proof*	*Clinical proof*
Interactions with morphological alterations of microangiopathic vessels			
Ginkgo biloba	Stabilizing of cellular membrane	No	No
Anthocyanosides	Decrease in basement membrane thickening	Yes	No
ACE-inhibitors	Retinal renin–angio tensin system	Yes	In part unpublished
Improvement of haemostasis			
Aspirin	Inhibition of platelet aggregation	Yes	No
Ticlopidine	Like aspirin	Yes	Doubtful
Calcium dobesilate	Like aspirin Inhibition of sorbitol production	Yes	Doubtful
Medical treatment of diabetic maculopathy			
Carbonic anhydrase Inhibitors	Receptor interaction in RPE cells	Yes	No
Inhibitors of protein kinase C	Inhibition of vascular leakage	Yes	Not evaluated
Pharmacological interaction with sorbitol pathway			
Sorbinil	Inhibition of aldose reductase	Yes	No
Pharmacological interaction with endocrinological mechanisms			
Inhibitors of protein kinase C	Inhibition of vascular leakage	Yes	Not evaluated

and prevent the progression to late stages. So far such an ideal medical treatment is given only via a superb control of the diabetic metabolism in combination with optimal control of any incidental systemic hypertension. The efficacy of this–in most instances–pharmacological treatment for the prevention of diabetic microvascular eye disease has been proven by several large studies.[5–7]

Therefore, before any pharmacological treatment is even considered, optimal metabolic control of diabetes should have been achieved. Specifically, a variety of different groups of pharmacological substances for the treatment of diabetic retinopathy is offered by the pharmaceutical industry (Table 5.1). The theoretical effect is mostly based on an improvement in haemodynamics. In recent years, the results of biochemical and metabolic research have offered promising means of influencing the development and progression of retinal vascular changes in diabetes. Nevertheless, scientific evidence for the efficacy of any such treatment so far is scarce. One reason for this lack of knowledge is the variety of retinal changes and the differences in the natural course of the disease which make significant and reliable investigations difficult. Lately, some multicentre collaborative clinical trials have begun which will investigate new and promising aspects of medical treatment of diabetic retinopathy.

This chapter will describe the groups of substances that are suggested for medical treatment of diabetic retinopathy and will discuss critically their theoretical and clinical effects on diabetic retinopathy.

PHARMACOLOGICAL SUBSTANCES

Vitamins A and E

Vitamins A and E are essential for the synthesis of rhodopsin. These vitamins are prescribed for a wide variety of retinal and macular disorders. To our present knowledge there is no relationship between pathological changes of the synthesis of rhodopsin and diabetic retinopathy. Therefore, there is no rationale for a theoretically proposed effect. In the literature no hint could be found concerning an effect on diabetic retinopathy.

Ginkgo biloba extract

Ginkgo biloba is the extract of the only species of the ginkgo trees (*Ginkgo biloba*) existing today. Ginkgo biloba is said to have a stabilizing effect on cellular membranes. Theoretically, in endothelial cells such a membrane-stabilizing effect could prevent the breakdown of the blood–retinal barrier and might therefore slow down the progression of diabetic maculopathy or even the process of neovascularization. To our knowledge this has never been proven. Lanthony and Cosson carried out a double-blind clinical trial in 29 subjects with early diabetic retinopathy.[8] They found differences between diabetic subjects treated by ginkgo biloba and the placebo group. The functional criterion was the colour vision sensitivity, studied by the desaturated Panel D-15 and the 100-Hue Farnsworth test. The significance of the results is limited by the short follow-up of 6 months and the small number of 29 subjects.

Anthocyanosides

In the presence of persistent hyperglycaemia glucose chemically attaches to proteins non-enzymatically to form a stable product (ketoamine or Amadori product). After a series of reactions the development of advanced glycosylation end products (AGEs) occurs. AGEs are resistant to degradation and continue to accumulate indefinitely on long-lived proteins by participation in protein cross-linking. This could lead to trapping of albumin and immunoglobulin G within the basement membrane resulting in irreversible thickening[9] (*Fig. 5.2*).

Anthocyanosides are an extract of the wild bilberry (*Vaccinium myrtillus*). In 1974 Romani described a decrease of capillary basement membrane thickening in diabetics treated with anthocyanosides.[10] Boniface and Robert showed a significant decrease of protein biosynthesis activity in 12 diabetics treated with 600 mg anthocyanosides per day for 2 months.[11] They

Glucose + proteins

↓

Ketoamine (Amadori product)

↓

Advanced glycosylation end products (AGEs)

Figure 5.2
Persistent hyperglycaemia activates non-enzymatic glycosylation. After a series of reactions advanced glycosylation end products (AGEs) occur, that are resistent to degradation and accumulate indefinitely on long-lived proteins by participation in protein cross-linking.

Glucose

↓

Aldose reductase

↓

Sorbitol

↓

Sorbitol dehydrogenase

⊥

Fructose

Figure 5.3
Persistent hyperglycaemia activates the aldose reductase. Because of the inhibition of sorbitol dehydrogenase, sorbitol cannot be converted to fructose. The intracellular accumulation of sorbitol is toxic related to osmotic and oxidative stress.

investigated samples of gingivae tissue taken before and after treatment. Using radioactive labelled amino acids they measured the radioactivity as an indicator of protein biosynthesis activity. Huismans performed a multicentre collaborative clinical trial which enrolled 266 subjects with non-proliferative diabetic retinopathy over a period of 1 year.[12] He observed a reduction in microaneurysms in 23%, in intraretinal haemorrhage in 15%, and in perivascular exudates in 14%. On the other hand, 75% showed no changes with respect to microaneurysms, 82% no reduction in intraretinal haemorrhage, and 83% no reduction in exudates. The author himself points out the difficulties of investigation of a slowly progressive and widely variable disease reflecting the natural course of diabetic retinopathy.

Repossi et al studied 40 subjects with focal macular oedema and hard exudates in a circinate arrangement and found a decrease of macular oedema and hard exudates in 15% of the subjects treated with anthocyanosides compared with 10% of the placebo group.[13] In 60% of the treated diabetics and in 50% of the untreated subjects no change could be observed. The significance of the results is limited by the lack of any quantification and the small number of 40 subjects at all. At the moment there is no proof of any protective effect of anthocyanosides concerning diabetic retinopathy.

Sorbinil

In the sorbitol or polyol pathway the enzyme aldose reductase converts glucose to sorbitol. Persistent hyperglycaemia activates the aldose reductase. Because of the inhibition of sorbitol dehydrogenase, sorbitol cannot be converted to fructose. The intracellular accumulation of sorbitol is toxic, related to osmotic and oxidative stress[9] (*Figs 5.3 and 5.4*).

Inhibition of aldose reductase (e.g. by sorbinil) could reduce the increased sorbitol production and slow down the elevated flux through the polyol pathway. In animal studies this approach has been shown to prevent microangiopathy successfully.[14] But results in humans have been disappointing so far. Although the Sorbinil Retinopathy Trial Research Group was able to find a slightly slower progression rate

Accumulation of AGEs and sorbitol

↓ ↓

Capillary basement membrane thickening and osmotic and oxidative stress

↓

Damage of endothelial cells and pericytes

↓

Deterioration of capillary function

↓

Microaneurysms leakage capillary closure

Figure 5.4
Capillary basement membrane thickening and osmotic and oxidative stress caused by intracellular accumulation of sorbitol damage endothelial cells and pericytes. Abnormal capillary function and haemodynamics result in the development of microaneurysms, leakage and capillary closure.

in the microaneurysm count, they could not observe a clinically important effect of sorbinil on the course of retinopathy in adults with insulin-dependent diabetes of moderate duration.[15]

Carbonic anhydrase inhibitors

Acetazolamide, a carbonic anhydrase inhibitor, can influence the active transport of ions of the retinal pigment epithelium by receptor interaction.[16] Cox et al succeeded in a reproducible resolution of chronic macular oedema in patients with retinitis pigmentosa treated with acetazolamide.[17] But the therapeutic effect did not occur in patients with primary retinal vascular disorders, such as branch or central retinal vein occlusion. Paresthesia, nausea, altered taste, and mild depression occurred as side effects in almost all patients.

Calcium dobesilate

Beside the morphological vascular changes of capillary basement membrane thickening and endothelial dysfunction and pericyte damage, abnormalities of haemostasis are well described in diabetics, causing a microthrombotic tendency. In combination with reduced endothelial cell production of prostacyclin (PGI_2) and decreased concentrations of the activators of fibrinolysis, increased platelet aggregation and increased concentrations of factors V and VIII, fibrinogen, and thromboxane A_2 promote microthrombus formation and small vessel occlusion[9,18] (*Figs 5.5 and 5.6*). Although improvement of haemodynamics may not be

Increased concentration of factor V, VIII, fibrinogen | Decreased concentration of plasminogen activator

⇓

Microthrombotic tendency

⇑

Increased platelet aggregation and adherence to the vascular wall

Decreased concentration of prostacyclin

Increased concentration of thromboxane-A_2

Figure 5.5
Abnormabilities of haemostasis in diabetic patients resulting in microthrombotic tendency.

Nonenzymatic glycosylation in erythrocytes

↓

Accumulation of AGEs

↓

Increased rigidity

↓

Damage to the vascular wall

Figure 5.6
Interaction of erythrocytes with the vascular wall.

causative, it is an interesting additional therapeutic approach.

Calcium dobesilate (Doxium) has been shown to induce the synthesis and release of nitric oxide in endothelial cell cultures and may play a major role in endothelial relaxation by stimulating the release of endothelium-dependent relaxation factor (EDRF).[19,20] Furthermore, calcium dobesilate is suggested to have antioxidant properties, protecting the endothelium from oxidative stress and reducing vascular leakage by stabilizing endothelial cell function.

Some authors have investigated the effect of calcium dobesilate on the improvement of blood viscosity and protection of the blood–retinal barrier.[21–23] No favourable effect on diabetic maculopathy and visual acuity is reported by Adank and Körner, who compared 54 patients receiving on average 650 mg calcium dobesilate per day for 6–30 months, with 54 subjects of the control group.[21] In cases of moderate background retinopathy, the effect of calcium dobesilate was statistically significant by reducing the number of microaneurysms, haemorrhages, and hard exudates, using a scoring system. Regression of microaneurysms count and reduction of vascular leakage is described by several authors.[22,24–27]

Schmidt and Michal report on an inhibiting effect of calcium dobesilate on the polyol pathway in erythrocytes.[28] It seems doubtful and unlikely that calcium dobesilate could be protective in this way. As shown above, direct inhibitors of aldose reductase (e.g. sorbinil) did not have a clinically important effect on the course of diabetic retinopathy.[15]

In order to elucidate the alleged efficacy of calcium dobesilate on the prevention of diabetic macular oedema a multicentre study is under way. Due to the protocol, which involves a follow-up of several years, the results of this study will not be presented for 4 years.

Aspirin

The hypothesis that aspirin protects against diabetic retinopathy was developed in part from the observation that arthritic diabetic patients taking aspirin had less diabetic retinopathy.[29] Aspirin inhibits platelet aggregation by acetylization of the enzyme cyclooxygenase.[30] By reducing the production of thromboxane-A_2, haemodynamics might be improved. Investigating the effect of aspirin on platelet aggregation in a normal population and in older patients with diabetes, Khosla et al found a greater rate and degree of platelet aggregation with collagen and arachidonic acid in patients with diabetic retinopathy.[31]

The Groupe d'Etude DAMAD found a retarding effect of aspirin alone or in combination with dipyridamole–a dilatator of coronary arteries–on the development of microaneurysms.[32] No effect could be observed on the development of neovascularization. However, the ETDRS could not find any difference between patients treated with photocoagulation alone and patients treated with aspirin additionally compared with the placebo group.[2] Investigating 1370 of 9283 patients enrolled in the Wisconsin Epidemiologic Study of Diabetic Retinopathy, Klein et al found no association between the severity of diabetic retinopathy and having used aspirin daily for at least 3 months.[33] Therefore, at the moment there is no hint of a protecting effect of aspirin on the development and progression of diabetic retinopathy.

Ticlopidine

Ticlopidine hydrochloride, originally developed as an inhibitor of platelet aggregation in cases of intolerance of aspirin, should improve haemodynamics in a similar way to aspirin. Measuring the mean yearly increase in microaneurysms by fluorescein angiography, a French group found a statistically significant slower progression rate of nonproliferative diabetic retinopathy in a randomized, double-blind, placebo-controlled trial in 435 patients over a period of 3 years (Ticlopidine Microangiopathy of Diabetes (TIMAD) Study Group).[34] No effect on the development of neovascularization could be observed. No severe side effects are reported. It remains unclear why the ETDRS Research Group and the TIMAD Study Group came to different results concerning the same operative mechanism of aspirin and ticlopidine.

Inhibitors of angiotensin-converting enzyme

Beside their antihypertensive effect, angiotensin-converting enzyme inhibitors protect against the development and progression of diabetic nephropathy. This has been proven in some randomized, placebo-controlled trials[35–37] to occur as a result of reducing microalbuminuria in normotensive patients with diabetic nephropathy. Reduction of glomerular capillary hydraulic pressure was thought to be the major mechanism.[38]

The damaging effect of arterial hypertension on the blood–retinal barrier has been demonstrated in patients with essential hypertension without diabetes as well as in insulin-dependent diabetics with hypertension.[39,40] Interestingly, the protecting effect of antihypertensive treatment is much more marked in diabetics than in non-diabetics.[39,40] This observation emphasizes the major role of elevated blood pressure in damaging diabetic capillaries by dysfunctional autoregulation.

Retinal vessels show angiotensin II receptors.[41] In 1988 Sramek et al demonstrated immunohistochemically the presence of prorenin in the pars plicata corporis ciliaris, suggesting that the ciliary body synthesizes renin, which might be part of an ocular renin–angiotensin II system.[42] Thus, besides the improvement in haemodynamics as a result of reducing systemic blood pressure, there might be some more pharmacological means for angiotensin-converting enzyme inhibitors to interact with diabetic vessels with damaged autoregulation in a protective way.

Larsen et al report on a protective effect of captopril on the blood–retina barrier in normotensive insulin-dependent diabetic patients with nephropathy and background retinopathy.[43] In a prospective, randomized, placebo-controlled study of 20 subjects over a period of 18 months, fluorescein leakage remained nearly unchanged in the captopril-treated group, whereas the permeability increased significantly in the control group. The authors emphasize that metabolic control, reflected by blood glucose and glycosylated haemoglobin, did not change significantly during the study, 'although a trend towards improved control was noted in both patient groups'.[43] It remains unclear whether the protective effect is determined by reducing systemic blood pressure alone or by receptor-induced interactions with retinal autoregulation. There was no difference or change of arterial blood pressure in either of the two patient groups.

Implementing a double-blind, placebo-controlled protocol, Chase et al report on an improvement of background retinopathy in two subjects treated with captopril over a period of 2 years.[44] None of the controls improved. Three patients of the control group and one treated patient deteriorated 'significantly'. But the small number of patients makes it impossible to achieve statistically significant results. The study enrolled subjects with no visible diabetic retinal changes as well as one patient with proliferative retinopathy. Because of the differences in natural course of the disease, such a broad variety of retinal changes does not permit reliable results.

Persistent hyperglycaemia

↓

Diactlglycerol

↓

Protein kinase C isoform βII

Figure 5.7
Persistent hyperglycaemia increases diacylglycerol production and activates preferentially protein kinase C isoform βII.

VEGF

↓

Protein kinase C isoform β

↓

Vascular leakage

Figure 5.8
Vascular endothelial growth factor (VEGF) rapidly activates protein kinase C in vivo. This effect appears to be mediated predominantly by the β-isoform of protein kinase C.[50–51] VEGF is highly potent in increasing vascular permeability.[49]

Inhibitors of protein kinase C

Persistent hyperglycaemia increases diacylglycerol mass and activates protein kinase C (*Fig.* 5.7). This was demonstrated in mesangial cell cultures and in glomerula of diabetic rats.[45,46] Shiba et al characterized protein kinase C activity biochemically and functionally in the rat retina.[47] In this model, hyperglycaemia-independent activation of protein kinase C isoform βII by vitreal injection of phorbol dibutyrate mimicked the abnormal blood circulation observed in diabetic rats. In diabetes, hyperglycaemia-induced elevated diacylglycerol levels activate predominantly one of the 11 isoenzymes, protein kinase C isoform βII, measured in the aorta and hearts of diabetic rats and in bovine cell culture.[48] Thus it might be possible that protein kinase C isoform βII plays a major role in vascular regulation in diabetic retinopathy.

Vascular endothelial growth factor (VEGF) is highly potent in increasing vascular permeability, 50 000 times more potent than histamine in dermal microvasculature.[49] Intravitreal injection of VEGF increases retinal permeability, demonstrated in vivo by fluorophotometry in non-diabetic rats.[50] At concentrations observed clinically, VEGF rapidly activates protein kinase C in vivo.[50] In vitro, the increase in protein kinase C activation is concentration- and time-dependent.[51] Interestingly, in vitro and in vivo, this effect of VEGF appears to be mediated predominantly by the β-isoform of protein kinase C[50,51] (*Fig.* 5.8). In 1997 Aiello et al could demonstrate the inhibition of a VEGF-induced increase in permeability by an orally effective β-isoform-selective inhibitor (*Fig.* 5.9).[50]

DISCUSSION

On the basis of the pharmacological mechanisms the effects of medical treatment of diabetic retinopathy will be elucidated and the efficacy reported in the literature will be discussed.

Interactions with morphological alterations of retinal capillaries

Persistent hyperglycaemia causes an increase in non-enzymatic glycosylation, resulting in the development of advanced glycosylation end products (AGEs). Because of their resistance to degradation, AGEs accumulate indefinitely on long-lived proteins, causing capillary basement membrane thickening, 'the histological hallmark of microangiopathy' in diabetes.[9] Heparan sulphate normally hinders the filtration of negatively charged proteins

Persistent hyperglycaemia → ↓ → Protein kinase β → ⊥ → Permeability

VEGF → ↓ → Protein kinase β → ⊥ → Permeability

[←β-isoform-selective→] inhibitor of protein kinase

⇓

Decreased vascular leakage

Figure 5.9
Aiello et al demonstrated the inhibition of a VEGF-induced increase in permeability by an orally effective β-isoform-selective.[50] Therefore a β-isoform-selective inhibitor of protein kinase C might inhibit the hyperglycaemia-induced activation of protein kinase C as well as the VEGF-mediated increase in permeability.

such as albumin. Endothelial cell damage impairs the synthesis of proteoglycans and leads to abnormal packing of the peptide chains, producing excessive leakiness of the membrane.[9] The pathognomonic loss of pericytes impairs capillary autoregulation. Elevated blood flow damages the vascular wall. Microaneurysms, endothelial cell loss, and capillary closure follow.

Stabilizing the cellular membrane is suggested to be a mechanism of ginkgo biloba. To our knowledge reliable biochemical studies do not exist. The clinical trial of Lanthony and Cosson, who report on differences between treated and untreated subjects concerning colour vision sensitivity studied by the desaturated Panel D-15 and the 100-Hue Farnsworth test, is limited by the short follow-up of 6 months and the small number of subjects.[8] Furthermore, it seems doubtful whether such small differences in macular function could be evaluated by a screening test like Panel D-15 and 100-Hue Farnsworth.[52]

Reducing capillary basement membrane thickening in dermal histology sections seems to be an effect of anthocyanosides.[10] Using radiolabelled amino acids, Boniface and Robert demonstrated a significant reduction in the biosynthesis activity of gingivae connective tissue–especially polymeric collagen and structure glycoproteins–by anthocyanoside medication.[11] Similar results might be possible in retinal capillaries, but this has not been proven yet. Thus, at the moment, there is no proven clinical effect of ginkgo biloba and anthocyanosides until a prospective, randomized, controlled study might show a benefit.

Impaired capillary autoregulation increases the damaging effect of elevated blood pressure to the vascular wall. Best possible control of blood pressure and glucose metabolism is without doubt a causal approach to slowing down the progression of vascular damage.[5–7] Beside their antihypertensive effect, angiotensin-converting enzyme inhibitors protect against development and progression of diabetic nephropathy.[35–37] Larsen et al report on a protective effect of captopril on the blood–retina barrier in normotensive insulin-dependent diabetic patients with nephropathy and background retinopathy, studied in a large and reliable prospective, randomized, placebo-controlled trial.[43] Orally reported results of the EURODIAB controlled trial of lisinopril in insulin dependent diabetes (EUCLID) study concerning the protective effect of lisinopril on diabetic retinopathy are encouraging and deserve a critical evaluation of the published data. At the moment it remains unclear whether the protective effect is determined by reducing systemic blood pressure alone or by receptor-induced interactions with the postulated ocular renin–angiotensin II system.

Improvement of haemostatasis

Most of the pharmacological substances available and prescribed today interfere with the abnormalities of haemostasis described above. According to the trials mentioned before, aspirin, ticlopidine, and calcium dobesilate reduce blood viscosity and therefore improve haemodynamics. Most of the studies report on a slower progression rate or reduction of microaneurysm count as investigated by fluorescein angiography. Undoubtedly microaneurysm count reflects the severity of early diabetic retinopathy.[53] But it remains doubtful whether changes in angiographic visibility over time might be used for follow-up assessment.[52] A decrease in angiographically visible microaneurysms, for example, by thrombosis, must not be interpreted as reflecting restoration of normal vascular architecture.[52] The ETDRS Research Group and the Wisconsin Epidemiologic Study could not find a positive effect of aspirin with respect to the progression of non-proliferative diabetic retinopathy and the development of neovascularization. Nor did resorption of vitreous haemorrhage accelerate.[2,33]

Medical treatment of diabetic maculopathy

None of the pharmacological substances for improvement of haemodynamics previously mentioned has an influence on diabetic macular oedema. The therapeutic effect of acetazolamide in partially or completely resolving chronic macular oedema in patients with retinitis pigmentosa, reported by Cox et al in 1988, did not occur in patients with primary retinal vascular disorders.[17] Obviously, the concept of deep leakage from the retinal pigment epithelium is not affected in diabetic retinopathy. As mentioned above there have been no reliable clinical studies investigating the effect of ginkgo biloba and anthocyanosides. Inhibition of protein kinase C might be an interesting and promising mechanism to reduce leakage of retinal capillaries. Further studies must be performed to investigate the effect of β-selective inhibitors of protein kinase C in reducing diabetic macular oedema.

Pharmacological interaction with the polyol pathway

The effect of aldose reductase inhibitors to prevent microangiopathy successfully has only been proven in animal studies.[14] Results in humans have been disappointing so far.[15] The reason for this remains unclear. In the future chemical modification of the substances might perhaps show some benefit.[52] Because of the major importance of polyol pathway with respect to endothelial cell and pericyte damage, inhibition of aldose reductase is still of great interest for its causal approach.

Pharmacological interaction with endocrinological mechanisms

The influence of endocrinological alterations on the development and progression of diabetic retinopathy has been well known for a long time. Postpubertal children have a 4.8 times greater prevalence of retinopathy than those who are not sexually mature.[54] Men with type I diabetes show a higher risk of progression to proliferative retinopathy than women.[55] In pregnancy diabetic retinopathy often deteriorates.[56] Postpartum or postoperative pituitary insufficiency can reduce diabetic fundus alterations.[57] In growth-hormone-deficient dwarfs with diabetes, complications of diabetes including retinopathy do not occur.[57]

The increasing understanding of the relationship of endocrinological factors to the development from non-proliferative to proliferative retinopathy offers some interesting and promising aspects of medical treatment. Basic fibroblast growth factor levels in the vitreous are greater in patients with proliferative retinopathy.[58,59]

Vascular endothelial growth factor (VEGF) concentrations are higher in patients with active proliferative retinopathy and other ischaemic retinal diseases.[60] VEGF stimulates the growth of retinal endothelial cells in vitro and is highly potent in increasing vascular permeability.[49,60] Intravitreal injection of VEGF increases retinal permeability, demonstrated in vivo by fluorophotometry in non-diabetic rats.[50] At concentrations observed clinically, VEGF activates predominantly the β-isoform of protein kinase C in vivo.[50] Aiello et al were able to demonstrate the inhibition of a VEGF-induced increase in permeability by an orally effective β-isoform-selective inhibitor.[50]

Therefore, a β-isoform-selective inhibitor of protein kinase C might inhibit the hyperglycaemia-induced activation of protein kinase C as well as the VEGF-mediated increase in permeability. Each of these factors regarded alone, but especially their combination, represents a very promising approach to slowing down the progression of diabetic vascular changes and diabetic maculopathy. In the future the clinical efficacy must be proven by a reliable, prospective, and controlled study.

CONCLUSION

It remains true of all pharmacological substances mentioned for a possible treatment of diabetic retinopathy that their effect on this disease are at least still controversial. Most of the effects are not yet proven clinically in a reliable way. On the other hand, increasing understanding especially of endocrinological factors affecting the progression of diabetic retinopathy raises some interesting and promising questions. In the future inhibitors of angiotensin-converting enzyme as well as inhibitors of protein kinase C will have to prove their clinical efficacy in reliable trials.

Thus, best possible control of blood glucose including assessment of HbA_{1C} and blood pressure control, is still of major importance. Especially the Oslo Study and the Diabetes Control and Complication Trial Research Group reports the benefit of this.[6,7] Progress in transplantation techniques–for example, combined renal and pancreatic transplantation–may make it possible to achieve normoglycaemia and influence the course of diabetic retinopathy in a causal and preventive way.[61] The recent discovery of a biological activity of proinsulin C peptide in the prevention of vascular and neural dysfunction in diabetic rats may lead to an improvement in the therapy of diabetes by a combination of C peptide and insulin in a more physiological way.[62]

Today the best possible medical treatment of diabetes and correct and timely laser coagulation and vitreoretinal surgery determine the course of diabetic retinopathy. According to the results of the ETDRS Research Group and the Diabetic Retinopathy Vitrectomy Study Research Group diabetic patients can be protected from blindness to a high degree.[2,63]

REFERENCES

1. Diabetic Retinopathy Study Research Group, Preliminary report on effects of photocoagulation therapy, *Am J Ophthalmol* (1976) **81**:383–96.
2. Early Treatment Diabetic Retinopathy Study Research Group, Early treatment diabetic retinopathy study design and baseline patient characteristics, *Ophthalmology* (1991) **98**:741–56.
3. Kampik A, Ulbig M, Diabetic retinopathy, *Curr Opin Ophthalmol* (1990) **1**:161–6.
4. Ulbig M, Kampik A, Heidenkummer HP, Vitrektomie bei proliferativer diabetischer Retinopathie. Präoperative Faktoren für das operative Vorgehen und das postoperative Ergebnis, *Fortschr Ophthalmol* (1990) **87**:443–8.
5. KROC Collaborative Study Group, Blood glucose control and the evolution of diabetic retinopathy and albuminuria. A preliminary multicenter trial, *N Engl J Med* (1984) **311**:365–72.

6. Brinchmann-Hansen O, Dahl-Jorgensen K, Sandvik L, Hanssen KF, Blood glucose concentrations and progression of diabetic retinopathy: the seven year results of the Oslo Study, *BMJ* (1992) **304**:19.
7. The Diabetes Control and Complications Trial Research Group DCCT, The effect of intensive treatment of diabetes on the development and progression of long-term complications in insulin-dependent diabetes mellitus, *N Engl J Med* (1993) **329**:977–86.
8. Lanthony P, Cosson JP, Evolution de la vision des couleurs dans la rétinopathie diabétique débutante traitée par extrait de Ginkgo biloba, *J Fr Ophtalmol* (1988) **11**:671–4.
9. Barnett AH, Origin of the microangiopathic changes in diabetes, *Eye* (1993) **7**:218–22.
10. Romani JD, Le traitement de la microangiopathie diabétique évaluée à partir des lésions vasculaires cutanées, *La Médicine Practicienne* (1974) 556.
11. Boniface R, Robert AM, Einfluß von Anthocyanen auf den Bindegewebsmetabolismus beim Menschen, *Klin Monatsbl Augenheilkd* (1996) **209**:368–72.
12. Huismans H, Medikamentöse Behandlung der diabetischen Retinopathie in der augenärztlichen Praxis, *Der Augenspiegel* (1988) **6**:16–21.
13. Repossi P, Malagola R, De Cadilhac C, Der Einfluß der Anthocyanoside auf Gefäßkrankheiten mit veränderter Permeabilität, *Ann Ottalmol* (1987) **113**:1–6.
14. Robinson WG, Nagata M, Laver N, Kinoshita JH, Diabetic-like retinopathy in rats prevented with an aldose reductase inhibitor, *Invest Ophthalmol Vis Sci* (1989) **30**:2285–92.
15. Sorbinil Retinopathy Trial Research Group, A randomized trial of sorbinil, an aldose reductase inhibitor, in diabetic retinopathy, *Arch Ophthalmol* (1990) **108**:1234–44.
16. Wolfensberger TJ, Carter ND, Wistrand PJ, Bird AC, Expression of membrane-bound carbonic anhydrase in human RPE and choriocapillaris: significance for acetazolamide treatment of cystic macular edema, *Invest Ophthalmol Vis Sci (ARVO Suppl)* (1992) **33**:922.
17. Cox SN, Hay E, Bird AC, Treatment of chronic macular edema with acetazolamide, *Arch Ophthalmol* (1988) **106**:1190–5.
18. Janka HU, Standl E, Stiegler H, Standl R, Angiopathien bei Diabetes mellitus. In: Mehnert H, Schöpfling H, Standl E, Usadel KH, eds, *Diabetologie in Klinik und Praxis* (Thieme: Stuttgart, 1994).
19. Suschek C, Kolb H, Kolb-VachofenV, Dobesilate enhances endothelial nitric oxide synthetase activity in micro- and microvascular endothelial cells, *Br J Pharmacol* (1997) **122**:1502–8.
20. Ruiz E, Lorente R, Tejerina T, Effects of calcium dobesilate on the synthesis of endothelium-dependent relaxing factor in rabbit isolated aorta, *Br J Pharmacol* (1997) **121**:711–16.
21. Adank AC, Körner F, Calcium dobesilate in diabetic retinopathy. A retrospective controlled study, *Ophthalmologica* (1985) **190**:102–11.
22. Leite EB, Mota MC, Faria de Abreu JR, Cunha-Vaz JG, Effect of calcium dobesilate on blood–retinal barrier in early diabetic retinopathy, *Int Ophthalmol* (1990) **14**:81–8.
23. Vojnikovic B, Hyperviscosity in whole blood, plasma, and aqueous humor decreased by Doxium (calcium dobesilate) in diabetics with retinopathy and glaucoma: a double-blind controlled study, *Ophthalmic Res* (1984) **16**:150–62.
24. Binkhorst PG, Van Bijsterveld OP, Calcium dobesilate versus placebo in the treatment of diabetic retinopathy: a double-blind cross-over study, *Curr Ther Res Clin Exp* (1976) **20**:283–8.
25. Freyler H, Sehorst W, Gefäßabdichtung bei diabetischer Retinopathie durch Kalziumdobesilat, *Klin Monatsbl Augenheilkd* (1974) **164**: 246–51.
26. Freyler H, Microvascular protection with calcium dobesilate (Doxium) in diabetic retinopathy, *Ophthalmologica* (1974) **168**:400–16.
27. Salama Benarroch I, Nano H, Pérez H et al, Assessment of calcium dobesilate in diabetic retinopathy, a double-blind clinical investigation, *Ophthalmologica* (1977) **174**:47–51.
28. Schmidt M, Michal M, Inhibition of sorbitol formation in human erythrocytes by calcium

dobesilate, *Arzneimittelforschung* (1989) **39**: 493–5.

29. Powell EDU, Field RA, Diabetic retinopathy in rheumatoid arthritis, *Lancet* (1964) **2**:17–18.
30. Forth W, Henschler D, Rummel W, *Allgemeine und spezielle Pharmakologie und Toxikologie* (Wissenschaftsverlag: Mannheim, 1987) 324–5.
31. Khosla PK, Seth V, Tiwari HK, Saraya AK, Effect of platelet aggregation in diabetes mellitus, *Diabetologia* (1982) **23**:104–7.
32. Groupe d'Etude DAMAD, Essai controllé de l'aspirine et de l'association aspirine eldipyridamole sur l'évolution de la rétinopathie diabétique, II. protocole ophtalmologique, *Diabetes Metab* (1982) **8**:307–11.
33. Klein BE, Klein A, Moss ES, Is aspirin usage associated with diabetic retinopathy? *Diabetes Care* (1987) **10**:600–3.
34. TIMAD Study Group, Ticlopidine treatment reduces the progression of nonproliferative diabetic retinopathy, *Arch Ophthalmol* (1990) **108**:1577–83.
35. Lewis EJ, Hunsicker LG, Bain RP, Rhode RD, The effect of angiotensin-converting-enzyme inhibition on diabetic nephropathy, *N Engl J Med* (1993) **329**:1456–62.
36. Viberti G, Mogensen CE, Groop LC, Pauls JF, Effect of captopril on progression to clinical proteinuria in patients with insulin-dependent diabetes mellitus and microalbuminuria, *JAMA* (1994) **271**:275–9.
37. Euclid Study Group, Randomized placebo-controlled trial of lisinopril in normotensive patients with insulin-dependent diabetes and normoalbuminuria or microalbuminuria, *Lancet* (1997) **349**:1787–92.
38. Zatz R, Dunn BR, Meyer TW et al, Prevention of diabetic glomerulopathy by pharmacological amelioration of glomerular capillary hypertension, *J Clin Invest* (1986) **77**:1925–30.
39. Krogsaa B, Lund-Andersen H, Parving HH, Bjældager P, The blood–retinal barrier permeability in essential hypertension, *Acta Ophthalmol* (1983) **61**:541–4.
40. Parving HH, Larsen M, Hommel E, Lund-Andersen H, Effect of antihypertensive treatment on blood–retinal barrier permeability to fluorescein in hypertensive type 1 (insulin-dependent) diabetic patients with background retinopathy, *Diabetologia* (1989) **32**:440–4.
41. Ferrari-Dileo G, Davis EB, Anderson DR, Angiotensin binding sites in bovine and human retinal blood vessels, *Invest Ophthamol Vis Sci* (1987) **28**:1747–51.
42. Sramek SJ, Wallow IHL, Day RP, Ehrlich EN, Ocular renin–angiotensin: immunohistochemical evidence for the presence of prorenin in eye tissue, *Invest Ophthalmol Vis Sci* (1988) **29**:1749–52.
43. Larsen M, Hommel E, Parving HH, Lund-Andersen H, Protective effect of captopril on the blood–retina barrier in normotensive insulin-dependent diabetic patients with nephropathy and background retinopathy, *Graefes Arch Clin Exp Ophthalmol* (1990) **228**:505–9.
44. Chase HP, Garg SK, Harris S, Hoops S et al, Angiotensin-converting enzyme inhibitor treatment for young normotensive diabetic subjects: a two year trial, *Ann Ophthalmol* (1993) **25**:284–9.
45. Ayo SH, Radnik R, Garoni JA et al, High glucose increases diacylglycerol mass and activates protein kinase C in mesangial cell cultures, *Am J Physiol* (1991) **261**:F571–7.
46. Craven PA, DeRubertis FR, Protein kinase C is activated in glomeruli from streptozotocin rats. Possible mediation by glucose, *J Clin Invest* (1989) **83**:1667–75.
47. Shiba T, Inoguchi T, Sportsman JR et al, Correlation of diacylglycerol level and protein kinase C activity in rat retina to retinal circulation, *Am J Physiol* (1993) **265**:E783–93.
48. Inoguchi T, Battan R, Handler E et al, Preferential elevation of protein kinase C isoform βII and diacylglycerol levels in the aorta and heart of diabetic rats: differential reversibility to glycemic control by islet cell transplantation, *Proc Natl Acad Sci USA* (1992) **89**:11059–63.
49. Ferrara N, Houck KA, Jakeman LH, Leung DW, Molecular and biological properties of the vascu-

lar endothelial growth factor family of proteins, *Endocr Rev* (1992) **13**:18–32.
50. Aiello LP, Bursell SE, Clermont A et al, Vascular endothelial growth factor-induced retinal permeability is mediated by protein kinase C in vivo and suppressed by an orally effective β-isoform-selective inhibitor, *Diabetes* (1997) **46**:1473–80.
51. Xia P, Aiello LP, Ishii H et al, Characterization of vascular endothelial growth factor's effect on the activation of protein kinase C, its isoforms, and endothelial cell growth, *J Clin Invest* (1996) **98**:2018–26.
52. Ulbig M, Kampik A, Pharmakologische Therapie bei diabetischer Retinopathie, *Z Prakt Augenheilkd* (1993) **14**:379–87.
53. Kohner EM, Sleightholm M, The KROC Collaborative Study Group: Does microaneurysm count reflect severity of early diabetic retinopathy? *Ophthalmology* (1986) **93**:586–9.
54. Murphy RP, Nanda M, Plotnik L et al, The relationship of puberty to diabetic retinopathy, *Arch Ophthalmol* (1990) **108**:215–18.
55. Haffner SM, Klein R, Dunn JF et al, Increased testosterone in type I diabetic subjects with severe retinopathy, *Ophthalmology* (1990) **97**:1270–4.
56. Klein BE, Moss SE, Klein R, Effect of pregnancy on progression of diabetic retinopathy, *Diabetes Care* (1990) **13**:34–40.
57. Merimee TJ, A follow-up study of vascular disease in growth-hormone-deficient dwarfs with diabetes, *N Engl J Med* (1978) **298**:1217–22.
58. Sivalingam A, Kenney J, Brown GC et al, Basic fibroblast growth factor levels in the vitreous of patients with proliferative diabetic retinopathy, *Arch Ophthalmol* (1990) **108**:869–72.
59. Hanneken AJ, De Juan E, Lutty GA et al, Altered distribution of basic fibroblast growth factor in diabetic retinopathy, *Arch Ophthalmol* (1991) **109**:1005–11.
60. Aiello LP, Avery RL, Arrigg PG et al, Vascular endothelial growth factor in ocular fluid of patients with diabetic retinopathy and other retinal disorders, *N Engl J Med* (1994) **331**:1480–7.
61. Ulbig M, Kampik A, Thurau S et al, Long-term follow-up of diabetic retinopathy for up to 71 months after combined renal and pancreatic transplantation, *Graefes Arch Clin Exp Ophthalmol* (1991) **229**:242–5.
62. Ido Y, Vindigni A, Chang K et al, Prevention of vascular and neural dysfunction in diabetic rats by C-peptide, *Science* (1997) **277**:563–6.
63. Diabetic Retinopathy Vitrectomy Study Research Group, Early vitrectomy for severe vitreous hemorrhage in diabetic retinopathy. Four-year results of a randomized trial: DRVS Report No 5, *Arch Ophthalmol* (1990) **108**:958–64.

6 Treatment of neovascularization of the retina and iris

Rosario Brancato and Francesco Bandello

DEFINITION

Proliferative diabetic retinopathy (PDR) is characterized by a proliferation of fibrovascular tissue on the retinal surface and inside the vitreous cavity. In the late stage of the disease, proliferation may also occur on the iris, as well as in the anterior chamber angle.[1]

The proliferation begins with the formation of new vessels with very little fibrous component. They arise from primitive mesenchymal elements that differentiate into vascular endothelial cells. The newly formed vascular channels then undergo fibrous metaplasia; i.e. the angioblastic cells are transformed into fibrous tissue.[1]

PATHOGENESIS

Proliferative diabetic retinopathy is secondary to retinal ischaemia or hypoxia.[2] Apparently, the presence of living tissue is essential for neovascularization, since new vessels only seldom appear when total anoxia occurs as, for example, in central retinal artery occlusion. It is important to stress that a strict cause–effect relationship links retinal ischaemia to the appearance of new vessels and, for this reason, elimination of retinal ischaemia is essential for inducing regression of new vessels.

EPIDEMIOLOGY

Diabetic retinopathy is one of the first four causes of blindness in the United States and it is the leading cause among subjects aged 20–64 years.[3] In an epidemiological study carried out in Lombardy, a region of north-western Italy, some years ago, the prevalence of diabetic retinopathy was 37.3%; the prevalence of non-proliferative retinopathy was 29.7% and that of proliferative retinopathy 7.6%.[4]

DIAGNOSIS

On examining a diabetic patient, before dilation, it is important to examine the iris accurately using high magnification on the slit lamp. New vessels may already be present at the pupillary border. In case of doubt, it is useful to perform fluorescein angiography of the iris. This examination is more sensitive than biomicroscopy for recognizing new vessels in the iris.[5] In addition, fluorescein angiography of the iris yields valuable information on retinal status owing to the strict relationship between iridopathy and retinopathy in diabetes:[6,7] when neovascularization of the iris is detected in an eye in which it is impossible to evaluate the fundus because of cataract, concomitant advanced retinopathy must be presumed, and great care must be taken in its management;

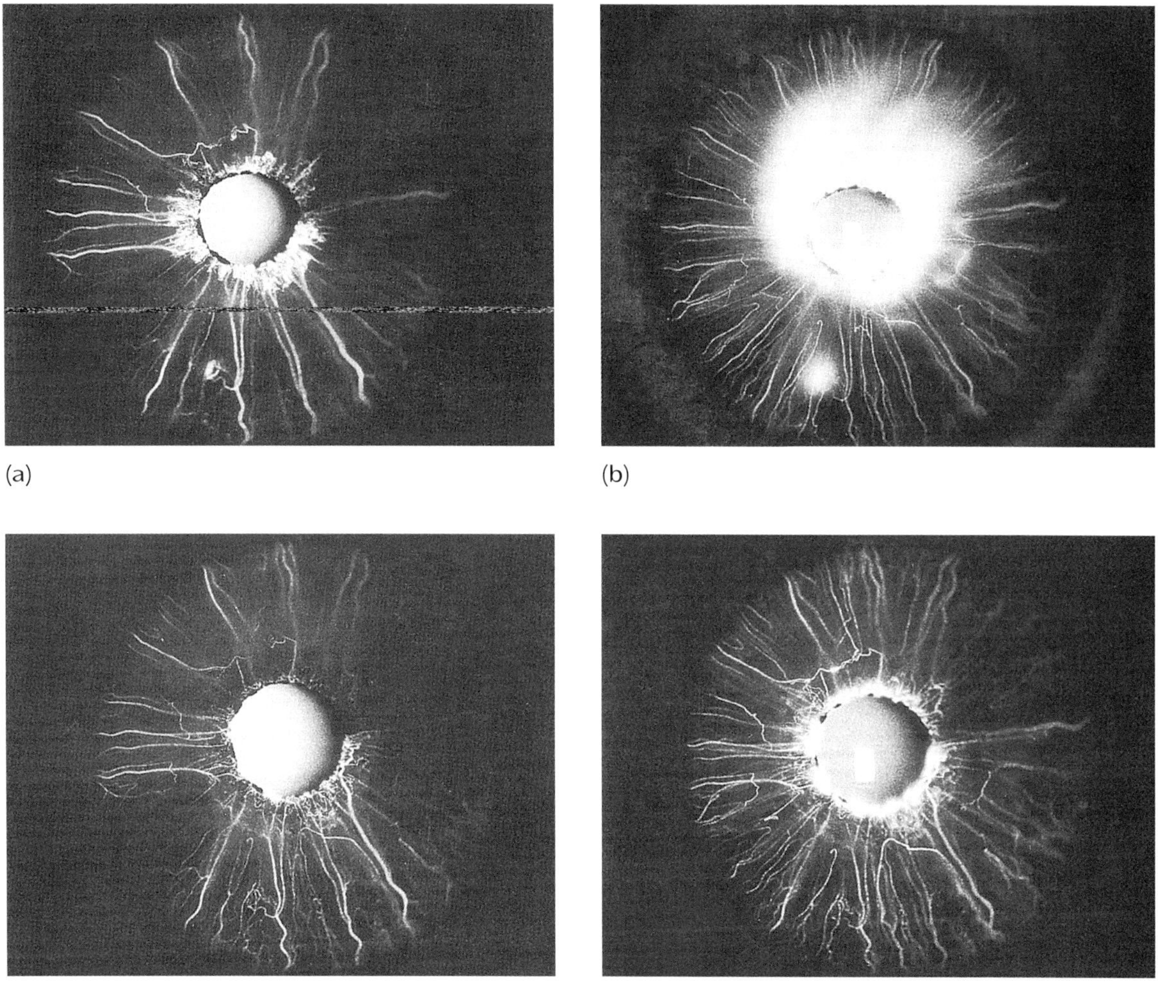

(a) (b) (c) (d)

Figure 6.1
Iris new vessels before (a), (b) and after (c), (d) laser treatment of retinal ischaemia. The iris angiograms show very well the regression of rubeosis iridis.

before surgery, cryocoagulation or transscleral photocoagulation must be performed to destroy the non-perfused peripheral areas of the retina. When at 2–3 months control, angiography of the iris shows the regression of new vessels in the iris, cataract removal may be performed (*Fig. 6.1*). If a photographic slit lamp is not available, it might be useful to use the fundus camera.

Ophthalmoscopic identification of retinal ischaemia, which is the cause of new vessels, is usually difficult. In some cases it appears with a pale colour and crossed by white vessels. At the edge of these areas, intraretinal microvascular abnormalities, cotton wool spots, and haemorrhages are frequently present. Neovascularization at the disc or elsewhere begins as minute budding from one small vessel; this budding later develops into a network of delicate vessels that can be seen only by the higher magnification of the slit lamp. Later, new vessels tend to grow far into the vitreous, accompanied by marked glial proliferation. As the neovascular frond matures, the glial tissue component increases, and the percentage of neovascularization decreases. Older intravitreal fronds can be heavily gliotic and have little neovascularization in or on the surface of the glial tissue.

The condition of the vitreous body must be accurately analysed in this phase. Knowing the state of the vitreous and the relationship of the posterior hyaloid to the retina is most significant for determining the type of photocoagulation treatment that should be employed, as well as the ultimate prognosis for a particular eye.

The diagnosis of early PDR is much easier if retinal fluorescein angiography is carried out. It is possible to identify new vessels because they leak dye early and profusely. The diffusion is secondary to the lack of tye-junctions at the level of the endothelial cells in newly formed vessels. Furthermore, fluorescein angiography makes it possible to define the extent of ischaemic areas because they appear hypofluorescent.

Usually, retinal ischaemia is located in the midperiphery. Therefore, it is always important to extend the evaluation not only to the posterior pole, but also to all the midperipheral quadrants; in such a way fluorescein angiography will by the basis for performing an accurate laser treatment (*Fig. 6.2*).

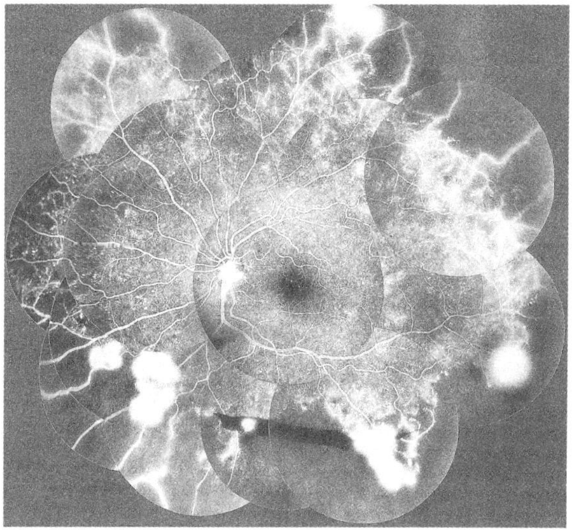

Figure 6.2
Fluorescein angiography allows better identification of new vessels, which appear as hyperlfuorescent areas, and retinal ischaemia, which appears hypofluorescent. In this case, it is possible to identify a hypoflourescence in the inferior sectors secondary to the masking effect of vitreous haemorrhage.

TREATMENT

The Diabetes Control and Complications Trial demonstrated that a good metabolic control could delay the advent or, at least, improve the evolution of retinal complications in diabetes.[8] Intensive insulin treatment was shown to reduce the risk of developing proliferative or severe nonproliferative retinopathy and to decrease the risk of requiring laser surgery by approximately 50%. However, some intensively treated patients may experience early worsening of the retinopathy, but thereafter a reduced risk of progression will occur. Therefore, while close control of blood glucose as well as blood pressure is encouraged, it is important to monitor carefully any patient undergoing correction of poorly controlled blood glucose levels. Following the first studies carried out by Aiello,[9] and James and L'Esperance[10] in the early 1970s, two multicentre studies, the

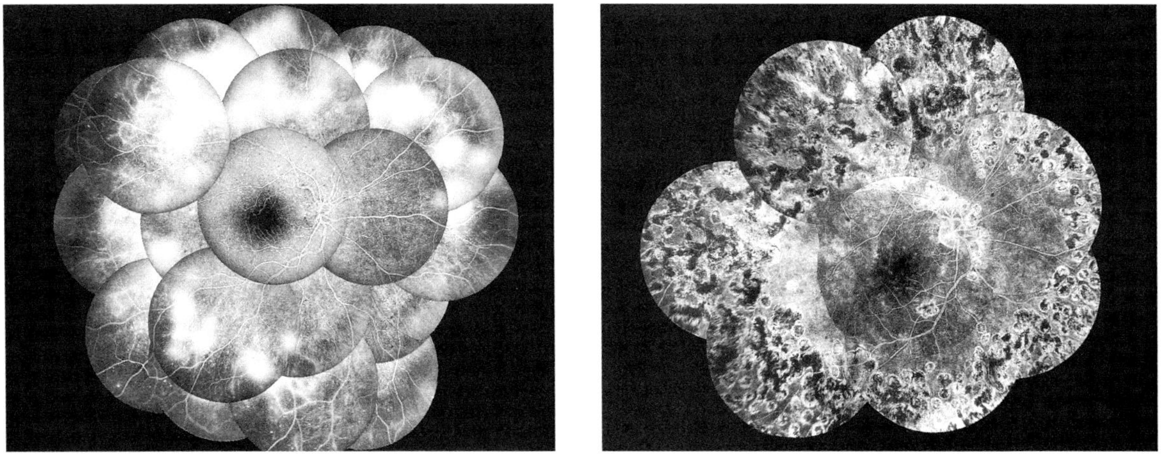

(a) (b)

Figure 6.3
Laser treatment performed to destroy all areas of retinal ischaemia (b) allowed in this case the regression of new vessels elsewhere (a).

Diabetic Retinopathy Study and the British Multicentre Study, were undertaken to evaluate the efficacy of laser treatment for PDR.

The Diabetic Retinopathy Study (DRS) began in 1971 and enrolled more than 1700 patients at 15 centres.[11] One eye of each patient was randomly assigned to either argon laser or xenon arc lamp therapy and the other served as a control. The treatment consisted of panretinal photocoagulation, focal treatment of new vessels elsewhere and, in the argon laser group, treatment of disc new vessels.

The British Multicentre Study (BMS) was carried out in Great Britain and included 99 patients affected by PDR. One eye was assigned to xenon arc treatment, while the other was used as control.[12]

Both trials demonstrated that photocoagulative treatment is effective in improving the evolution of PDR. The DRS results revealed a rate of blindness in non-treated patients three times higher than in the treated ones (16.3% vs 6.4%). The DRS also identified as risk factors, predictive of severe visual loss, new vessels that had already produced vitreous haemorrhages, and huge new vessels.[13] The use of laser treatment on eyes showing these characteristics reduced blindness by more than 50% after 4 years of follow-up. Similar results were reported by the BMS.

The goal of retinal photocoagulation is to cause regression of existing neovascular tissue and to prevent new vessel formation in the future. Laser treatment must be applied to ischaemic areas, which are responsible for new vessel formation. Photocoagulation must be carried out on the basis of a panretinal fluorescein angiography (*Fig. 6.3*)

The indications for the treatment of eyes with severe non-proliferative retinopathy are still being debated. Data from the Early Treatment Diabetic Retinopathy Study (ETDRS)[14] demonstrate that early laser treatment of eyes with severe non-

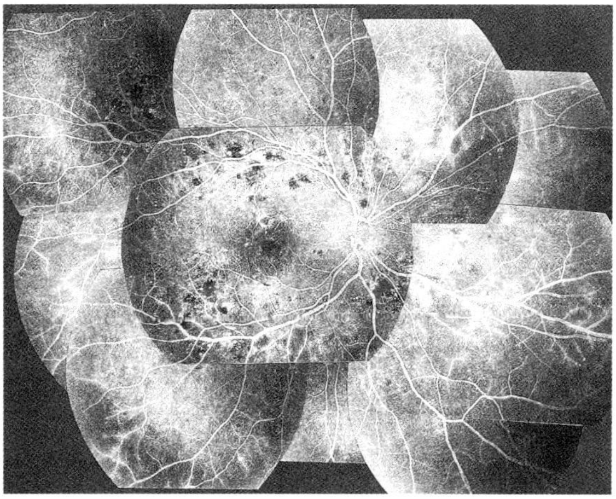

(a)

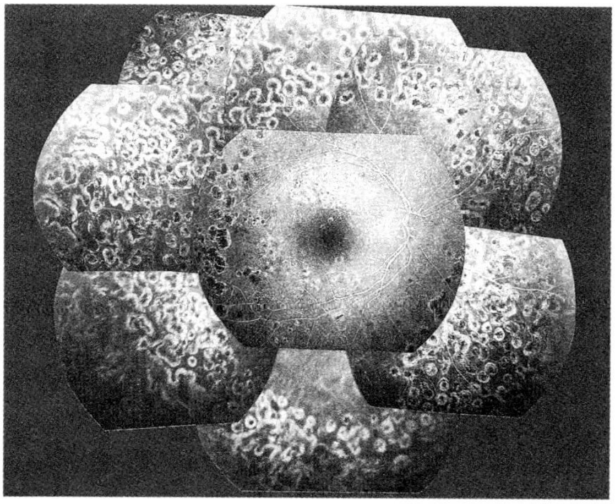

(b)

Figure 6.4
In some cases of severe non-proliferative retinopathy (a), it is useful to perform a laser treatment of retinal ischaemia (b). In this case, no worsening of macular oedema was noted after laser therapy.

proliferative diabetic retinopathy reduces the risk of severe visual loss as well as the rates of progression to high-risk PDR. Nevertheless, guidelines for treatment are not well codified; ETDRS results, in fact, stem from patients affected by both severe non-proliferative retinopathy and early PDR.

In cases of severe non-proliferative retinopathy, some systemic factors must be considered in scheduling laser photocoagulation, such as:

1. Patient compliance: follow-up frequency, distance of the patient's home from the ophthalmic department, etc. Laser treatment may be postponed in patients willing to undergo regular controls; in negligent patients, however, early photocoagulation must be performed.
2. Presence of renal failure and/or actual or scheduled pregnancy, because these conditions may accelerate progression of retinopathy.
3. Presence of developing cataract owing to the progression of lens opacity may impair future laser treatment or mask the onset of retinal new vessels. In addition, previous treatment of retinal ischaemia is useful in avoiding postoperative neovascular complications in diabetic patients scheduled for cataract extraction.

Laser treatment: in these cases, must be strictly limited to the areas of retinal ischaemia, sparing all the well-perfused zones[15] (*Fig 6.4*).

The laser sources generally employed to perform retinal photocoagulation are the traditional continuous wave gas ion lasers: argon blue-green (488–514 nm), monochromatic argon green (514 nm), krypton red (647 nm), krypton yellow (577 nm), and the newer solid-state lasers: diode (810 nm) and double-frequency Nd:YAG (532 nm).

All these lasers have been applied to perform treatment of PDR.[16–22] Even though the different absorption spectra of the ocular pigments (melanin of the retinal pigmented epithelium and of the choroid, blood haemoglobin of the retinal vessels and macular xanthophyll) should theoretically allow selective photocoagulation, argon, krypton, double-frequency Nd:YAG, and diode lasers appear to have similar effects in current clinical practice, though with some exceptions. Argon blue-green should be avoided, owing to the possibility of damage in the inner retinal layers as well as in the macular xanthopyll and to undesired effects on the operator's eyes.[23] Moreover, since blood haemoglobin absorbs yellow and green light, in eyes with vitreous haemorrhages or also cataract, it is preferable to use krypton red or diode lasers.

TECHNIQUE

The guidelines for laser treatment are already codified. The panretinal photocoagulation (PRP) can begin from two to three disc diameters from the centre to the periphery, or in a centripetal pattern, from the periphery to the centre, or otherwise in a sequence of quadrants.

In order to avoid unintentional photocoagulation inside the temporal vascular arcades, it is preferable to delimit the posterior pole by two to three rows of impacts. The spots must be contiguous but not confluent. In general 1500–2500 spots are enough to complete the PRP.

Spot diameter is 500–1000 μm in size at the periphery and 200 μm nearer the centre.

The laser burns must be moderately intense.

The number of spots delivered is generally 600–800 for each episode; in particular situations this number can be increased. The intervals between sessions range from 3 to 10 days or more. The PRP is performed through a contact lens, either a Goldmann three-mirror, or a Quadraspheric Volk or even a Mainster wide-field lens.

Almost all cases require only topical anesthaesia, while retrobulbar injection is seldom necessary.

When media opacities preclude photocoagulation, it is possible to perform a cryoablation or a transsceral photocoagulation by diode or continuous wave Nd:YAG laser.[24]

Failure of the new vessels to regress, increasing neovascularization, and vitreous haemorrhage must be regarded as indications for treatment. Additional treatments consist of other burns among scars, or over small areas of residual ischaemia, also near the posterior pole.

SIDE EFFECTS

Some side effects are associated with PRP, including loss of night and peripheral vision and a slight reduction in central visual acuity.[25] Macular oedema, if present, may worsen. It is better, for this reason, to treat macular oedema 20–30 days before PRP. In the event of macular oedema secondary to PRP and detected fluorangiographically some months later, its early treatment is advisable in order to avoid chronic evolution and functional effects.[26] Choroidal detachment may also occur and it is secondary to laser overdose. Usually its resolution is spontaneous.

PARS PLANA VITRECTOMY

The Diabetic Retinopathy Vitrectomy Study (DRVS) randomized diabetic patients with dense vitreous haemorrhages to early (1–6 months) vs later (12 months) vitrectomy.[27] The greatest benefit of early vitrectomy was in type I diabetic patients with duration of diabetes for less than 20 years. However, there was no difference between early and later vitrectomy among type II diabetic patients and type I diabetic patients with duration of diabetes for 20 years or longer.

Current indications for pars plana vitrectomy in diabetic patients can be summarized as follows:

1. Vitreous haemorrhage for more than 2–3 months, or recurrence of vitreous haemorrhage. The major goals of vitrectomy in this case are to remove the opaque vitreous gel and to perform endophotocoagulation.
2. Tractional retinal detachment, with macular involvement and visual acuity reduction. The goals are then to release anterior and posterior vitreoretinal traction, to release tangential retinal traction, and to perform endophotocoagulation.
3. Fibrovascular proliferation at the disc with vitreoretinal traction, without involvement of the posterior pole. The goals are then to remove fibrovascular tissue, to release tractions, and to perform endophotocoagulation.
4. Fibrovascular proliferation with vitreoretinal traction, macular ectopia. The goals are then to remove fibrovascular tissue, to release vitreoretinal traction, to reattach the retina, and to perform endophotocoagulation.
5. Macular oedema secondary to thickening and/or traction of posterior hyaloid. The major goals of vitrectomy are then to separate posterior hyaloid from the retina and to remove it.

NEOVASCULARIZATION OF THE IRIS

Neovascularization of the iris surface and anterior chanber angle is one of the more serious complications of PDR. Panretinal photocoagulation is useful in successfully dealing with the early phases of the angle neovascularization.[28,29] The early sign of developing new vessels in the iris is mild anterior chamber flare. This sign indicates increased permeability of the abnormal new anterior segment vessels. In early cases, variable and unpredictable intraocular pressure measurements may be associated with the minimal anterior chamber flare. At this time, new vessels may be seen gonioscopically or at the pupillary border. Fluorescein angiography of the iris gives a precise picture of the morphology and vascular dynamic of iris vessels; it shows up vascular anomalies and alterations to permeability that are hard to assess biomicroscopically.[7]

Further research is still needed to clarify the pathogenesis of rubeosis iridis, but various theories have been proposed. The most plausible one suggests that a causal factor is a vasoactive substance produced by the retina in conditions of hypoxia.[30] Shulze postulates that it is ischaemia not of the retina but of the iris itself that causes the neovascularization of the iris.[31] It is sometimes possible by iris fluorescein angiography to identify a process of ischaemia of the iris accompanying the neovascularization. Other investigations of diabetic iridopathy, however, have failed to find any such unperfused areas in the iris.[32]

The main therapeutic approach to new vessels in the iris is prevention, by panretinal photocoagulation of the causal elements. There is no known medical or surgical therapy that affects the natural history of rubeosis iridis. The eye tolerates the neovascularization of the iris until neovascular glaucoma arises. Once the angle is closed no medical therapy has any effect.

If carried out before neovascular glaucoma arises, photocoagulation can obliterate the new vessels and achieve regression of the lesions of the iris. The fluorescein angiogram of the iris after laser treatment of retinal ischaemic areas shows less vascular congestion and less dye leakage into radial vessels and residual new vessels.

REFERENCES

1. Apple DJ, Pathology. In: L'Esperance FA, James WA, eds, *Diabetic Retinopathy. Clinical Evaluation and Management* (CV Mosby: St Louis, 1981) 38–57.
2. Little HL, Pathogenesis. In: L'Esperance FA, James WA, eds, *Diabetic Retinopathy. Clinical Evaluation and Management* (CV Mosby: St Louis, 1981) 58–88.
3. American Academy of Ophthalmology, *Retina and Vitreous. Basic and Clinical Course*, Section 12 (American Academy of Ophthalmology, San Francisco, 1994) 51–63.
4. Garancini P, Micossi P, Valsania P et al, Prevalence of retinopathy in diabetic subjects from out-patient clinics in Lombardy (Italy), and associated risk factors. A multicentre epidemiologic study, *Diabetes Res Clin Pract* (1989) **6**:129–38.
5. Bandello F, Brancato R, Lattanzio R et al, Biomicroscopy versus fluorescein angiography of the iris in the detection of diabetic iridopathy, *Graefes Arch Clin Exp Ophthalmol* (1993) **231**:444–8.
6. Bandello F, Brancato R, Lattanzio R et al, Relation between iridopathy and retinopathy in diabetes, *Br J Ophthalmol* (1994) **78**:542–5.
7. Brancato R, Bandello F, Lattanzio R, The role of iris fluorescein angiography in clinical practice, *Surv Ophthalmol* (1997) **42**:41–70.
8. Diabetes Control and Complications Trial Research Group, The effect of intensive treatment of diabetes on the development and progression of long-term complications in insulin-dependent diabetes mellitus, *N Engl J Med* (1993) **329**:977–86.
9. Aiello LM, Ruby laser photocoagulation in diabetic retinopathy, *Isr J Med Sci* (1972) **8**:293–6.
10. James WA, L'Esperance FA, Treatment of diabetic optic nerve neovascularization by extensive retinal photocoagulation, *Am J Ophthalmol* (1974) **78**:939–44.
11. The Diabetic Retinopathy Study Research Group, Photocoagulation treatment of proliferative diabetic retinopathy: clinical application of Diabetic Retinopathy Study (DRS) findings, DRS Report no. 8, *Ophthalmology* (1981) **88**:583–600.
12. British Multicentre Study Group, Proliferative diabetic retinopathy treatment with xenon-arc photocoagulation, *BMJ* (1977) **81**:739–41.
13. The Diabetic Retinopathy Study Research Group, Four risk factors for severe visual loss in diabetic retinopathy: the third report from the Diabetic Retinopathy Study, *Arch Ophthalmol* (1979) **97**:654–5.
14. Early Treatment Diabetic Retinopathy Study Research Group, Early photocoagulation for diabetic retinopathy. ETDRS Report no. 9, *Ophthalmology* (1991) **98**:761–74.
15. Brancato R, Bandello F, Lattanzio R, Laser treatment of proliferative diabetic retinopathy: why, when, how? In: Belfiore F, Bergman RN, Molinatti GM, eds, *Current Topics in Diabetes Research. Front Diabetes* (Karger: Basel, 1993) 221–6.
16. Brancato R, Menchini U, Bandello F, Pece A, Comparative study on the treatment of diabetic retinopathy with blue-green argon laser vs. krypton and dye (Rhodamine 6G) laser. In: Proceedings of the 25th International Congress of Ophthalmology, Rome, May 1986. (Kugler & Ghedini: Amsterdam, 1987) 304–7.
17. McHugh JDA, Marshall J, ffytche TJ et al, Initial clinical experience using diode laser in the treatment of retinal vascular diseases, *Eye* (1989) **3**:516–27.
18. Bandello F, Brancato R, Trabucchi G et al, Diode vs. argon-green laser panretinal photocoagulation in proliferative diabetic retinopathy: a randomized study in 44 eyes with a long follow-up time, *Graefes Arch Clin Exp Ophthalmol* (1993) **231**:491–4.
19. Bandello F, Brancato R, Lattanzio R et al, Double-frequency Nd:YAG laser versus argon-green laser in the treatment of proliferative diabetic retinopathy: randomized study with long-term follow-up, *Lasers Surg Med* (1996) **122**:494–501.
20. Brancato R, Bandello F, New laser modalities for posterior segment treatment, *Curr Opin Ophthalmol* (1991) **2**:299–305.

21. Brancato R, Bandello F, Trabucchi G, Does wavelength matter when photocoagulating eyes with macular degeneration or diabetic retinopathy? *Arch Ophthalmol* (1994) **112**:156–7.
22. Puliafito CA, Semiconductor diode laser photocoagulation in retinal vascular diseases, *Lasers Surg Med* (1990) **2**:67–70.
23. Gunduz K, Arden GB, Changes in colour contrast sensitivity associated with operating argon lasers, *Br J Ophthalmol* (1989) **73**:241–6.
24. Brancato R, Carassa RG, Value of ultrasound biomicroscopy for cyclodestructive procedures, *Curr Opin Ophthalmol* (1996) **7**:87–92.
25. Little HL, Complications of argon laser photocoagulation in the treatment of diabetic retinopathy. In: Little HL, Jack RL, Patz A, Forsham PH, eds, *Diabetic Retinopathy* (Thieme Stratton: New York, 1983) 285–96.
26. Early Treatment Diabetic Retinopathy Study Research Group, Photocoagulation for diabetic macular edema: Report no. 1, *Arch Ophthalmol* (1985) **103**:1796–806.
27. The Diabetic Retinopathy Vitrectomy Study Research Group, Early vitrectomy for severe proliferative diabetic retinopathy in eyes with useful vision. Results of a randomized trial. Diabetic Retinopathy Vitrectomy Study Report no. 3, *Ophthalmology* (1988) **95**:1307–20.
28. Little HL, Rosenthal AR, Dellaporta A, The effect of panretinal photocoagulation on rubeosis iridis, *Am J Ophthalmol* (1976) **81**:804–8.
29. Jacobson DR, Murphy RP, Rosenthal AR, Treatment of angle neovascularization with panretinal photocoagulation, *Ophthalmology* (1979) **86**: 1270–5.
30. Patz A, Clinical and experimental studies on retinal neovascularization, *Am J Ophthalmol* (1982) **94**: 715–43.
31. Schulze RR, Rubeosis iridis, *Am J Ophthalmol* (1967) **63**:487–90.
32. Laatikainen L, Development and classification of rubeosis iridis in diabetic eye disease, *Br J Ophthalmol* (1979) **63**:150–4.

7 Complications of photocoagulation

Fred Hendrikse and Ellen C La Heij

INTRODUCTION

Photocoagulation for the different forms of diabetic retinopathy is well established. It is very effective in preventing and treating proliferative diabetic retinopathy and iris neovascularizations, as well as stabilizing or improving their condition in the majority of patients with non-proliferative diabetic retinopathy. It has, however, several potential complications. The ophthalmologist must have knowledge of these complications in order to balance the beneficial effect and potential complications, and to prevent these complications as far as possible. Furthermore, it is important to inform patients about possible complications to prevent later misunderstandings.

CORNEA

Iatrogenic epithelial defects may easily be caused by the laser contact lens, because the diabetic cornea is more susceptible to corneal erosion and has a significantly decreased sensitivity.[1]

IRIS/PUPIL ABNORMALITIES

Burns to the stroma of the iris may be caused by not carefully setting the focus on the retina.[2] Even posterior synechiae may result. Accommodative insufficiency and asthenopia amplitudes are well-known complications following panretinal photocoagulation.[2–4] Accommodative amplitudes in the Early Treatment Diabetic Retinopathy Study (ETDRS) patients were lower than normal[4] especially in older patients with a longer duration of diabetes. In addition, full scatter photocoagulation was found to give a transient additional reduction of 1/3 diopter in accommodative amplitude at the 4-month visit.[4]

Even partial sphincter palsies, cholinergic supersesnitivity, and light-near dissociation have been reported after panretinal photocoagulation.[2,5,6] These complications are thought to be the result of a heat transferral and resultant damage of the ciliary nerves in the suprachoroidal space.[5,7] Therefore, in applying scatter photocoagulation, the long posterior ciliary nerves along the horizontal meridians should be avoided if risk of the above-mentioned complications is to be reduced.

LENS

Focal lens burns (*Fig. 7.1*), with coagulation of lens proteins, resulting in non-progressive lens opacities, occur most often in eyes with nuclear sclerosis treated with argon blue-green light, because these wavelengths are especially

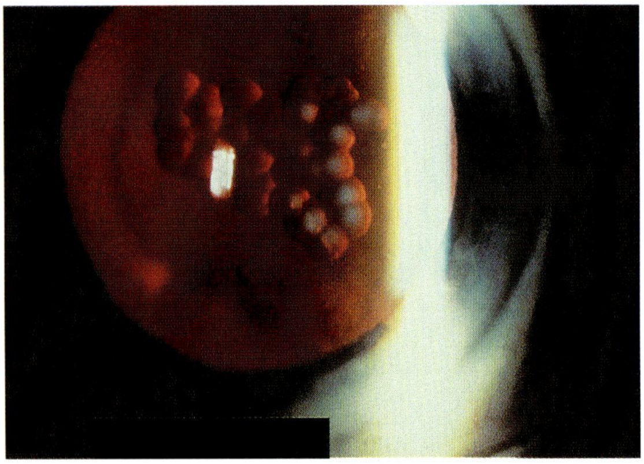

Figure 7.1
Lens burns after retinal laser treatment.

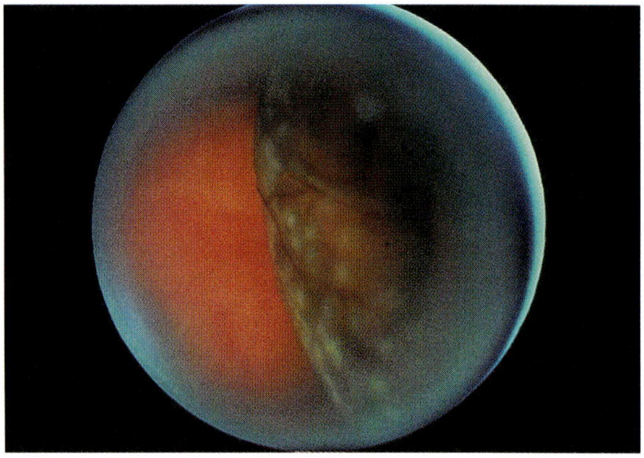

Figure 7.2
Choroidal detachment after panretinal laser treatment.

absorbed by the yellow cataract pigments.[8] Therefore, krypton red, which is minimally absorbed by these lens pigments, is recommended for use in patients with nuclear cataracts. In the presence of pigment on the anterior lens capsule, however, krypton red in particular may induce focal lens opacities.

INCREASED INTRAOCULAR PRESSURE

Intraocular pressure may rise immediately after panretinal photocoagulation.[9] This elevation is most often transient, and may last for several hours to days. Maximum elevation is approximately 1 day after photocoagulation and within 1 week pressure levels will be within the normal range. In most cases the anterior chamber angle remains open during such a transient attack, but a reduced outflow facility may be measured.[6] In some cases, however, ciliary body swelling and ciliochoroidal with detachment of the choroid after extensive photocoagulation (*Fig.* 7.2) may cause closure of the anterior chamber angle resulting in a rise in intraocular pressure.[10–13] Also, an annular and anterior rotation of the ciliary body has been described.[13] Usually this pressure elevation is self-limited, but sometimes medical treatment may be necessary. Laser iridotomy is not recommended.[10] A higher incidence of transient intraocular pressure rise[9,10,12] and choroidal detachment[14] has been reported after single-session panretinal scatter treatment. It is therefore recommended that panretinal photocoagulation be performed in multiple sessions, usually 2–3 weeks apart. No difference efficacy has been found when comparing single- to multiple-session treatment.[14]

MACULA

Macular oedema (*Fig.* 7.3) may result from panretinal photocoagulation, and preexisting macular oedema may worsen.[15–18] It is hypothesized that increased macular blood flow and inflammation induced by the laser treatment may be responsible for this oedema of the macular region.[5] To avoid this complication, macular grid laser photocoagulation may be performed before

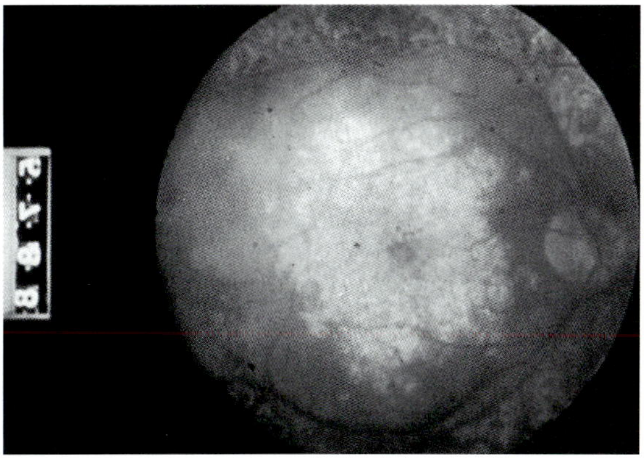

Figure 7.3
Macular oedema after panretinal laser treatment.

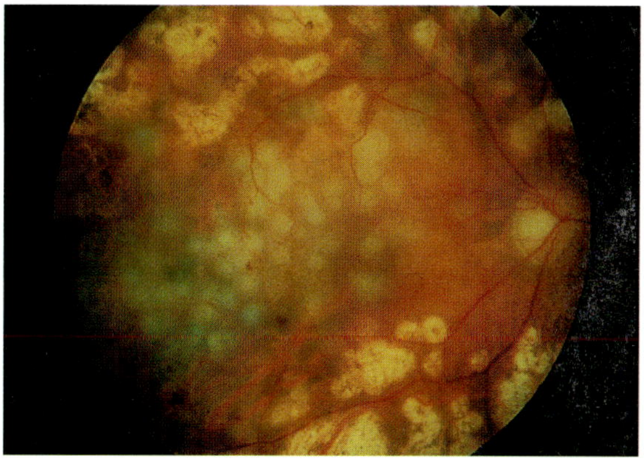

Figure 7.4
Accidentally coagulated macular area during panretinal laser treatment through a peripheral mirror of the Goldmann lens. The patient gazed to the side, unnoticed by the ophthalmologist.

applying full scatter photocoagulation. Also, a combined procedure of macular grid laser and panretinal photocoagulation of the inferior one-half of the retina in the first session, followed by a completion of panretinal laser treatment in the second session, is recommended.[7] By placing a more peripherally oriented pattern of scatter photocoagulation, one can also reduce the occurrence of macular oedema.

Even choroidal detachment and exudative macular detachment have been described following panretinal photocoagulation.[14,19,20] It is postulated that the choriocapillaris and the retinal pigmented epithelial cells (RPE cells) are damaged by photocoagulation; and that this dysfunction of RPE cells may result in an exudative retinal detachment.[21]

A rare but disastrous macular complication following panrtinal photocoagulation is macular hole formation as a direct result of an inadvertent central foveal burn (*Fig. 7.4*). This complication can be avoided by frequently checking and locating the fovea during treatment. One can demarcate the temporal border of the macula with a few rows of laser burns. Peripheral treatment can best be performed from posterior to anterior along the supero- and inferotemporal arcades. When using the Goldmann three-mirror contact lens, always check whether the macular area is in the central lens.

Iatrogenic choroidal neovascularization (*Fig. 7.5*) with chorioretinal anastomosis has been

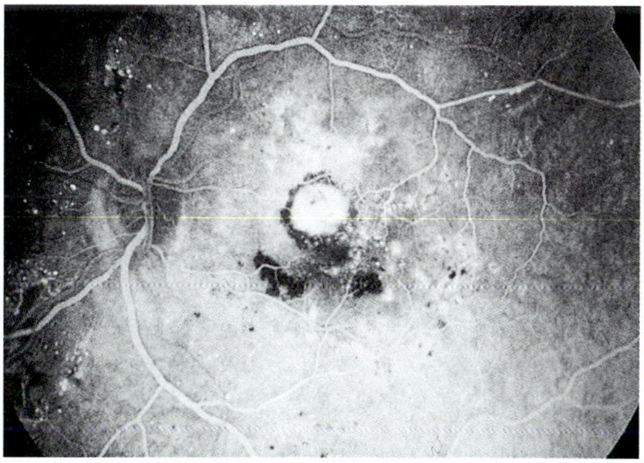

Figure 7.5
Submacular neovascularization after perifoveal laser treatment.

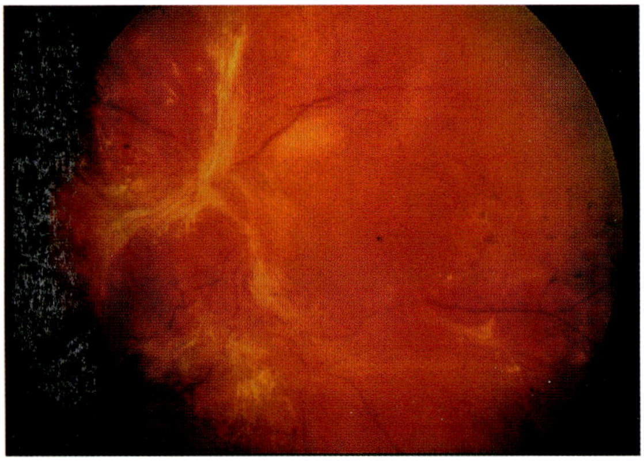

Figure 7.6
Contraction of epiretinal fibrosis with macular traction after laser treatment.

described in patients treated for macular oedema and proliferative diabetic retinopathy.[22,23] In these cases, the laser probably causes an iatrogenic break in Bruch's membrane. Sometimes a small haemorrhage is seen immediately after placing such a burn. Moreover, choriocapillaris endothelial budding and rupture of Bruch's membrane may be induced by laser treatment, even without a clinically evident break.[24] Even proliferations of new vessels from the choroid into the vitreous with vitreous haemorrhage through the atropic retina have been described following intense photocoagulation burns.[25,26] Especially high-intensity laser treatment with small spot sizes (50 μm) will cause a puncture of Bruch's membrane. This spot size should therefore be avoided when treating the macular area, and the least laser intensity necessary to create a light-grey burn should be used. Moreover, one should keep in mind that when spot size is reduced, the energy level should also be decreased, because energy density varies inversely with the spot area. Also, short-duration exposures (< 0.2 seconds) with long wavelengths and repeated applications to the same area should not be used if puncture of Bruch's membrane is to be avoided.

Distortion of the central retina after panretinal photocoagulation may be caused by contraction of a chorioretinal scar with traction lines extending into the fovea (*Fig. 7.6*). Retreating a previously photocoagulated area may be a risk factor in these cases. Also, epiretinal fibrosis and membranes may form, especially after laser treatment of retinal haemorrhages. These membranes may contact and eventually lead to macular distortion with metamorphopsia.[25]

VISUAL FIELD LOSS

Peripheral visual field

A modest visual field loss in the peripheral visual field occurs in up to 50% of the eyes treated,[27] more commonly after xenon arc than after argon laser treatment, as reported by the Diabetic Retinopathy Study.[28,29] Later, the ETDRS confirmed these findings and found that peripheral visual field loss is more often seen after confluent laser treatment and after repeated treatment of the same retinal area with greater risk for nerve fibre layer damage.[16,30] With mild, low-intensity, short-duration burns, the necrosis caused by laser treatment may involve only the RPE and outer segments, and regrowth may cause little or no functional loss in the area.[5,31] If the burn also involves the inner retina, including the passing nerve fibres supplying other retinal areas, the scotoma will be larger.

Central visual field

Intense laser treatment of the papillomacular bundle should be avoided. Full-thickness retinal burns should not be employed over more than four clock hours of the nerve fibre layer temporal to the optic disc if the risk of loss of central vision is to be avoided.[32] Laser treatment of the superior or inferior half of the central macula is less harmful for central visual function than laser burns of the temporal or nasal margin of the fovea. Reading vision is more likely to be disturbed when parafoveal burns are placed on the temporal side of the left eye and on the nasal side of the right eye.

After laser grid treatment for macular oedema, the photocoagulation scar may enlarge progressively, resulting in RPE atrophy and visual loss.[33] This is more frequently seen in myopic eyes. Schatz et al found in their study that 5% of the diabetic eyes treated with macular grid for oedema suffered from central vision loss.[33] Other authors, however, could not support their findings.[6] It has been demonstrated that diabetic patients with macular oedema and a paracentral scotoma have a 3–4 dB reduction of sensitivity of their central visual field per treatment session, regardless of the wavelength used for the macular grid treatment.[34] To avoid the complication of scar tissue enlargement, only the minimum of photocoagulation required should be used. Some paracentral scotomas become less apparent to the patient with time. A few reports have been published of visual loss after panretinal photocoagulation due to choroidal ischaemia. Especially patients with collagen vascular diseases may be susceptible to this ischaemic damage.[20,35]

OPTIC DISC

Rare reports in the literature describe the occurrence of permanent severe visual loss probably due to a thermal optic neuropathy by the placement of laser burns too close to the optic disc.[36] Also, nerve fibre bundle damage in the juxtapapillary retina or injury to the optic nerve head itself may produce a dramatic visual loss. It is recommended that treatment be applied no closer than one disc diameter to the optic nerve head, and that a neovascularization of the disc nerve be treated directly.

HAEMORRHAGE

Haemorrhage may occur as a complication of photocoagulation either immediately after treatment or as a delayed consequence (*Fig.* 7.7). As mentioned earlier, spot sizes of 50 μm with high energy and short-duration exposures may cause a break in Bruch's membrane with direct bleeding. When such a haemorrhage occurs, intraocular pressure should be raised by pressure with the contact lens. Often, it stops spontaneously within a few seconds. Direct laser treament of neovascular tufts are contraindicated because significant vitreous haemorrhage may result. Delayed haemorrhage may occur from iatrogenic choroidal neovascularization, as mentioned above.

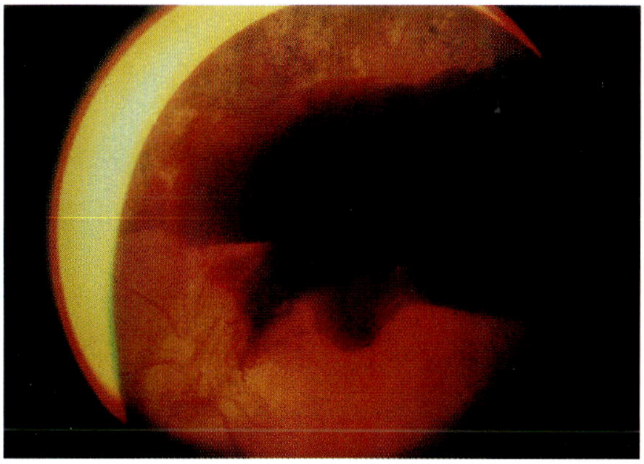

Figure 7.7
Vitreous haemorrhage after panretinal laser treatment.

CONTRACTION OF VITREORETINAL STRANDS

Progressive tractional retinal detachment may be seen in patients with marked pre-existing vitreoretinal traction.[37] It may worsen after treatment, and is more frequently seen after xenon photocoagulation than after argon laser treatment.[37]

PHYSICAL FUNCTIONS

Loss of hue discrimination and a tritan blue-yellow defect is more frequently seen in diabetic patients. It is increased after macular and panretinal photocoagulation. Dark adaptation, already increased in diabetic patients, may show a further increase after panretinal photocoagulation.[38] Furthermore, diabetic patients will experience worsening of their night vision (nyctalopia) and a loss of central light sensitivity after panretinal photocoagulation.[38,39]

REFERENCES

1. Ruben ST, Corneal sensation in insulin dependent and non-insulin dependent diabetics with proliferative retinopathy, *Acta Ophthalmol Copenh* (1994) **72**:576–80.
2. Lobes LAJR, Bourgon P, Pupillary abnormalities induced by argon laser photocoagulation, *Ophthalmology* (1985) **92**:234–6.
3. Lerner BC, Lakhanpal V, Schocket SS, Treatment myopia and accommodative paresis following cryotherapy and panretinal photocoagulation, *Am J Ophthalmol* (1984) **97**:704–8.
4. Braun CI, Benson WE, Remaley NA et al, Accommodative amplitudes in the Early Treatment Diabetic Retinopathy Study, *Retina* (1995) **15**:275–81.
5. Gass JDM, Complications of photocoagulation therapy of macular lesions. In: Craven D, ed, *Stereoscopic Atlas of Macular Diseases. Diagnosis and Treatment* (Mosby: St Louis, 1997).
6. Rogell GD, Internal ophthalmoplegia after argon laser panretinal photocoagulation, *Arch Ophthalmol* (1979) **97**:904–5.
7. Olk LJ, Lee CM, Complications and side effects of treatment. In: Papadopaulos D, ed, *Diabetic Retinopathy. Practical Management* (JB Lippencott: Philadelphia, 1993).
8. McCanna R, Chandra SR, Stevens TS et al, Argon laser-induced cataract as a complication of retinal photocoagulation, *Arch Ophthalmol* (1982) **100**:1071–3.
9. Bondeau P, Pavan PR, Phelps CD, Acute pressure elevation following panretinal photocoagulation, *Am J Ophthalmol* (1981) **99**:1239–42.
10. Mensher JH, Anterior chamber depth alteration after retinal photocoagulation, *Arch Ophthalmol* (1977) **95**:113–16.
11. Boulton PE, A study of the mechanism of transient myopia following extensive xenon arc photocoagulation, *Trans Ophthalmol Soc UK* (1974) **93**: 287–300.
12. Huamonte FU, Peyman GA, Goldberg MF, Locketz A, Immediate fundus complications after retinal scatter photocoagulation. I. Clinical picture and pathogenesis, *Ophthalmol Surg* (1976) **7**:88–99.
13. Phelps C, Angle closure glaucoma secondary to ciliary body swelling, *Arch Ophthalmol* (1974) **92**:286–90.
14. Doft BH, Blankenship GW, Single versus multiple treatment sessions of argon laser photocoagulation for proliferative diabetic retinopathy, *Ophthalmology* (1982) **89**:772–90.
15. Ferris FL, Podger MJ, Davis MD, The Diabetic Retinopathy Study Research Group, Report no. 12. Macular edema in diabetic retinopathy study patients, *Ophthalmology* (1987) **94**:754–60.
16. Early Treatment Diabetic Retinopathy Study Research Group, Report no. 9. Early photocoagulation for diabetic retinopathy, *Ophthalmology* (1991) **98**:766–85.
17. McDonald HR, Scharz H, Macular edema following panretinal photocoagulation, *Retina* (1985) **5**:5–10.

18. Meyers SM, Macular edema after scatter laser photocoagulation for proliferative diabetic retinopathy, *Am J Ophthalmol* (1980) **90**:210–16.
19. McDonald HR, Scharz H, Visual loss following panretinal photocoagulation for proliferative diabetic retinopathy, *Ophthalmology* (1985) **92**:388–93.
20. Kleiner RC, Elmann MJ, Murphy RP, Ferris FL, Transient severe visual loss after panretinal photocoagulation, *Am J Ophthalmol* (1988) **106**:298–306.
21. Pollack A, Heriot WJ, Henkind P, Cellular processes causing defects in Bruch's membrane following krypton laser photocoagulation, *Ophthalmology* (1986) **93**:1113–19.
22. Varley MP, Frank E, Purnell EW, Subretinal neovascularisation after focal argon laser for diabetic macular edema, *Ophthalmology* (1988) **95**:567–73.
23. Wallon I, Chorioretinal and choriovitreal neovascularisation after photocoagulation for proliferative diubetic retinopathy, *Ophthalmology* (1985) **92**:523–32.
24. Boulton PE, A study of the mechanism of transient myopia following extensive xenon arc photocoagulation, *Trans Ophthalmol Soc UK* (1974) **93**:287–300.
25. Gass JDM, Options in the treatment of macular diseases, *Trans Ophthalmol Soc UK* (1972) **92**:449–68.
26. Benson WE, Townsend RE, Pheasant TR, Chorioovitreal and subretinal proliferations: complications of photocoagulation, *Ophthalmology* (1979) **86**:283–9.
27. Russel PW, Sekuler R, Fetkenhour C, Visual function after panretinal photocoagulation: a survey, *Diabetes Care* (1985) **57**:57–63.
28. Diabetic Retinopathy Study Research Group, Photocoagulation treatment of proliferative diabetic retinopathy: the second report of diabetic retinopathy/vitrectomy study findings, *Am J Ophthalmol* (1978) **85**:82–106.
29. Diabetic Retinopathy Study Research Group, Report no. 8. Photocoagulation of proliferative diabetic retinopathy: clinical applications of DRS findings, *Invest Ophthalmol Vis Sci* (1981) **88**:583–600.
30. Frank RN, Visual field and electroretinopathy following extensive photocoagulation, *Arch Ophthalmol* (1975) **93**:591–8.
31. Roider J, Michaud NA, Flotte TJ, Birngruber R, Response of the retinal pigment epithelium to selective photocoagulation, *Arch Ophthalmol* (1992) **110**:1786–892.
32. Blair CJ, Gass JDM, Photocoagulation of the macula and papillomacular bundle in the human, *Arch Ophthalmol* (1972) **88**:167–71.
33. Scharz H, Maderia D, McDonald HR, Johnson RN, Progressive enlargement of laser scar following grid laser photocoagulation for diffuse macular edema, *Arch Ophthalmol* (1991) **109**:1539–51.
34. Jost BF, Olk RJ, Patz A et al, Anterior segment ischaemia following laser photocoagulation in a patient with systemic lupus erythematosus, *Br J Ophthalmol* (1988) **72**:11–16.
35. Striph GC, Hart WM, Olk RJ, Modified grid laser photocoagulation for diabetic macular edema. The effect on the central visual field, *Ophthalmology* (1988) **95**:1673–9.
36. Swartz M, Apple DJ, Greel D, Sudden severe visual loss associated with peripapillary burns during panretinal argon photocoagulation, *Br J Ophthalmol* (1983) **67**:517–19.
37. McMeel JW, Photocoagulation approach with various diabetic vitreoretinal problems. In: L'Esperance F, ed, *Current Diagnosis and Management of Chorioretinal Diseases* (CV Mosby: St Louis, 1977) 269.
38. Pender PM, Benson WE, Compton H, Cox GB, The effects of panretinal photocoagulation on dark adaptation in diabetics with proliferative retinopathy, *Am Acad Ophthalmol* (1981) **88**:635–8.
39. Russel PW, Schuler R, Fetkenhour C, Visual function after panretinal photocoagulation: a survey, *Diabetes Care* (1985) **8**:57–63.

8 Surgical management of diabetic eye disease

Chris Canning

INTRODUCTION

Diabetic retinopathy remains a blinding condition–the most common cause of severe visual loss in the working-age population of the developed world. The observation that diabetic eyes with pre-existing chorioretinal lesions had less neovascularization suggested that destruction of peripheral parts of the retina might save the central vision. This led to the development of light photocoagulation and ushered in an era of possible treatment.

It soon became apparent that only some diabetic eyes affected by neovascular complications responded to such treatment. The development of pars plana vitrectomy and the ability to manipulate intraocular tissues has meant that many of these devastating complications are now treatable.[1] Unfortunately, the fact remains that one is operating on a profoundly damaged structure–the cure of diabetic eye disease does not lie in vitreoretinal surgery, but rather with a cure for diabetes itself.[2]

This chapter will look at the techniques and potentials of vitreoretinal surgery. This can only be a snapshot of current practice–concepts will change, indications for surgery will follow, and surgical techniques will evolve.

SURGICAL PATHOPHYSIOLOGY

Surgery in diabetic eye disease can be sight-saving provided that the right operation is done at the right time. There is a huge potential for making things worse by inappropriate intervention, however. Three options are always available – no surgical intervention (medical treatment of diabetes only), laser photocoagulation, and vitreoretinal surgery.

The correct treatment option has to be based on an understanding of the pathophysiology. There are two primary processes in diabetic retinopathy that can be improved by surgery – haemorrhage and fibrovascular traction. There are other processes, such as diabetic macular oedema, where the role of surgery is still uncertain.

In essence, neovascularization commencing in the retinal venous vasculature proliferates on the posterior hyaloid. Tractional or shearing forces on these vessels cause haemorrhage, and attendant fibrous proliferation causes traction between points on the retina where vitreous is attached.

Haemorrhage

Haemorrhage is important because it obscures the patient's vision and prevents a view of the retina–proliferation and tractional detachment can progress under haemorrhage and not be noticed. Indeed, blood may act as a stimulus for further proliferation. Blood may be found between the retina and the hyaloid (subhyaloid) or within the vitreous.

Subhyaloid blood appears as a dense smooth obscuration of the retina that can, if it overlies the

Table 8.1

	Subhyaloid haemorrhage	*Intravitreal haemorrhage*
Effect on patient's vision	Severe visual loss	Some vision possible
Potential for unrecognized fibrovascular proliferation	Minimal	Significant
Delineation of vitreoretinal adhesions	Well defined	Not defined
Vitreoretinal separation that assists the surgeon	Present	Absent

macula, result in dramatic reduction in vision. The edges of such a collection of blood are usually very well demarcated and the surrounding retina may be seen as normal.

Such a haemorrhage may be helpful during surgery because it separates the vitreous from the retina, thus reducing the amount of dissection needed. It also clearly shows those areas where the vitreous still adheres to the retina. Since neovascularization needs the scaffolding of the posterior hyaloid, aggressive fibrovascular proliferation is unlikely to occur unobserved beneath such blood.

Blood in the vitreous, on the other hand, often does not result in such a sudden and complete drop in vision for the patient, but it may be more of a problem for the surgeon. The vitreous may still be attached to the retina beneath it so the potential for fibrovascular proliferation occurring unnoticed does exist. Such blood also provides no help for the surgeon during the operation.

Fibrovascular traction

Fibrovascular proliferation occurs when new vessels grow from the surface of the retina and adhere to the posterior hyaloid. This tissue tends to contact and force is applied to the points where the vessels are attached to the retina. The response of the retina to this force may be to split (tractional retinoschisis), detach (tractional detachment) or tear (combined traction/rhegmatogenous detachment). It can be difficult to distinguish between tractional schisis and detachment. In one study by Lincoff et al[3] schisis was clearly present in 20% and detachment in 48%, and the rest were equivocal.

Where the chemical stimulus for neovacularization is present and the posterior hyaloid is detached, abortive neovascular complexes may form on the surface of the retina.[4]

INDICATIONS FOR SURGERY

Always remember that surgery can make a patient dramatically worse. There is evidence, however, that surgery offers a better long-term prognosis than no surgery in certain conditions.

Haemorrhage

Vitrectomy can clear the blood, thus improving the patient's vision, whilst at the same time allowing a view of the underlying retina. Further surgical or laser treatment of underlying neovascularization can then take place.

Conventional wisdom has it that one should allow 6 months for blood to absorb spontaneously before considering surgery.[5] The Diabetic Retinopathy Vitrectomy Study has shown that early vitrectomy (within 1–4 months of the onset of symptoms) offers better long-term vision than delayed surgery in patients whose presenting acuity is 6/240 or less.[6–8] This is particularly so in insulin-dependent diabetics.

Other factors also influence the timing of surgery. Has there been a full panretinal photocoagulation before the haemorrhage? If there has been, aggressive proliferation is less likely to occur unnoticed under the blood.[9] What is the vision in the fellow eye? Poor vision in the fellow eye makes the need to restore vision in the haemorrhage eye more urgent.

Fibrovascular traction

Fibrovascular proliferation needs surgery either if it threatens to involve the macula or if it does involve the macula and has caused visual loss fairly recently (last 6–12 months).[10] A macula that has been detached for more than 1 year has little if any visual potential left. Combined traction-rhegmatogenous detachment often results in sudden visual loss. The presence of a break in the retina usually means that surgery will be necessary.

Good preoperative panretinal photocoagulation can be tremendously helpful at the time of surgery even if neovascularization persists. There is valid concern that laser given to an eye where fibrovascular traction is present may induce haemorrhage from further traction. By and large the benefits of laser outweight the risks–at worst the laser will only precipitate an operation that would have been necessary at some time anyway.

Vitreomacular traction is a unique type of fibrous traction where the vitreous separates from the posterior pole everywhere but at the macula. The collapsed gel then pulls on the macula inducing a macula schisis.

Diabetic macular oedema

The idea of surgery here is that an attached vitreous gel can assert traction on the retina and exacerbate macular oedema. Vitrectomy is only indicated, therefore, where there is no posterior vitreous detachment–the aim of surgery is to induce one. Some reports suggest benefits, but this indication has yet to reach mainstream clinical practice.[11]

PREOPERATIVE ASSESSMENT

The most important preoperative assessment is whether the patient has an indication for the operation. This requires a good history noting type, duration and control of the diabetes; the nature and duration of the visual symptoms; previous eye treatment; and general health. Poor diabetic control, uncontrolled hypertension, and cardiac or renal failure are all risk factors in giving an anaesthetic. They can all also affect the surgical result, as can anticoagulants and aspirin.

Examination includes best corrected visual acuity, intraocular pressure check, state of the anterior chamber looking particularly for iris neovascularization, and dilated fundoscopy using the slit lamp biomicroscope and indirect ophthalmoscope. It is wise to avoid putting a contact lens on the eye in the immediate preoperative period, as the corneal epithelium is prone to slough.

Ultrasound can be helpful if blood obscures the view of the fundus. It provides some information about the presence and extent of retinal detachment and vitreoretinal adhesions. Electroretinography and visual evoked potentials do have some prognostic value for final visual outcome, but they are not used routinely.[12,13]

SURGICAL TECHNIQUES

Anaesthesia

As with all intraocular surgery, there is a choice between local and general anaesthesia for diabetic eye disease.[14,15] Local anaesthetic is the preferred option in most cases for several reasons. Firstly, the surgery is usually exclusively intraocular – there is no need to isolate the extraocular muscles or place a scleral explant. The operation is therefore not very painful. Secondly, all patients have diabetes and many have other associated illnesses that increase the risk of general anaesthetic. Thirdly, patients can eat, drink and take insulin in their usual way with local anesthesia so the risk of peri-operative loss of control of the diabetes is minimized.

Table 8.2

Objective	*Technique*	
Clear the visual axis	Cornea[6,17]	• Avoid contact lens before surgery • Use as little mydriatic as possible • Keep the epithelium well watered during surgery or coat it with HPMC or viscoelastic • Remove the epithelium only as a last resort
	Lens[18,19]	• Pars plana lensectomy leaving the anterior capsule • Small incision phacoemulsification • IOL inserted at the end of vitreoretinal surgery if appropriate
	Vitreous haemorrhage[20]	• Two, three or four port pars plana vitrectomy • 'Chemical' vitrectomy (e.g. hyaluronidase) still under clinical trial
Relieve vitreoretinal traction[21]	• Core vitrectomy, then either the segmentation or en bloc dissection technique • Segmentation technique – excise the posterior hyaloid 360 degrees between the posterior pole and the vitreous base – 'isolate the posterior pole – cut around all neovascular stalks to separate them from each other • En bloc dissection technique – cut a hole in the posterior hyaloid in the upper quadrants – pass scissors through the hole and cut all neovascular stalks parallel to the plane of the retina – excise the freed posterior hyaloid	
Prevent re-bleeding	• Per-operative thrombin • Meticulous diathermy of all bleeding vessels • Clear as much vitreous as possible from the vitreous base and close the sclerostomies cleanly • Silicone oil as a last resort	
Close retinal breaks and reattach the retina	• Internal drain of sub-retinal fluid through the existing retinal hole • Internal tamponade with gas or oil (22) (the breaks are usually too posterior for external tamponade • Laser or cryopexy to the break	
Discourage re-proliferation	• Pan-retinal laser photocoagulation	

Standard peri- or retro-bulbar anaesthesia is quite adequate, although local anaesthetic infusion within the muscle cone using with a blunt tip cannula can be added. General anaesthesia is sometimes needed for patients who are unable to co-operate with the local.

Surgery

The objectives for surgery in proliferative diabetic eye disease are straightforward – achieving them is more difficult. They are to get a clear view of the retina by removing whatever is preventing it, to relieve all vitreoretinal traction, to prevent rebleeding, to re-attach the retina and close any retinal breaks, and to discourage re-proliferation of new vessels on the retina of anterior segment. Each objective has a number of techniques that can be applied.

Vitrectomy has become standardized to the extent that almost all systems use a common 20-guage size. All ports are situated in the pars plana, about 3.5 mm from the limbus in a phakic eye and 3.0 mm in an aphakic one.

Three port vitrectomy is most frequently used. One port is for infusion of fluid and is most commonly placed in the infero-temporal quadrant. The infusion cannula has a length of 2.5 mm or 4 mm, both being long enough to get through the sclera and pars plana yet short enough to avoid touching the lens. One of the other ports will usually be for an endoillumination fibre optic light pipe whilst the other will be used for the vitrector or a variety of scissors, picks, forceps, diathermy tips or laser probes.

Four-port vitrectomy differs from three-port in that there are four ports fashioned, one in each quadrant. The technique may involve only using three ports at any one time but being able to move them around the eye, or the fourth port may be attached to a wide-angle illumination pipe.

Two-port vitrectomy uses the infusion cannula in one port and the active instrument in the other. Illumination then has to come via an indirect ophthalmoscope. The surgeon's second hand holds the condensing lens. This technique is suitable for clearance of vitreous blood and limited work close to the retina. It does not permit the use of both hands inside the eye and does not have the resolution needed for extensive preretinal dissection.

In three- or four-port vitrectomy the posterior segment of the eye can be visualized using an operating microscope and lens system. There is a big choice of lens systems now–hand-held irrigating contact lens, self-retaining contact lens, sew-on contact lens, wide-angle indirect contact lens or non-contact indirect lens. Sometimes a combination of systems works best in a given eye–a wide-angle system for doing the vitrectomy and relief of anteroposterior traction and a higher-resolution system for working on the posterior pole.

Cataract is frequently associated with proliferative eye disease. Whilst it is often quite possible to see adequately through it, removal of the lens is sometimes necessary. Intracapsular extraction with no retinal laser treatment promotes iris neovascularization. Extracapsular/phaco techniques do not seem to do this, particularly if the retina is fully treated with laser. It is usually helpful to delay putting in the lens implant until all the posterior segment surgery has been completed. A corneal wound can leak during vitrectomy, resulting in a flat anterior chamber, and the view of the far retinal periphery may be compromised by the edge of the lens.

Perfluorocarbon liquids, introduced to vitreoretinal surgery a decade ago by Stanley Chang, have a limited role in diabetic surgery. The liquid will flatten erstwhile detached retina and allow laser treatment to be applied. It can also show up and stabilize areas of residual vitreoretinal adhesion during the operation, but its low surface tension means it can flow through breaks in the retina.

Silicone oil is a very useful adjunct to surgery. It holds the upper half of the retina in place, tamponades superior breaks and prevents postoperative ooze from retinal vessels from filling the vitreous cavity. There are also problems associated with its use, however. It induces about +6 dioptres of hypermetropia, it is very likely to cause a cataract, it can cause secondary glaucoma and it needs to be removed as another operative procedure.

Very occasionally subhyaloid blood or focal vitreoretinal traction can be treated with the Nd:YAG laser, without the need for vitrectomy. The laser can create a hole in the posterior hyaloid to allow blood into the vitreous body, whence its absorption can occur more quickly.[23] Laser can also cut isolated vitreous adhesion bands.

PROGNOSIS

The result of surgery depend largely on preoperative and operative findings. Indeed, the presence of such severe eye disease reduces the long-term survival of the patient.[24] Eyes with vitreous haemorrhage and no retinal detachment do especially well–over 80% have improved vision with a stable anatomical result. Significantly better results are obtained where the preoperative visual acuity is 6/240 or better and no iris neovascularization or neovascular glaucoma are present. Eyes also do well if at least a quarter of the retina had been treated with laser before the haemorrhage occurred, and where a clear lens is retained at surgery.[25]

Traction retinal detachment with macular involvement will have anatomical improvement in 65–80% and some visual improvement in 26–70% of cases, influenced by the duration of macular traction, the extent of capillary non-perfusion at the posterior pole, and whether vitreous haemorrhage coexists.

Combined traction and rhegmatogenous detachments do less well. Overall visual acuity improves in about a half of operated eyes, with around 60% having an acuity of 6/240 or better.

COMPLICATIONS AND THEIR MANAGEMENT

Postoperative complications include persistent or re-bleeding, retinal detachment, endopthalmitis, cataract and glaucoma.

Persistent or re-bleeding

In the immediate postoperative period, there is often a little blood in the vitreous cavity. This should clear within the first week or two. Persistent haemorrhage or re-bleeding can occur in up to one-third of eyes that had haemorrhage to start with. Clearance of blood is assisted when there is a channel from the posterior segment to the anterior chamber. This can be achieved by stripping anterior hyaloid from the back surface of the lens. It is not usually possible to strip more than one quadrant, but this is sufficient. Seeing red blood cells in the anterior chamber postoperatively is a good not a bad sign–the blood should clear quite quickly.

Re-bleeding may come from a vessel on the surface of the retina that has either not been cauterized adequately or has persistent traction on it. Less commonly, haemorrhage may come from fibrovascular proliferation in the vitreous base.[26] Occasionally, fibrin may be more prominent than blood. Injection of tissue plasminogen activator has been tried in this situation with limited success.[27]

It is wise to wait 2 or 3 months for blood to clear. Regular checks during the time of waiting should include intraocular pressure measurement, biomicroscopy of the anterior chamber to ensure no iris proliferation is developing, and ultrasound examination of the posterior segment to ensure that the retina remains attached. If the pressure goes up (glaucoma secondary to red cells in the anterior chamber), the iris becomes vascularized or the retina detaches, then further vitrectomy is needed.

Once the cause of the problem is identified it can be treated.

Vitreous base proliferation is difficult to treat. The aim of surgery is to shave as much vitreous off the vitreous base as possible, then treat the base with laser photocoagulation. This often requires removal of the lens. Sometimes, with recurring bleeding from this source, silicone oil is the only way to get control.

Retinal detachment

A hole in the retina is likely to lead to retinal detachment if there is persistent traction on it from residual membranes or retinal shortening. Such breaks may predate the surgery, but more commonly result from manipulation of the retina. They are usually posterior and not amenable to external tamponade. The only treatment is reoperation using an internal approach. The aim is to relieve traction, apply laser or cryopexy and provide an internal tamponade. Gas works best when the traction is relieved completely, whilst silicone oil may be needed otherwise.

Endophthalmitis

Although diabetes is a risk factor for infections generally, endophthalmitis is fortunately rare. When it occurs, the management is not different from other cases of post-vitrectomy endophthalmitis. It is easy to obtain a good vitreous fluid sample without needing to use a vitrector, and identification of the infecting organism is vital. Similarly, injection of intracameral antibiotics is an easy matter. The diabetes must be well controlled during this period.

Cataract

Cataract is unfortunately very common after all vitrectomy procedures, including those in diabetics. Patient need to be warned about cataract before their original surgery. Some factors need to be remembered before cataract surgery. The iris might not dilate well if early neovascularization is present. Pigment tends to be less well attached than normal to the iris and may come loose in quantities during surgery. The lack of the vitreous can cause alarming excursions of the lens during the phaco procedure. Aim for a clean capsulorrhexis and full mobilization of the cortex and nucleus before starting the phaco. Be prepared for the lens/iris diaphragm to drop right back when the fluid infusion starts–relax, the lens is unlikely to disappear completely![28] Aggressive neovascularization can complicate cataract surgery with new vessels growing on the lens capsule.[29]

Glaucoma

There are four mechanisms at least for post-vitrectomy glaucoma–steroid response, red cells obstructing the drainage angle, ghost cell obstruction and neovascularization. It is important to distinguish between these to manage the patient correctly.

Pressure rise from steroids is no more common in diabetics than others, but it is easy to overlook this mechanism. The treatment is withdrawal of steroids–they are not needed for long after vitrectomy anyway, as there is little manipulation of extraocular tissues.

In cases where a lot of blood remains in the posterior segment, or re-bleeding has occurred, the anterior chamber can become overloaded with red cells. Simply washing the anterior chamber out (two 25 gauge needles are inserted through the cornea near the limbus, one connected to a balanced salt solution reservoir and one open to the air) will often sort out the problem. If the glaucoma recurs then the posterior segment will need washing out too.

Ghost cells are the result of long-standing vitreous haemorrhage. Red cells eventually lose their haemoglobin and become spherical and rigid. These cells have a great potential for blocking the drainage angle, as they have difficulty getting out of the eye. Treatment is as for red cells–a quick washout of the anterior chamber drops the pressure rapidly and works far better than any medical treatment.

Iris and drainage angle neovascularization presents the most difficult glaucoma to manage. Full panretinal laser photocoagulation minimizes the chance of it occurring. In the early stages in a phakic or pseudophakic eye, there is some evidence that filling the posterior segment with silicone oil can cause regression.[30] Once it is established, however, then a combination of medical treatment, trabeculetomy with cytostatics, or tube drainage procedures will be needed. The visual prognosis is poor.

CONCLUSION

There are a number of 'take home messages' that appear in this chapter:

- Vitreoretinal surgery done for the right reason can save sight, done for the wrong reason it can cause blindness–preoperative evaluation of the eye is essential.
- Thorough laser panretinal photocoagulation can avoid the need for retinal surgery in many cases and will make surgery easier if it becomes necessary.
- The more the vitreous has separated from the retina before surgery, the easier the operation becomes.
- The full range of current vitreoretinal techniques can be applied to diabetic eyes–the surgeon needs to have mastered all of them.
- Complications from surgery are not uncommon, and the surgeon needs to be looking for them to treat them early.

REFERENCES

1. Algvere P, Franzen G, Wiklund P, Visual and social benefits of vitreous surgery in diabetics. A long-term follow-up evaluation, *Acta Ophthalmol (Copenh)* (1987) **65**:363–8.
2. Blankenship GW, Diabetic retinopathy, present and future. Conclusion of diabetic retinopathy symposium. *Ophthalmology* (1981) **88**:658–61.
3. Lincoff H, Serag Y, Chang S et al, Tractional elevations of the retina in patients with diabetes, *Am J Ophthalmol* (1992) **113**:235–42.
4. Wong HC, Sehmi KS, McLeod D, Abortive neovascular outgrowths discovered during vitrectomy for diabetic vitreous haemorrhage, *Graefes Arch Clin Exp Ophthalmol* (1989) **227**:237–40.
5. Michels RG, Rice TA, Rice EF, Vitrectomy for diabetic vitreous hemorrhage, *Am J Ophthalmol* (1983) **95**:12–21.
6. Diabetic Retinopathy Vitrectomy Study Research Group, Early vitrectomy for severe vitreous hemorrhage in diabetic retinopathy. Two-year results of a randomized trial. DRVS Report no. 2, *Arch Ophthalmol* (1985) **103**:1644–52.
7. Diabetic Retinopathy Vitrectomy Study Research Group, Early vitrectomy for severe proliferative diabetic retinopathy in eyes with useful vision. Results of a randomized trial. DRVS Report no. 3, *Ophthalmology* (1988) **95**:1307–20.
8. Diabetic Retinopathy Vitrectomy Study Research Group, Early vitrectomy for severe vitreous hemorrhage in diabetic retinopathy. Four-year results of a randomized trial. DRVS Report no. 5, *Arch Ophthalmol* (1990) **108**:958–64.
9. Favard C, Guyot-Argenton C, Assouline M et al, Full panretinal photocoagulation and early vitrectomy improve prognosis of florid diabetic retinopathy, *Ophthalmology* (1996) **103**:561–74.
10. Shea M, Young PW, Howcroft MJ, 'Early' vitrectomy for vasoproliferative retinopathy in patients with insulin-dependent diabetes mellitus, *Can J Ophthalmol* (1982) **17**:150–2.
11. Tachi N, Ogino N, Vitrectomy for diffuse macular edema in cases of diabetic retinopathy, *Am J Ophthalmol* (1996) **122**:258–60.

12. Algvere P, Persson HE, Wanger P, Preoperative electroretinograms and visual evoked cortical potentials for predicting outcome of vitrectomy in diabetics, *Retina* (1985) 5:179–83.
13. Gribomont AC, Guerit JM, Prognostic value of preoperative flash and pattern visual evoked potentials for diabetic retinopathy vitrectomy, *Eur J Ophthalmol* (1994) 4:218–22.
14. Raucoules-Aime M, Roussel LJ, Rossi D et al, Effect of severity of surgery on metabolic control and insulin requirements in insulin-dependent diabetic patients, *Br J Anaesth* (1995) 74:231–3.
15. Oikkonen M, Diabetic autonimic neuropathy and the haemodynamic actions of vecuronium and pancuronium during vitrectomy, *Acta Anaesthsial Scand* (1995) 39:352–5.
16. Friend J, Thoft RA, The diabetic cornea, PMID: 6500867, UI: 85053821, *Int ophthalmol Clin* (1984) 24:111–23.
17. Chung H, Tolentino FI, Cajita VN et al, Re-evaluation of corneal complications after closed vitrectomy, *Arch Ophthalmol* (1988) 106:916–19.
18. Haimann MH, Abrams GW, Prevention of lens opacification during diabetic vitrectomy, *Ophthalmology* (1984) 91:116–21.
19. Blankenship GW, Posterior chamber intraocular lens implantation during pars plana lensectomy and vitrectomy for diabetic complications, *Graefes Arch Clin Exp Ophthalmol* (1989) 227:136–8.
20. Chaudhry NA, Lim ES, Saito Y et al, Early vitrectomy and endolaser photocoagulation in patients with type I diabetes with severe vitreous hemorrhage, *Ophthalmology* (1995) 102:1164–9.
21. McLeod D, Microsurgical management of neovascularization secondary to posterior segment ischaemia, *Eye* (1991) 5:252–9.
22. Treatment of retinal detachment by vitrectomy and injection of silicone oil. Long-term results and complications in 105 cases, *J Fr Ophthalmol* (1984) 7:11–18.
23. Raymond LA, Neodymium:YAG laser treatment for hemorrhages under the internal limiting membrane and posterior hyaloid face in the macula, *Ophthalmology* (1995) 102:406–11.
24. Gollamudi SR, Smiddy WE, Schachat AP et al, Long-term survival rate after vitrectomy surgery for complications of diabetic retinopathy, *Ophthalmology* (1991) 98:18–22.
25. Summanen P, Significance of various systemic and ocular parameters in the long-term prognosis after diabetic vitrectomy, *Int Ophthalmol* (1989) 13:311–19.
26. Lewis H, Abrams GW, Foos RY, Clinicopathologic findings in anterior hyaloid fibrovascular proliferation after diabetic vitrectomy, *Am J Ophthalmol* (1987) 104:614–18.
27. Dabbs CK, Aaberg TM, Aguilar HE et al, Complications of tissue plasminogen activator therapy after vitrectomy for diabetes, *Am J Ophthalmol* (1990) 110:354–60.
28. McDermott ML, Puklin JE, Abrams GW, Eliott D, Phacoemulsification for cataract following pars plana vitrectomy, *Ophthalmic Surg Lasers* (1997) 28:558–64.
29. Eifrig DE, Hermsen V, McManus P, Cunningham R, Rubeosis capsulare, *J Cataract Refract Surg* (1990) 16:633–6.
30. Azzolini C, Brancato R, Camesasca FI, Codenotti M, Influence of silicone oil on iris microangiography in diabetic vitrectomized eyes, *Ophthalmology* (1993) 100:1152–8.

9 Cataract surgery in diabetes

Jonathan Dowler and AM Peter Hamilton

INTRODUCTION

Diabetes is the commonest risk factor for cataract in Western countries, with a three- to fourfold excess prevalence in diabetic patients under 65, and up to twofold in older patients.[1] Cataract is also an important cause of visual loss in patients with diabetes, in some populations the principal cause of blindness in older-onset diabetics, and the second commonest cause in younger-onset diabetics.[2] The incidence of cataract surgery reflects this; estimates of the 10-year cumulative incidence of cataract surgery exceed 27% in younger-onset diabetics (≥ 45 years of age), and 44% in older-onset diabetics (≥ 75 years of age).[3]

The visual outcome of such surgery, however, depends on the severity of retinopathy and may be poor.[4] Cataract may prevent the recognition or treatment of sight-threatening retinopathy before surgery, and after surgery vision may be impaired by severe fibrinous uveitus,[5] capsular opacification,[6] anterior segment neovascularization,[7] macular oedema[8] and deterioration of retinopathy.[9] Appropriate management of cataract in the diabetic therefore represents a process incorporating meticulous pre- and postoperative monitoring and treatment of retinopathy, carefully timed and executed surgery and measures to preserve postoperative fundus view. Close co-operation between retinal specialist, diabetologist and cataract surgeon is essential.

PREOPERATIVE MANAGEMENT

Cataract surgery in eyes with sight-threatening diabetic retinopathy is associated with poor post-operative visual acuity,[4] and it is imperative that laser therapy for clinically significant macular oedema or high-risk proliferative retinopathy be applied before surgery. Even minor cataract may, however, impede clinical recognition of retinal thickening or neovascularization, and degrade angiographic images. Furthermore, even if sight-threatening retinopathy can be diagnosed, lens opacity may obstruct laser therapy. If so, it may be necessary to use a longer wavelength, for example, dye yellow (577 nm), or doide infrared (810 nm), better suited to penetrating nuclear cataract than argon green (514 nm). Panretinal photocoagulation may also be easier to apply with the indirect ophthalmoscope or trans-scleral diode probe. In eyes with proliferative retinopathy and cataract sufficiently dense to prevent any preoperative laser, if ultrasound reveals vitreous haemorrhage or traction macular detachment, a combination of cataract extraction, vitrectomy and endo-laser may be required. By contrast, if ultrasound reveals no indication for vitrectomy, it may be necessary to apply indirect laser panretinal photocoagulation during cataract surgery,[10] since this may reduce the incidence and severity of surgical complications. We, however, contend that surgery should where possible be undertaken

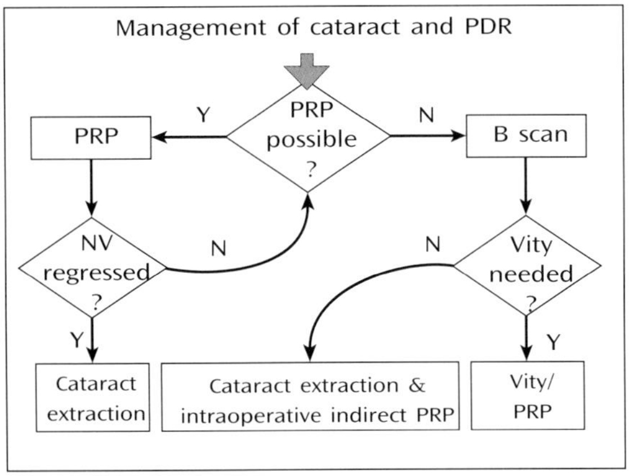

Figure 9.1
Algorithm for the management of proliferative diabetic retinopathy in the presence of cataract. PRP, panretinal photocoagulation; B-scan, B-scan ultrasound; NV, new vessels; Vity, vitrectomy.

before cataract precludes diagnosis and treatment of retinopathy (*Fig. 9.1*).

SURGERY: INDICATIONS AND TIMING

Symptomatic visual loss or disturbance is the major indication for cataract surgery in the non-diabetic. In diabetics, however, the need to maintain surveillance of retinopathy, and where necessary to carry out laser treatment, represents an additional indication. The high morbidity and poor postoperative visual acuity described in association with cataract surgery in diabetics have led some authors to recommend that surgery should be deferred until visual acuity has deteriorated to at least 6/30,[8] or not be undertaken at all.[11] At these levels of visual acuity, however, cataract is likely to be so dense as to preclude recognition or treatment of sight-threatening retinopathy prior to surgery, and the outcome of surgery may therefore be poor. By contrast, if surgery is undertaken before the cataract reaches the point where diagnosis and treatment of retinopathy are significantly impeded, it may be possible to maintain uninterrupted control of retinopathy, and the outcome of surgery may thereby be improved. We believe cataract surgery should be performed early in the diabetic.

SURGICAL TECHNIQUE AND INTRAOCULAR LENS SELECTION

Posterior segment complications frequently determine visual acuity after cataract extraction in diabetes, and thus surgical technique and the choice of intraocular lens is governed by the need to maintain postoperative fundus visualization. Rigid, large optic diameter polymethylmethacrylate (PMMA) lenses permit peripheral retinal visualization which may be valuable if panretinal photocoagulation or vitreoretinal surgery is required. They also allow wide posterior capsulotomy early in the postoperative course, important in eyes with more severe retinopathy, in which the risk of retinopathy progression[5] and capsular opacification is greatest.[6] They tend, however, to accumulate surface deposits,[12] and require a large incision, which may delay refractive stabilization and exacerbate postoperative inflammation. Foldable silicone lenses can be implanted through a small incision, but plate haptic designs may not be sufficiently stable to permit early capsulotomy, and the incidence of anterior capsular aperture contracture appears high.[13] All silicone lenses have the disadvantage that if vitrectomy surgery is required, fundus visualization may be compromised by droplet adherence, temporarily during fluid–gas exchange,[14] or more permanently by silicone oil.[15] Acrylic lenses, which may also be implanted through a small incision, appear stable,

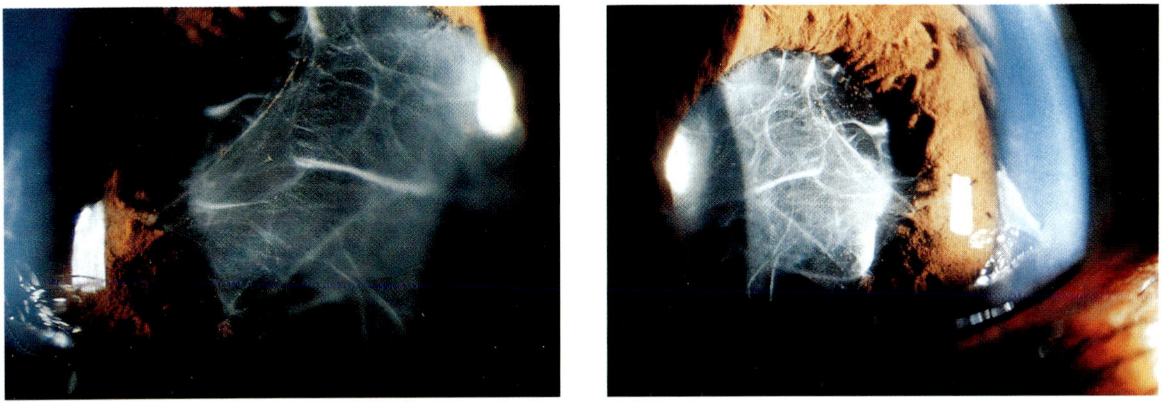

(a) (b)

Figure 9.2
Fibrin reaction following cataract surgery in a patient with proliferative retinopathy: (a) fibrin clot in anterior chamber; (b) iris bombe through pseudophakic pupil block.

show less adherence of silicone oil,[16] have a reduced incidence of stenosis of the anterior capsular aperture,[13] and may be associated with a reduced incidence of capsular opacification, although limited data are available regarding their use in diabetics.

Extracapsular cataract surgery using can-opener capsulotomy eliminates the risk of anterior capsular aperture stenosis but the tissue damage associated with a large incision and nucleus expression may further exacerbate the tendency in diabetic eyes to severe postoperative inflammation. A randomized paired eye comparison of phacoemulsification with foldable silicone lens vs extracapsular surgery with 7-mm PMMA lens in 46 diabetic patients[17] identified a higher incidence of early postoperative inflammation in eyes undergoing extracapsular surgery, and a higher incidence of capsular opacification. No significant difference was identified between eyes undergoing phacoemulsification and those undergoing extracapsular surgery in respect of incidence of clinically significant macular edema (CSME), requirement for macular laser therapy, severity or progression of retinopathy, requirement for panretinal photocoagulation or proportion of patients achieving 6/12 at 1 year.

POSTOPERATIVE MANAGEMENT

Anterior segment complications

Diabetic eyes appear especially susceptible to severe fibrinous uveitis after cataract surgery.[18] Iris vascular permeability is increased in proportion to retinopathy severity in diabetics, and cataract surgery may permit larger proteins such as fibrinogen to enter the anterior chamber. Fibrin membranes may form on the intraocular lens, anterior hyaloid face, posterior capsule or across the pupil, giving rise to pseudophakic pupil block glaucoma (*Fig. 9.2*). Capsular opacification is commoner in diabetics, its incidence appearing to correlate with the severity of retinopathy (*Fig. 9.3*).[6] Neovascularization derived from the anterior segment may encroach

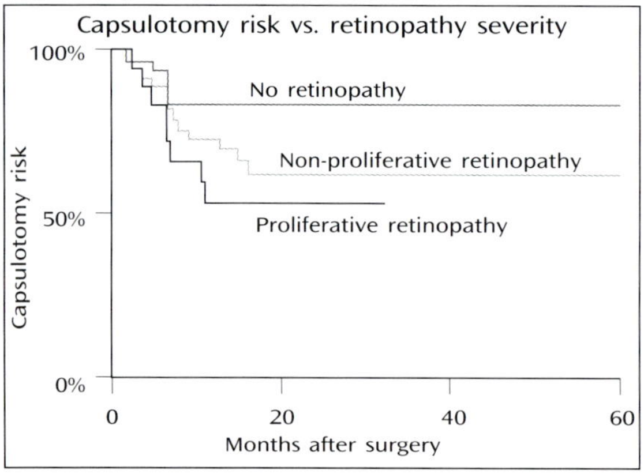

Figure 9.3
Relationship between severity of retinopathy and risk of capsulotomy.[6]

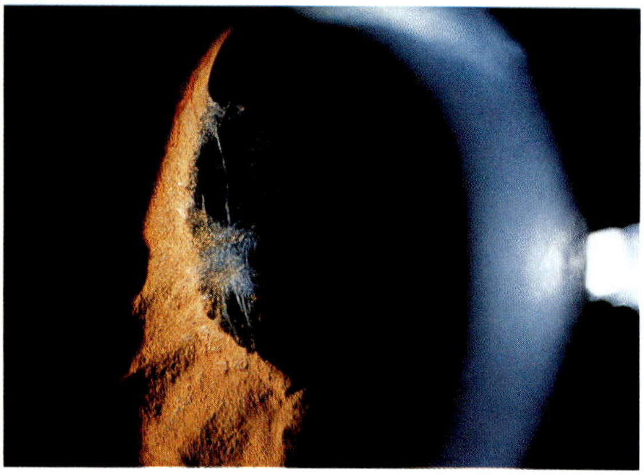

Figure 9.4
Rubeosis iridis following cataract surgery; note vessel running down iris at edge of illuminated area.

over the iris–rubeosis iridis (*Fig. 9.4*), the anterior surface of the posterior lens capsule–rubeosis capsulare,[19] or more rarely, new vessels derived from the posterior segment may arborize over the posterior surface of the posterior lens capsule–anterior hyaloidal fibrovascular proliferation (*Fig. 9.5*).[7] These complications may result from the action of soluble retina-derived factors, such as vasoactive endothelial growth factor (VEGF), which leave the eye

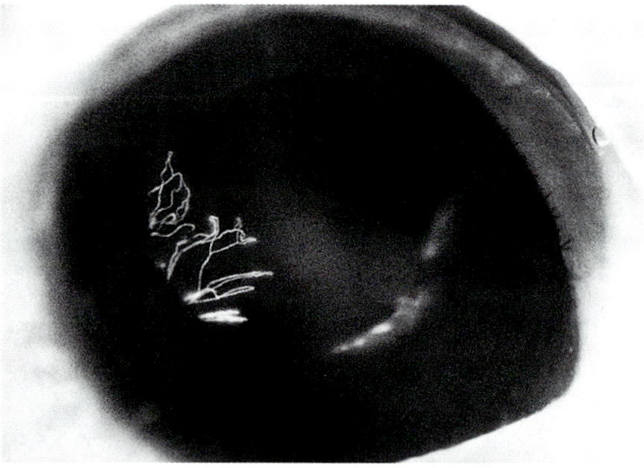

(a)

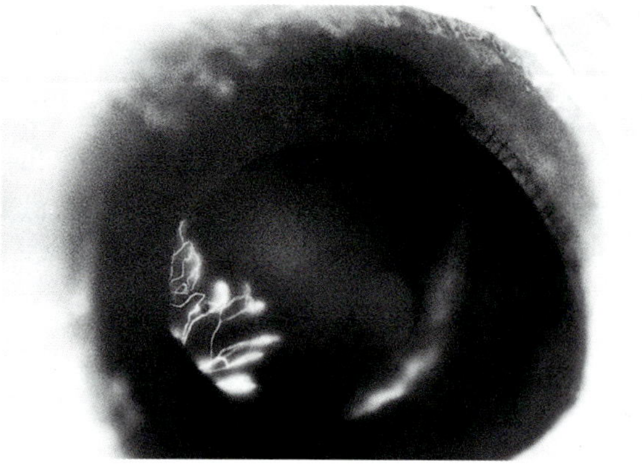

(b)

Figure 9.5
Anterior segment fluorescein angiogram of anterior hyaloidal fibrovascular proliferation, the aborization of vessels from anterior retina over the anterior hyaloid face: (a) early phase showing dye filling the vessels; (b) later phase showing dye leakage from vessels.

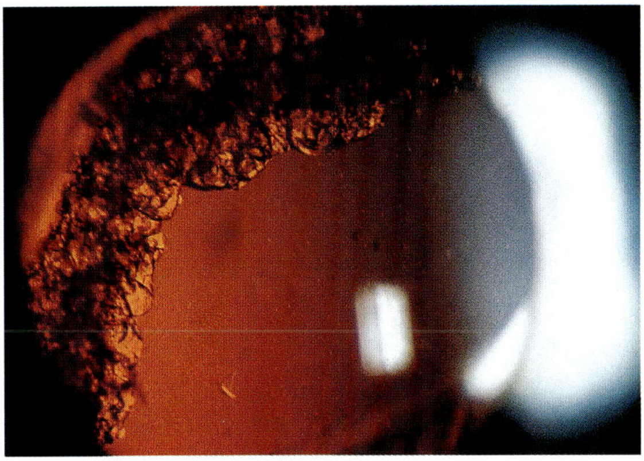

Figure 9.6
Massive proliferation of lens epithelial cells following capsulotomy in an eye with proliferative diabetic retinopathy.

through the trabecular meshwork but en route may stimulate neovascularization, cellular proliferation of the posterior capsule and increased iris vascular permeability. Postoperative uveitis may require intensive therapy with topical or periocular steroid, non-steroid anti-inflammatory agents, atropine, and tissue plasminogen activator if fibrin is prominent. Capsular opacification requires examination with retroillumination to exclude anterior hyaloidal fibrovascular proliferation, and as early and wide capsulotomy as is consistent with intraocular lens stability, since marginal cellular proliferation (*Fig. 9.6*) may subsequently compromise fundus visualization. Neovascular complications necessitate urgent panretinal photocoagulation, since both anterior and posterior segment neovascularization may progress extremely rapidly and secondary neovascular glaucoma is commonly refractory to treatment. If anterior hyaloidal fibrovascular proliferation is present, associated capsular opacification may preclude panretinal photocoagulation, and capsulotomy in this context may precipitate haemorrhage. Direct closure of anterior hyaloidal vessels with argon laser may permit safe capsulotomy and panretinal photocoagulation.

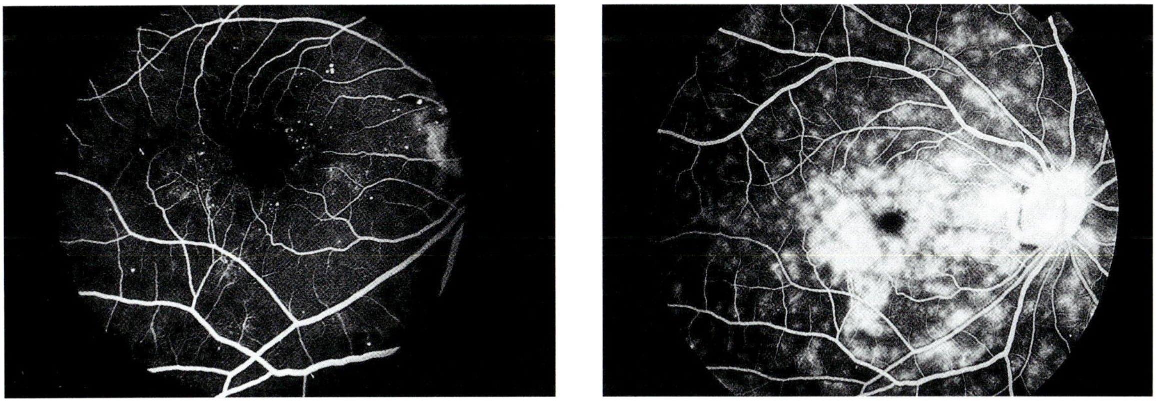

(a) (b)

Figure 9.7
Macular oedema following cataract surgery in diabetes. (a) Intraoperative fluorescein angiogram–minimal macular hyperfluorescence. (b) Angiogram 3 months after surgery–profuse macular and optic disc hyperfluorescence.

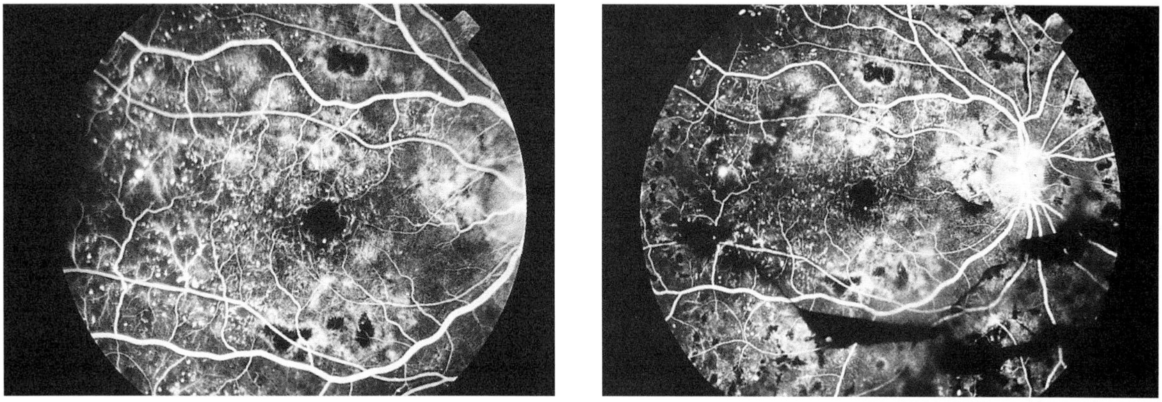

(a) (b)

Figure 9.8
Progression of diabetic retinopathy following cataract surgery. (a) Early postoperative fluorescein angiogram. (b) Angiogram 6 months after surgery demonstrating multiple flat-topped retrohyaloid haemorrhages indicating progression to high-risk proliferative retinopathy.

Posterior segment complications

Macular oedema is a common cause of poor visual acuity after cataract surgery in diabetes (*Fig. 9.7*).[8] It may represent diabetic macular oedema present at the time of surgery but unrecognized or untreated because of the presence of cataract, diabetic macular oedema precipitated or exacerbated by cataract surgery, or the typically self-limiting Irvine–Gass type macular oedema which occurs in a high proportion of both diabetics and non-diabetics after cataract surgery. This presents a therapeutic conundrum, since laser therapy appropriate to diabetic macular oedema present at the time of surgery or developing afterwards is inappropriate to Irvine–Gass macular oedema, where spontaneous resolution may be anticipated. In recent studies,[20] no patient with clinically significant macular oedema in the immediate postoperative period showed spontaneous resolution of oedema over the subsequent year, and thus it would seem reasonable to consider treatment in such patients. By contrast clinically significant macular oedema, which developed de novo at some point after surgery in half the patients studied, resolved within 6 months of surgery in half, and by 1 year in three-quarters of these. Spontaneous resolution was commoner in eyes with less severe retinopathy at the time of surgery, and in eyes showing angiographic improvement by 6 months. In such eyes a conservative approach seems justified.

Progression of retinopathy after cataract surgery (*Fig. 9.8*) is best documented by paired eye comparisons; one such study showed progression of non-proliferative retinopathy in 74% of operated and 37% of unoperated fellow eyes.[9] Deterioration appears particularly common in eyes with severe non-proliferative or proliferative retinopathy at the time of surgery, and preoperative or intraoperative panretinal photocoagulation may be considered. If high-risk proliferative retinopathy develops after surgery, panretinal photocoagulation should be applied as soon as possible, since progression of

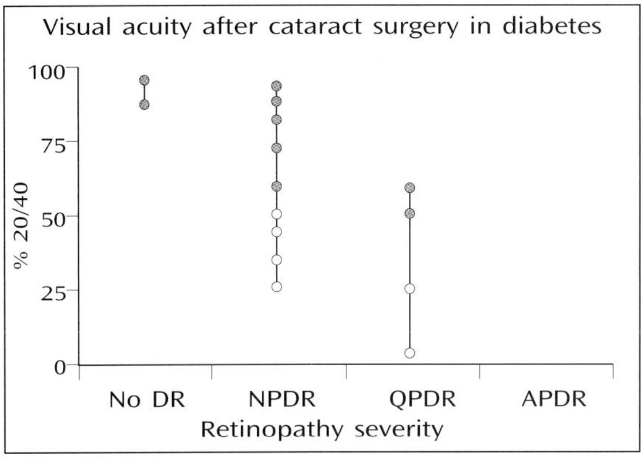

(a)

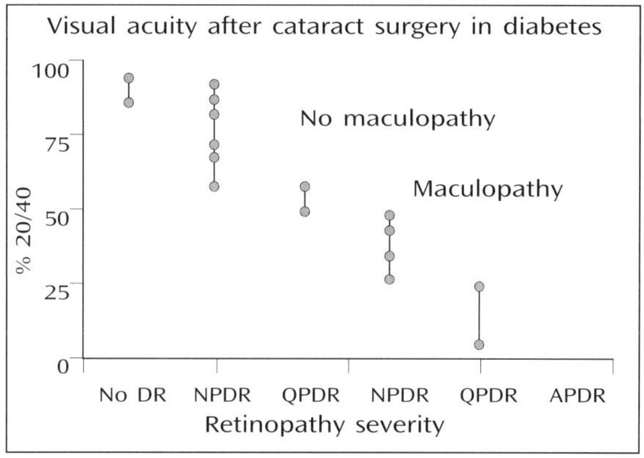

(b)

Figure 9.9
Meta-analysis of visual acuity following cataract surgery in diabetes: (a) proportion of patients in different retinopathy subgroups achieving postoperative visual acuity ≥6/12 (b) effect of presence or absence of maculopathy. No DR = No diabetic retinopathy, NPDR = Non-proliferative diabetic retinopathy, QPDR = Quiescent proliferative diabetic retinopathy, APDR = active proliferative diabetic retinopathy.

retinopathy may be rapid. This may, however, prove difficult because of photophobia, therapeutic contact lens intolerance, poor mydriasis, intraocular lens deposits and edge effects, capsulorrhexis stenosis or capsular opacification. If high-risk proliferative retinopathy and clinically significant macular oedema develop after surgery it seems appropriate to apply both macular and panretinal laser, since the latter carries the risk of exacerbating macular oedema. Close postoperative surveillance of the retina is essential in all patients with diabetic retinopathy undergoing cataract surgery, and close co-operation between retinal specialist and cataract surgeon should be encouraged to optimize management of macular oedema and visual outcome.

POSTOPERATIVE VISUAL ACUITY

A meta-analysis carried out in 1995 demonstrated an inverse relationship between the severity of diabetic retinopathy at the time of extracapsular cataract surgery, and postoperative visual acuity, and an association between poor visual outcome and the presence of maculopathy (*Fig. 9.9*).[4] In this study between 0 and 80% of eyes with diabetic retinopathy achieved a postoperative visual acuity ≥ 20/40.[4] More recent studies,[17,21,22] however, have demonstrated > 80% patients achieving a postoperative visual acuity ≥ 6/12. A number of possible factors may account for this improvement, including earlier intervention since the advent of phacoemulsification, recognition of the importance of glycaemic control and careful preoperative and postoperative management of retinopathy.

THE FUTURE

Much information about cataract surgery in diabetes has yet to be gathered. The optimal timing of surgery, the ideal surgical technique, the most appropriate intraocular lens, the role of glycaemic and blood pressure control in postoperative deterioration of retinopathy and the optimal management of postoperative macular oedema remain uncertain. Significant research effort is currently being devoted to the elucidation of these problems. These efforts must, however, be accompanied by more widespread recognition of the need to offer diabetics undergoing cataract surgery the pre- and postoperative care appropriate to their condition, rather than that afforded to the bulk of patients with age-related cataract, whose need is much less. Only through an appreciation of the unique problems of cataract surgery in diabetes can good results be obtained.

REFERENCES

1. Ederer F, Hiller R, Taylor HR, Senile lens changes and diabetes in two population studies, *Am J Ophthalmol* (1981) **91**:381–95.
2. Klein R, Klein BE, Moss SE, Visual impairment in diabetes, *Ophthalmology* (1984) **91**:1–9.
3. Klein BE, Klein R, Moss SE, Incidence of cataract surgery in the Wisconsin Epidemiologic Study of Diabetic Retinopathy, *Am J Ophthalmol* (1995) **119**:295–300.
4. Dowler JG, Hykin PG, Lightman SL, Hamilton AM, Visual acuity following extracapsular cataract extraction in diabetes: a meta-analysis, *Eye* (1995) **9**:313–17.
5. Hykin PG, Gregson RM, Hamilton AM, Extracapsular cataract extraction in diabetics with rubeosis iridis, *Eye* (1992) **6**:296–9.
6. Ionides A, Dowler JG, Hykin PG et al, Posterior capsule opacification following diabetic extracapsular cataract extraction, *Eye* (1994) **8**:535–7.
7. Ulbig MR, Hykin PG, Foss AJ et al, Anterior hyaloidal fibrovascular proliferation after extracapsular cataract extraction in diabetic eyes, *Am J Ophthalmol* (1993) **115**:321–6.
8. Pollack A, Leibe H, Bukelman A, Oliver M, Cystoid macular oedema following cataract extraction in patients with diabetes, *Br J Ophthalmol* (1992) **76**:221–4.
9. Jaffe GJ, Burton TC, Progression of nonproliferative diabetic retinopathy following cataract extraction, *Arch Ophthalmol* (1998) **106**:745–9.
10. Dowler JG, Hykin PG, Hamilton AM, The management of proliferative diabetic retinopathy in the presence of cataract, *Asia Pacific J Ophthalmol* (1995) **7**:2–4.
11. Schatz H, Atienza D, McDonald HR, Johnson RN, Severe diabetic retinopathy after cataract surgery, *Am J Ophthalmol* (1994) **117**:314–21.
12. Borgioli AM, Coster DJ, Fan RFT, Henderson J, Effect of heparin surface modification of polymethylmethacrylate intraocular lenses on signs of postoperative inflammation after extracapsular cataract extraction, *Ophthalmology* (1992) **99**: 1248–55.
13. Hayashi K, Hayashi H, Nakao F, Hayashi F, Reduction in the area of the anterior capsule opening after polymethylmethacrylate, silicone, and soft acrylic intraocular lens implantation, *Am J Ophthalmol* (1997) **123**:441–7.
14. Francese JE, Christ FR, Buchen SY et al, Moisture droplet formation on the posterior surface of intraocular lenses during fluid/air exchange, *J Cataract Refract Surg* (1995) **21**:685–9.
15. Apple DJ, Federman JL, Krolicki TJ et al, Irreversible silicone oil adhesion to silicone intraocular lenses. A clinicopathologic analysis, *Ophthalmology* (1996) **103**:1555–61.
16. Apple DJ, Isaacs RT, Kent DG et al, Silicone oil adhesion to intraocular lenses: an experimental study comparing various biomaterials, *J Cataract Refract Surg* (1997) **23**:536–44.
17. Dowler JG, Hykin PG, Hamilton AM, Phakoemulsification versus extracapsular cataract surgery in diabetes, *Ophthalmology* (1998) Submitted:
18. Hykin PG, Gregson RM, Stevens JD, Hamilton PA, Extracapsular cataract extraction in proliferative diabetic retinopathy, *Ophthalmology* (1993) **100**:394–9.

19. Eifrig DE, Hermsen V, McManus P, Cunningham R, Rubeosis capsulare, *J Cataract Refract Surg* (1990) **16**:633–6.
20. Dowler JG, Sehmi KS, Hykin PG, Hamilton AM, The natural history of macular oedema after cataract surgery in diabetes, *Ophthalmology* (1998) In press.
21. Henricsson M, Heijl A, Janzon L, Diabetic retinopathy before and after cataract surgery, *Br J Ophthalmol* (1996) **80**:789–93.
22. Wagner T, Knaflic D, Rauber M, Mester U, Influence of cataract surgery on the diabetic eye: a prospective study, *Ger J Ophthalmol* (1996) **5**:79–83.

10 Special investigations in diabetic retinopathy

Jean-Jacques De Laey and Bruno Vincke

Our understanding of the pathological mechanisms involved in diabetic retinopathy has greatly improved since the introduction of fluorescein angiography. This has led to better treatment strategies. However, a number of more recent techniques such as optical coherence tomography and infrared angiography or psychophysiological tests such as colour vision, contrast sensitivity and electrophysiology, may enhance our analysis of the pathological phenomena which are associated with diabetic retinopathy. Some of these tests may also have predictive value for the future progression of retinopathy. In this chapter the value of these various tests in the diagnosis and follow-up of diabetic retinopathy will be discussed.

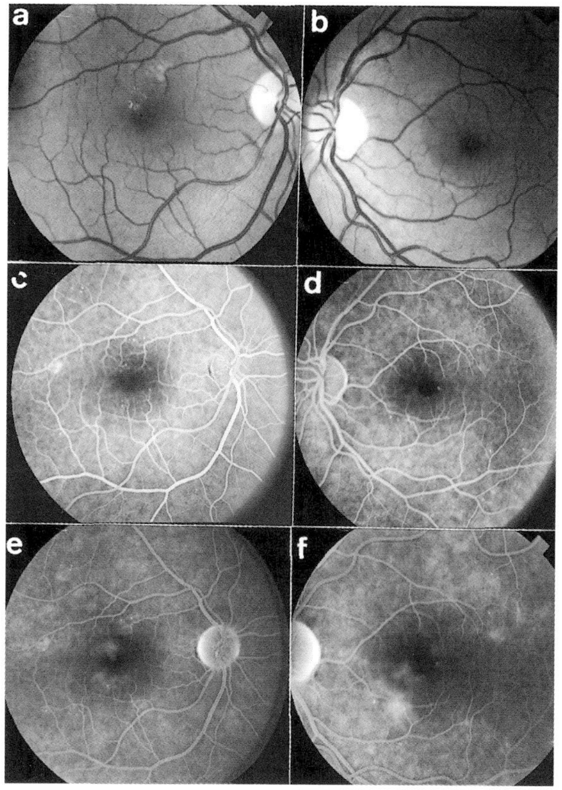

Figure 10.1
Red-free photographs (a), (b) and fluorescein angiographies (c)–(f) of a 44-year-old diabetic man. A few lipoid exudates and microaneurysms are seen on the red-free photographs, especially in the right eye. Fluorescein angiography does not show obvious capillary closure. The late staining is more marked than could be expected from the numbers of microaneurysms, suggesting a possible disruption of the outer blood–retinal barrier.

MORPHOLOGICAL ANALYSIS OF DIABETIC RETINOPATHY

Fluorescein angiography

Fluorescein angiography has shown a greater sensitivity in assessing diabetic microangiopathy than either ophthalmoscopy or fundus photography.

*Microaneurysms (*Figs 10.1 *and* 10.2*)*

The microaneurysm is supposedly the first ophthalmoscopic sign of diabetic retinopathy. Microaneurysms commonly cluster around focal areas of capillary non-perfusion (*Fig. 10.3*). This suggests that microaneurysms could be the

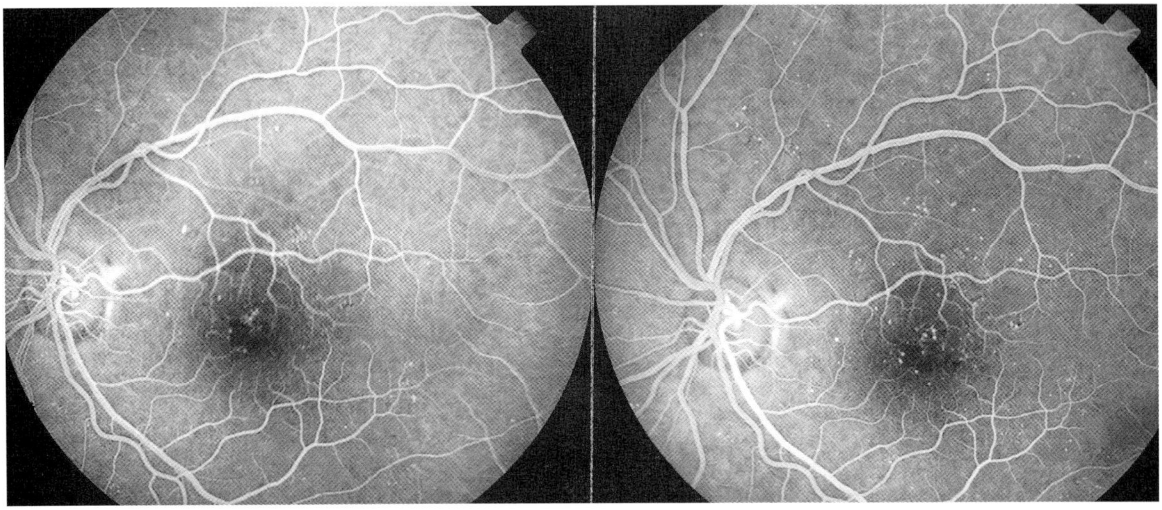

(a) (b)

Figure 10.2
(a), (b) Fluorescein angiographies of the left eye of a 59-year-old adult-onset diabetic woman. The two pictures were taken with a 9-month interval. Increasing numbers of microaneurysms are found on follow-up as well as an increase in size of the foveal avascular zone.

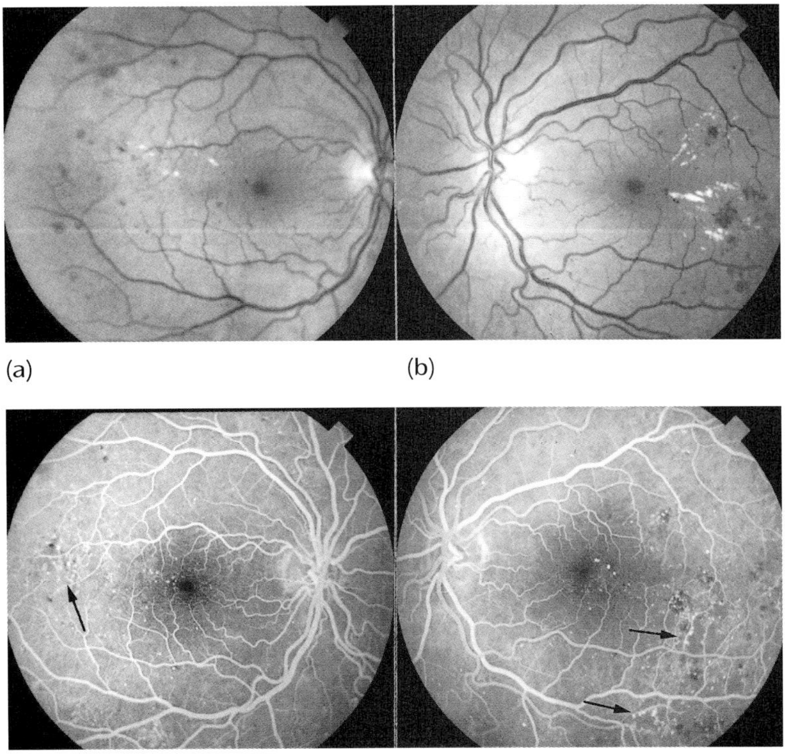

(a) (b) (c) (d)

Figure 10.3
Red-free photographs (a), (b) and fluorescein angiographies (c), (d) of 29-year-old insulin-dependent diabetes mellitus patient. Numerous microaneurysms, especially around areas of capillary non-perfusion, temporal to both maculas (arrows).

consequence of capillary closure. Microaneurysms can also be detected without visible non-perfusion. In a study for the first signs of retinopathy in 161 diabetic children the following features were found in decreasing order of frequency: microaneurysms, focal capillary dilatation, generalized capillary dilatation, leakage, retinal haemorrhages, areas of capillary non-perfusion and capillary remodelling. Whereas microaneurysms were found in more than 50% of the cases, focal areas of capillary closure were found only in 8%. The first lesions were seen in patients of at least 12 years of age and with a duration of diabetes of minimum 3 years. Microaneurysms were found relatively earlier than capillary closure.[1]

Microaneurysms are focal dilatations of the vessel wall. According to the Early Treatment Diabetic Retinopathy Study (ETDRS) red spots with a largest dimension of less than 125 μm (corresponding to the width of an average major vein at the disc margin) and with sharp margins should be considered as microaneurysms. Larger spots most probably represent haemorrhages unless they display typical features such as a round shape, smooth margins and a central light reflex.[2]

On fluorescein angiography microaneurysms are hyperfluorescent. Hellstedt and colleagues[3] found corresponding microaneurysms in the fluorescein angiography for about 50% of the red dots considered to be microaneurysms on colour or red-free photographs. These missing microaneurysms could be small intraretinal haemorrhages or thrombosed aneurysms.

In another study, they showed that 33% of the microaneurysms were visualized only in the early phase of the angiography, 31% in the late phase and 36% in both phases.[4] The microaneurysms frequently changed their phase of appearance during follow-up and 55–80% of the microaneurysms had disappeared after a 26–month follow-up period.[5] The total count of microaneurysms nevertheless increased with the duration of diabetes. Microaneurysm disappearance rate did not correlate with diabetic control, although in patients with satisfactory glucose control ($H_6A_1C \leq 7.5$ mmol) the microaneurysm formation rate tended to decrease.

The foveal avascular zone and capillary closure

The foveal avascular zone (FAZ) can be identified on fluorescein angiography. This is due to the higher content of melanin in the pigmented epithelium at the level of the fovea, which blocks the underlying choroidal fluorescence and thus allows for a better visualization of the retinal capillaries and also because the retinal capillary bed forms a monolayer.[6]

Normally its shape is oval, with a diameter varying from 0 to perhaps 1.000 μm, usually about 500–600 μm.

Bresnick et al[7] measured the FAZ in fluorescein angiograms from 36 diabetic patients and 20 non-diabetic controls. The median values for longest diameter, mean diameter and circumference were significantly greater in diabetics than in the control group. The FAZ dimensions were strongly correlated with the severity of capillary non-perfusion and with the presence of proliferative diabetic retinopathy, but not with fluorescein leakage. A definite correlation between increased FAZ and perifoveal area and decreased visual acuity could be found in macular ischaemia.[8–10]

The EDTRS[11] graded the FAZ as follows:

Grade 0: < 300 μm
Grade 1: $= 300$ μm
Grade 2: > 300 μm and < 500 μm
Grade 3: $>$ or $= 500$ μm
Grade 4: cannot grade.

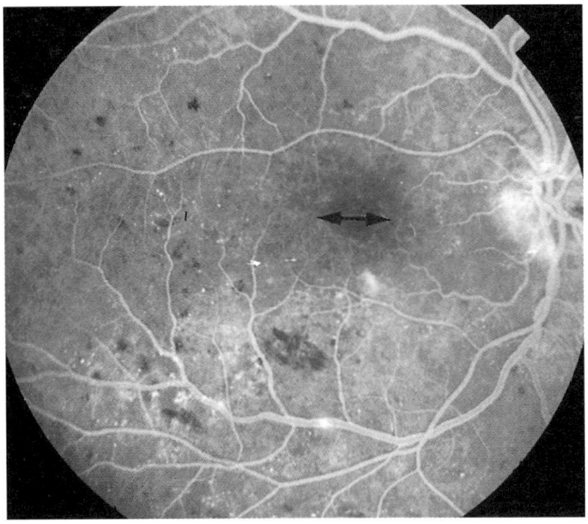

Figure 10.4
Enlarged foveal avascular zone with irregular contours in a 64-year-old diabetic man with proliferative retinopathy.

There is a marked variability of the size of the FAZ in normals. On the other hand, grading of the FAZ may be difficult in many angiograms, especially in older patients. Therefore, other characteristics may be of importance. Abnormalities in diabetic retinopathy include irregular contours, capillary beading into the FAZ and augmented perifoveal intercapillary areas[12] (*Figs 10.4* and *10.5*).

Capillary closure is often accompanied by dilatation of the adjacent capillary bed and by microaneurysm formation. Cotton wool spots or soft exudates are small infarcts of the inner retinal layers. On fluorescein angiography they block the underlying choroidal fluorescence (*Fig. 10.6*).

Intraretinal microvascular abnormalities (IRMAs)

Intraretinal microvascular abnormalities (IRMAs) is a term used to describe changes within areas of capillary closure and more specifically the telangiectatic shunt channels between arterioles and venules.[6] They are a sign of preproliferative retinopathy, although the term IRMAs should not be used to describe new vessels on the surface of the retina.

*Macular oedema (*Figs 10.7 *and* 10.8*)*

Macular oedema is the main cause of visual loss in non-proliferative diabetic retinopathy. Macular

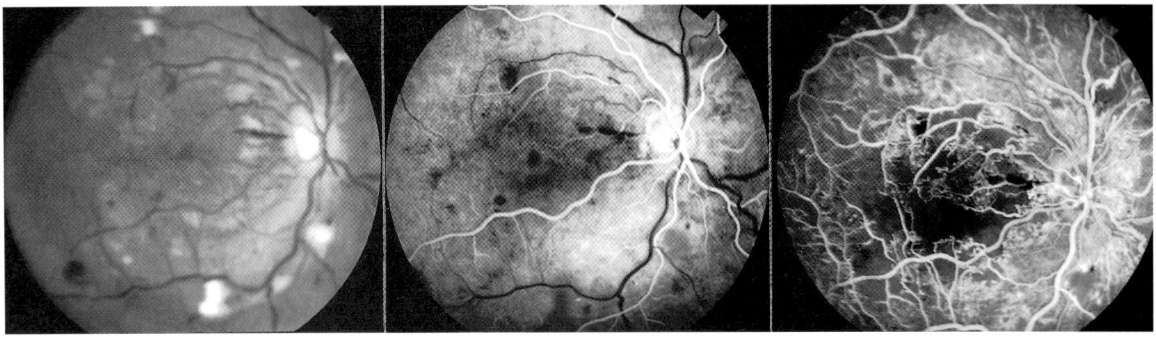

(a) (b) (c)

Figure 10.5
Thirty-two-year-old insulin-dependent diabetes mellitus patient with proliferative diabetic retinopathy. Extensive closures of the capillary bed in the posterior pole.

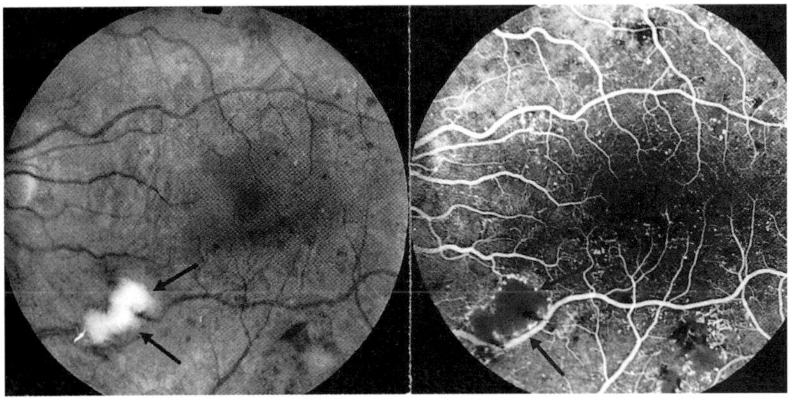

(a) (b)

Figure 10.6
(a), (b) Cotton wool spot blocking the underlying choroidal fluorescence and surrounded by capillary dilatations and microaneurysms (arrow).

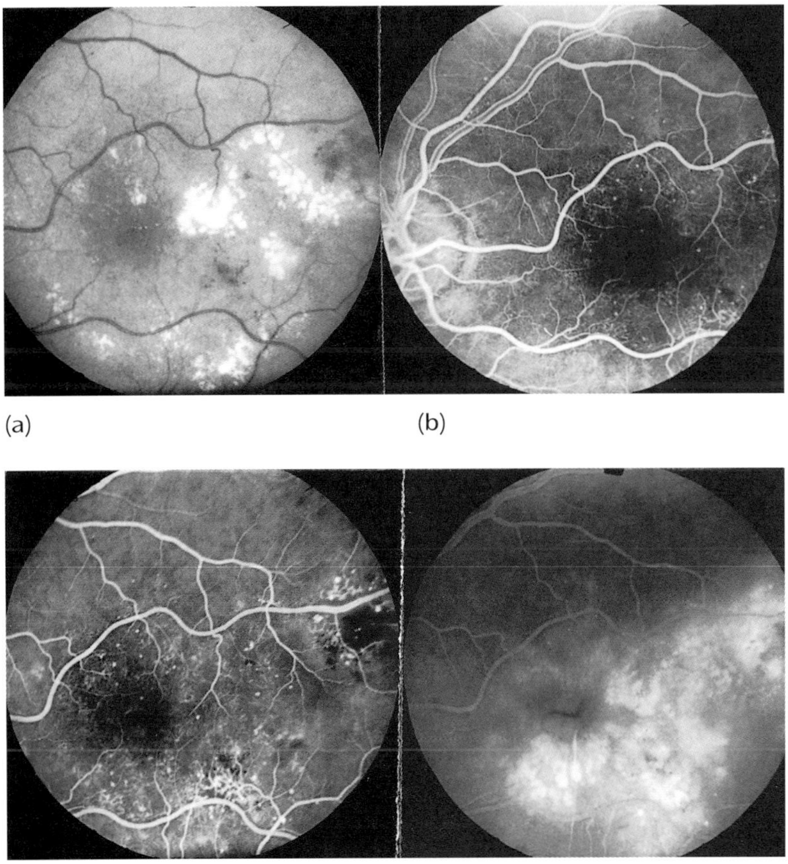

(c) (d)

Figure 10.7
Diffuse macular oedema in a 54-year-old diabetic man. The red-free photograph shows marked lipoid exudates and a foveal cyst (a). On the late fluorescein angiographic picture (d) a classic aspect of cystoid macular oedema is seen.

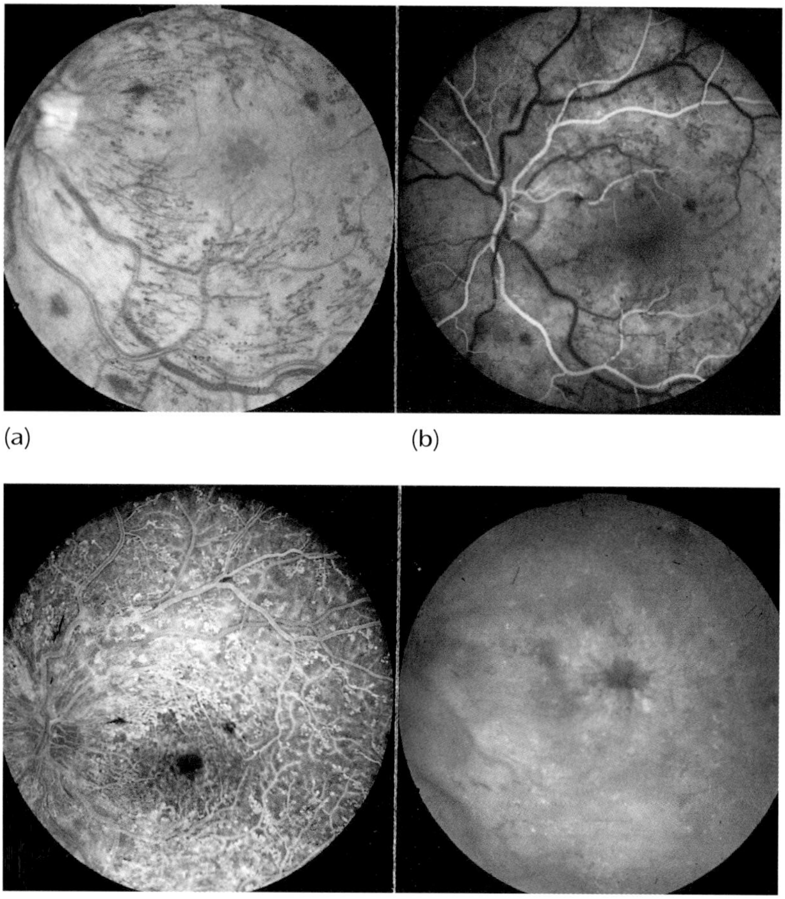

(a) (b) (c) (d)

Figure 10.8
Massive oedema of the posterior pole in an 18-year-old diabetic with florid diabetic retinopathy. Note the marked capillary dilatation on the red-free picture (a) and on fluorescein angiography (c). The foveal avascular zone is enlarged. Diffuse retinal oedema and cystoid macular oedema (d).

oedema can be focal or diffuse. In focal oedema clusters of microaneurysms leak fluorescein. This is often associated with hard exudates which sometimes form a circinate ring surrounding the area of leakage. Diffuse or cystic macular oedema is characterized on fluorescein angiography by an increased visibility of the capillary bed and by a progressive staining of the posterior pole region, with late pooling of dye within cystoid spaces. This is the result of a breakdown of the inner blood–retinal barrier at the level of the retinal capillary endothelial cells, although there is also evidence of involvement of the outer blood–retinal barrier (at the level of the retinal pigment epithelial cells). The importance of leakage accross the retinal pigment epithelium (RPE) barrier is difficult to assess with fluorescein angiography because of the marked diffusion from the retinal capillaries. Macular oedema is mainly diagnosed with fundus biomicroscopy, stereoscopic imaging and optical coherence tomography. Fluorescein angiography is of importance to assess the site of leakage and to determine the treatment strategy.

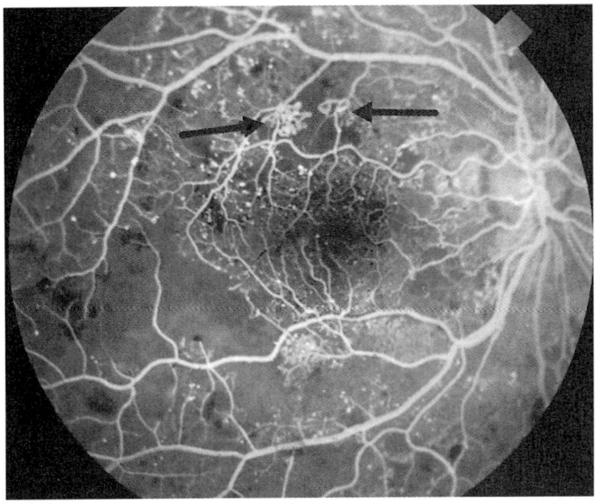

Figure 10.9
Extensive capillary closures close to the macula and early neovascularization (arrows).

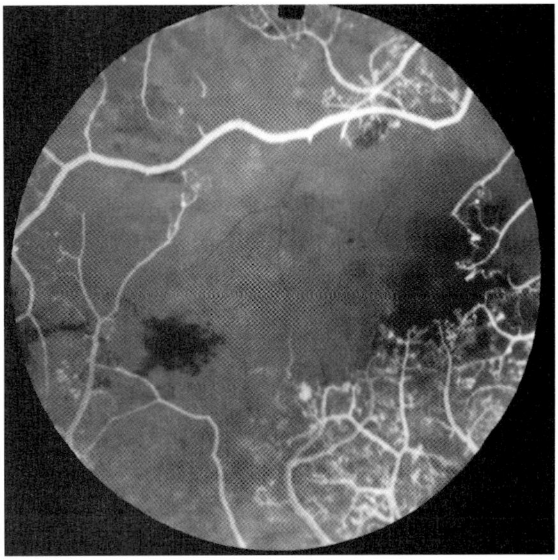

Figure 10.10
Massive infarction of the macular region in a 65-year-old non-insulin-dependent diabetes mellitus patient.

In the ETDRS clinically significant macular oedema was defined as either: (1) retinal thickening at least one disc diameter in extent, part of which is within one disc diameter of the macula; or (2) retinal thickening or hard exudates, extending to within 500 μm of the centre of the macula.[2]

Fluorescein leakage outside the fovea is usually but not necessarily related to increased retinal thickness. Leakage, as shown on fluorescein angiography, is a poor indicator of the amount of fluid accumulation in the retina.[13]

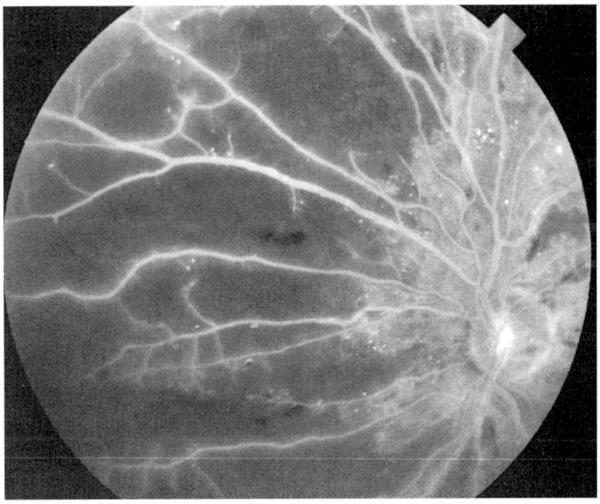

Figure 10.11
Extensive arteriolar closure with capillary non-perfusion nasally to the optic disc.

*Retinal ischaemia (*Figs 10.9, 10.10, 10.11 *and* 10.12*)*

Arteriolar occlusions with resulting retinal ischaemia will lead to neovascularization in the retina and at the optic disc. Capillary non-perfusion worsens as the diabetic retinopathy progresses and may herald evolution to proliferative diabetic retinopathy.[14] Wide-field fluoroangiographic studies have shown the importance of retinal non-perfusion in the midperiphery of the retina and its relation with neovascularization.[15,16] Although intraretinal manifestations

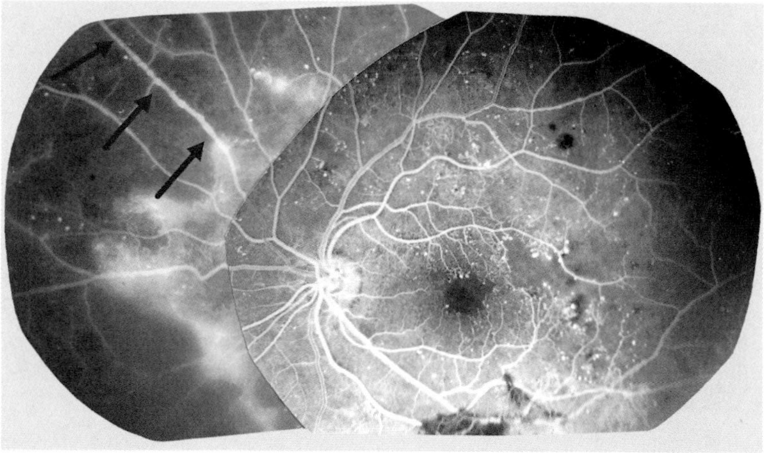

Figure 10.12
Composite large-field angiography in a 53-year-old diabetic patient. The foveal avascular zone is enlarged. Extensive arteriolar closures are seen temporally to the macula and nasally to the disc. Beading of the superonasal vein (arrow).

such as arteriolar narrowing and pruning, vascular anomalies such as venous beading and loop formation (*Figs 10.12* and *10.13*) and IRMAs may betray the existence of capillary non-perfusion, fluorescein angiography remains important in assessing the extent of retinal ischaemia.

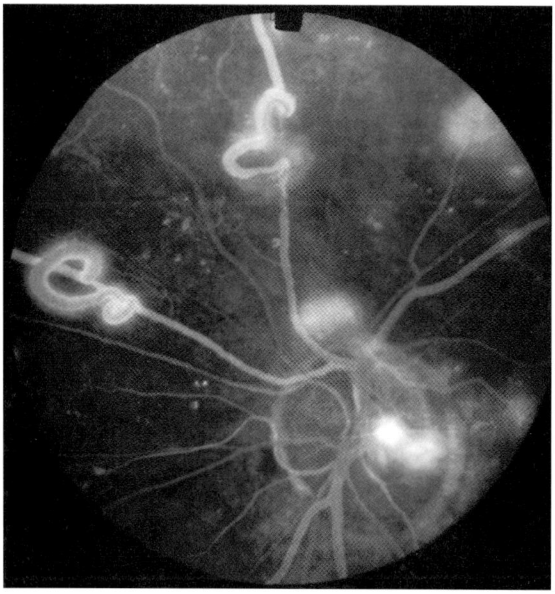

Figure 10.13
Venous loop formations, in proliferative diabetic retinopathy.

Neovascularization

The role of fluorescein angiography is usually limited to the detection of early retinal or optic disc neovascularization and in its differentiation from collaterals. Neovascularization can sufficiently be appreciated using direct ophthalmoscopy, stereo-fundus photographs and fundus biomicroscopy. These techniques also allow the study of fibrous proliferation, of vitreoretinal adhesions and of the extent of posterior vitreous detachment.

Fluorescein angiography is essential in the analysis of various components of diabetic retinopathy and in the understanding of the mechanisms involved in the progression of the disease. It also provides accurate documents for the follow-up and for the study of the influence of therapeutic measures. It has an important role in teaching residents. However, its role in the decision of treatment strategies is essentially limited to the treatment of diabetic maculopathy. In those cases it may help in deciding between a grid-like laser treatment or a more focal approach.

Fluorescein angiography may be extremely helpful in localizing the foveal region, especially in cases with marked and diffuse macular oedema.

Indocyanine-green angiography (ICG-A)

In contrast with the vast literature on diabetic retinopathy, relatively little is known on the influence of diabetes on the choroid. Indian ink injections of diabetic eyes have shown an irregular filling of the choroidal bed and the presence of aneurysmal dilatations in areas with poor or with adequate filling as well as calibre irregularity of the choroidal vessel.[17,18] Fryczkowski et al[19] studied with scanning electron microscopy vascular casts of autopsy eyes from patients with long-standing insulin-dependent diabetes mellitus. They noted tortuosity of the choriocapillaris, dilatations and narrowing of the vascular lumen and deformation of the interlobular vascular structures. These changes were most marked in the area between the equator and ora serrata.

Indocyanine-green angiography is less sensitive than fluorescein angiography in detecting retinal vascular anomalies, especially microaneurysm, retinal capillary non-perfusion and retinal neovascularization.[20] It has, however, shown irregular and delayed filling of the choroid in patients with diabetic retinopathy.[21] After photocoagulation, ICG angiography shows areas of destruction of the choriocapillaries corresponding to the laser scars and a remodelling of the choroidal vascular bed.[22]

Up to now ICG angiography has thus not proved to be of major clinical significance in diabetic eye disease.

Iris angiography

Iris neovascularization and neovascular glaucoma are feared complications of diabetic retinopathy. Iris fluorescein angiography, using a modified photo slit lamp, showed a correlation between diabetic iridopathy and the retinal angiopathy.[23]

Bandello et al[24] studied 225 eyes of 117 diabetic patients with clear media, both with iris and retinal fluorescein angiography. In eyes with diabetic iridopathy (non-proliferative or proliferative) the positive predictive value for (pre)proliferative retinopathy was 92.8% and the negative value 31.0%, whereas the positive predictive value for preproliferative or proliferative diabetic retinopathy became 100% in eyes with iris neovascularization and the negative value 65%.[24]

One of the problems of iris fluorescein angiography in diabetics is the sometimes profuse dye leakage. In heavily pigmented eyes also, the iris vascular pattern is difficult to demonstrate. In such cases ICG iris angiography appears superior to fluorescein iris angiography as the infrared light penetrates pigmented irides better and the dye does not extravasate readily, thus allowing a more detailed study of the fine vessel structures.[25]

When iris neovascularization is detected in eyes where the fundus cannot be examined, a serious concomitant retinopathy must be suspected and the necessary measures (either cryocoagulation or transscleral coagulation) must be considered before cataract extraction or vitrectomy. Endophotocoagulation during vitrectomy or photocoagulation can be performed in the days following surgery, as the surgical intervention may precipitate both the retinopathy and the iris neovascularization.[26,27]

Fluorophotometry

The method used for the study of the blood–retinal barriers is discussed in full detail in Chapter 12.

Assessment of macular oedema

Macular oedema is a major cause of blindness in diabetic retinopathy.[28] According to the ETDRS, macular oedema is a clinical diagnosis, based mainly on the analysis of stereophotographs with good stereoscopic effect.[2] Macular oedema can be clinically judged using fundus biomicroscopy.

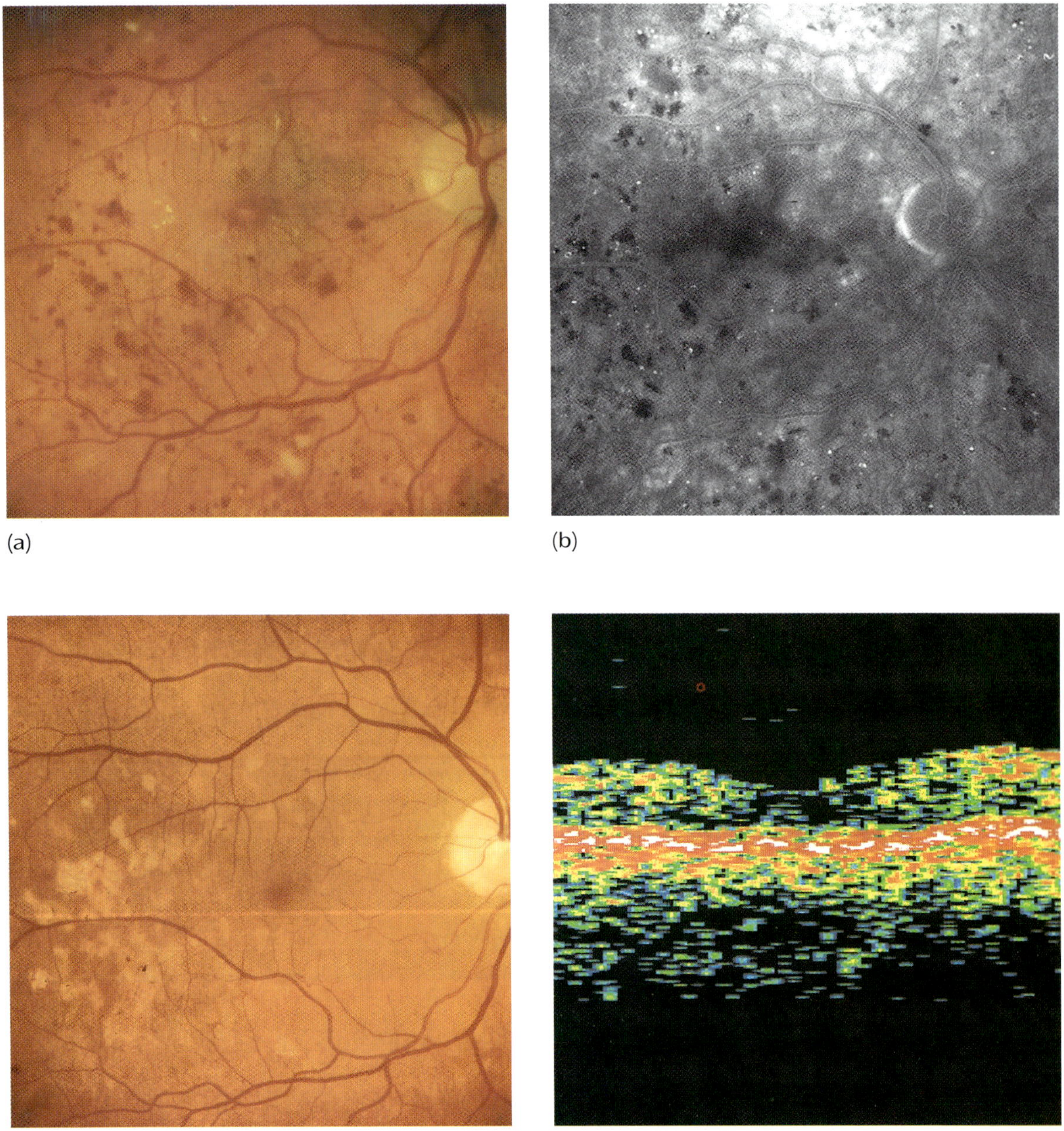

(a) (b) (c) (d)

Figure 10.14
A 42-year-old patient having had insulin-dependent diabetes mellitus for 20 years. (a) Colour photograph showing a marked background retinopathy. (b) Fluorescein angiography taken the same day as (a) indicating diffuse macular oedema. (c) Colour photograph taken 7 years after focal laser treatment. Regression of the macular oedema. (d) Optical coherence tomography taken the same day as (c). Normal thickness of the macula, with foveal depression. (Courtesy of Professor A Leys, MD, Catholic University of Leuven, Belgium.)

Zeimer and colleagues[29] used a green helium–neon laser operating at 543 nm with slit lamp biomicroscopy and obtained fundus images together with a narrow beam at 12°. The images were analysed using microdensitometry. The separation between the intersection of the laser with the vitreoretinal interface and the sensory retina–retinal pigment epithelial face is proportional to the retinal thickness. These authors were able to measure retina with a thickness as low as 80 μm and with a reproducibility varying between 6 and 15%.

The same group[30] employed this technique to assess quantitatively diabetic macular oedema and compared the results with those obtained with slit lamp biomicroscopy, stereophotography, fluorescein angiography and fluorophotometry. Slit lamp biomicroscopy detected in 80% of the cases a thickening of the retina of more than twice normal but failed to identify locations of the retina with an average thickness of 1.5 times normal. Stereophotographies could detect thickening greater than 1.6 times normal. Fluorescein leakage was not always associated with marked fluid accumulation, suggesting that fluorescein angiography is a poor indicator of the amount of fluid in the retina. Vitreous fluorophotometry showed a poor correlation with foveal thickening, which is not surprising as it measures the importance of fluorescein leakage in the various compartments of the eye and that leakage does not necessarily correlate with fluid accumulation.

Optical coherence tomography (OCT) is a recent technique which uses infrared light at 843 nm and low-coherence interferometry. Retinal tomography is performed in a manner similar to indirect ophthalmoscopy, using a 60-dioptre condensing lens and a slit lamp biomicroscope. Cross-sectional images are constructed with 10 μm of longitudinal resolution.[31] Optical coherence tomography makes it possible to demonstrate normal variation in retinal thickness and to discriminate morphological features of retina, optic disc and vitreoretinal interface. In patients with cystoid macular oedema OCT images can identify cystic changes and the development of a macular cyst to a lamellar hole (*Figs 10.14–10.17*). Retinal hard exudates appear as local regions of high

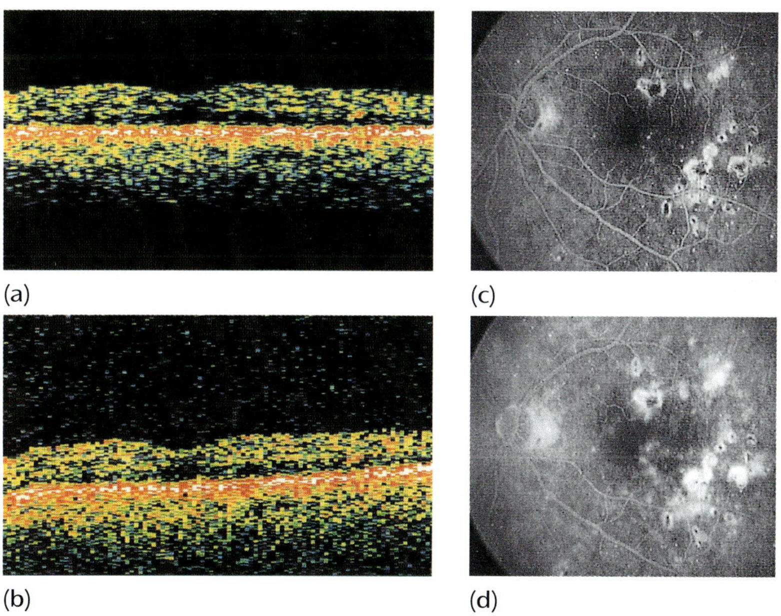

Figure 10.15
A 58-year-old insulin-dependent diabetes mellitus patient, treated with focal laser photocoagulation for diabetic macular oedema. Although optical coherence tomography still shows a foveal depression (a), the region temporal to the macula is slightly thickened (b), corresponding to an area of leaking microaneurysms (c), (d). (Courtesy of Professor A Leys, MD, Catholic University of Leuven, Belgium.)

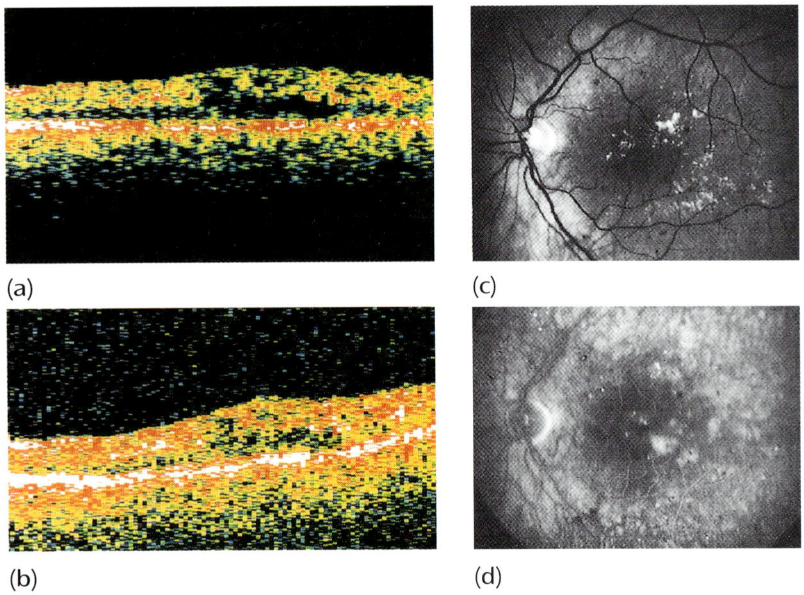

Figure 10.16
Macular oedema in a 50-year-old non-insulin-dependent diabetes mellitus patient. Optical coherence tomography shows a disappearance of the foveal region and thickening of the macula (a), (b). (Courtesy of Professor A Leys, MD, Catholic University of Leuven, Belgium.)

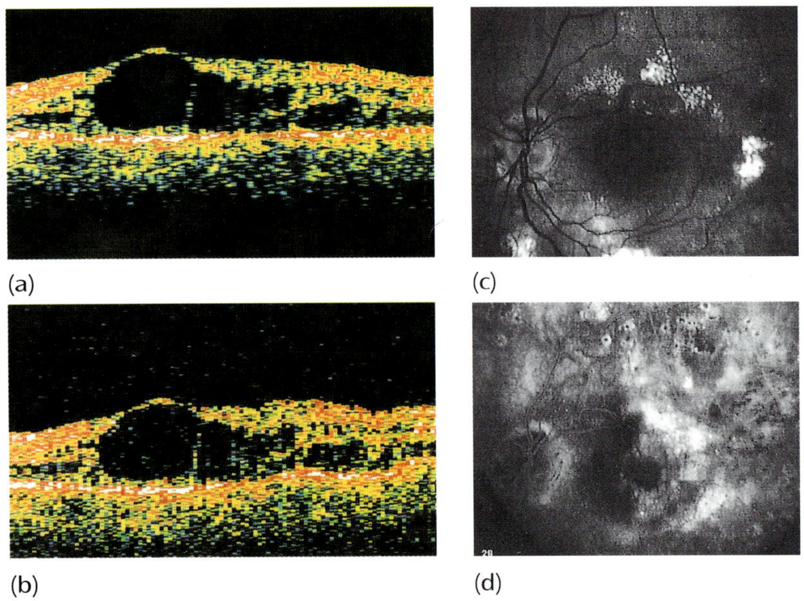

Figure 10.17
Optical coherence tomography (OCT) and fluoroangiography of a 69-year-old diabetic patient with cystoid macular oedema (c), (d). The cystoid spaces are highlighted on OCT (a), (b). (Courtesy of Professor A Leys, MD, Catholic University of Leuven, Belgium.)

optical reflectivity, but microaneurysms and vascular abnormalities are difficult to detect.[32] Optical coherence tomography is capable of quantifying macula thickness in diabetic macular oedema. Foveal thickness, as measured by OCT, correlated with visual acuity.[33] Optical coherence tomography even detected thickening in the absence of any abnormality on slit lamp examination.

Ultrasonography

Standardized ultrasonography combining A- and B-scan techniques is essential in the diagnosis of

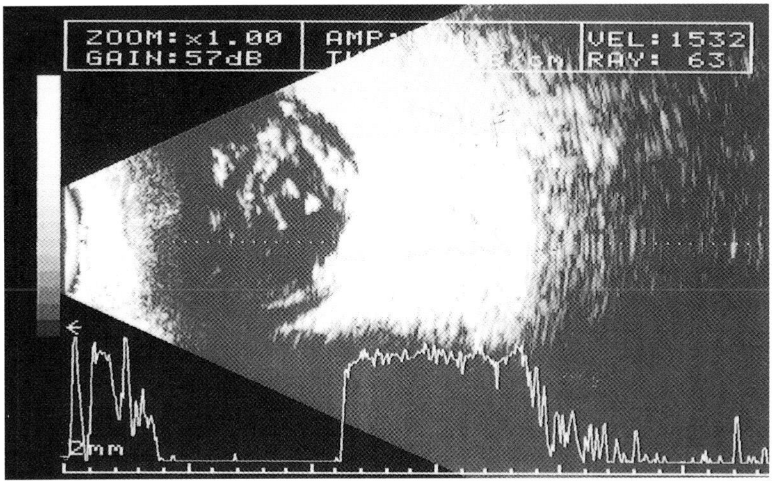

Figure 10.18
A- and B-scan echography in a case of long-standing diabetic vitreous haemorrhage, associated with retinal detachment.

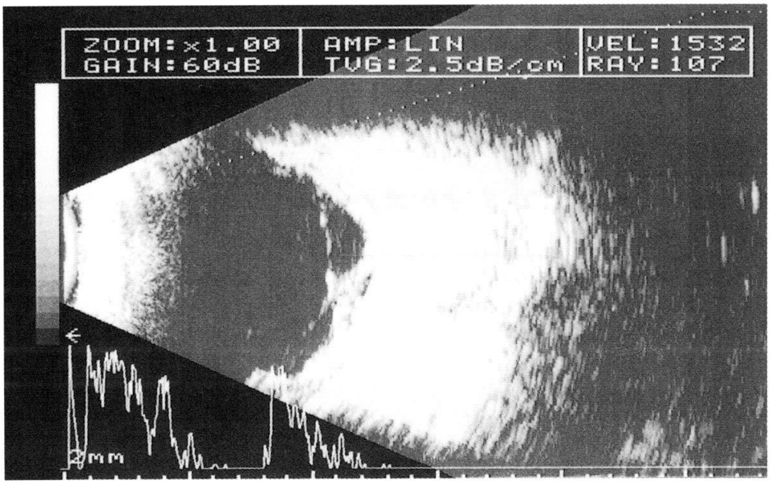

Figure 10.19
Tent-like retinal detachment, due to traction and localized vitreoretinal adherence.

vitreous traction and retinal detachment in the presence of opaque ocular media[34,35] (*Fig. 10.18*). Fresh haemorrhages in the vitreous produce echos which are variable in amplitude but may remain undetected on B-scan echography.[34,36,37] B-scan makes it possible to demonstrate posterior vitreous detachment by the presence of echos from the posterior hyaloid interface. Vitreous detachment may be complete or incomplete. Vitreoretinal adhesion, often stalk-like, can be demonstrated. Splitting of the outer posterior vitreous cortex is possible in patients with proliferative diabetic retinopathy. This so-called posterior vitreoschisis should be differentiated from posterior vitreous detachment. This is of importance, for failure to recognize this feature could

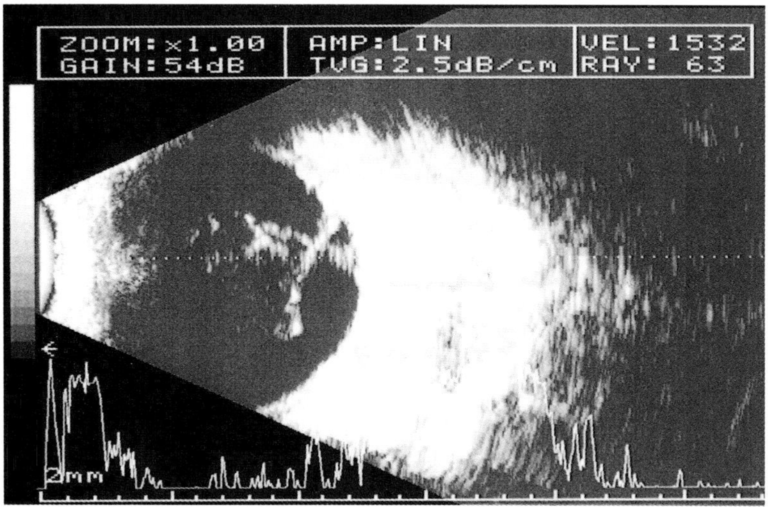

Figure 10.20
Tent-like retinal detachment.

result in an incomplete removal of the vitreous cortex. This in turn could serve as a scaffold for neovascular proliferation and contribute to further traction on the retinal surface.[38]

B-scan will also demonstrate the presence, the type and the extent of retinal detachment. Two main types of traction detachment are associated with proliferative diabetic retinopathy. The tent-like detachment (*Figs 10.19* and *10.20*) is the result of a localized vitreoretinal adherence, whereas the tabletop detachment has a broader vitreoretinal adherence and is usually more extensive[35] (*Fig. 10.21*). Ultrasonography is thus essential in the diagnosis, in the preoperative evaluation and in the planning of the surgical strategy when vitrectomy is considered.

STUDY OF RETINAL HAEMODYNAMICS IN DIABETIC RETINOPATHY

Retinal blood flow measurements have been performed using different techniques, such as fluorescein angiography with the scanning laser ophthalmoscope, blue field entoptoscopy, and especially bidirectional laser-doppler velocimetry. These measurements do not yet have clinical significance but allow a better understanding of the physiopathological changes mainly in early diabetic retinopathy.

Scanning laser ophthalmoscope

The scanning laser ophthalmoscope in combination with digital image analysis makes it possible to measure flow velocity in the perifoveal capillaries. The flow velocity is calculated by frame-to-frame analysis and is based on the transit time between two points separated by a known distance. In a study by Wolf et al the measured mean flow velocity was 3.28 ± 0.45 mm/second in healthy subjects and 2.89 ± 0.57 mm/second in diabetic patients without retinopathy or with background diabetic retinopathy.[39] This could be related to a reduction of the vascular autoregulation and increased plasma viscosity, whereas there was a slight but not significant decrease in perifoveal blood velocity level with more increasing severity of the diabetic retinopathy. The size

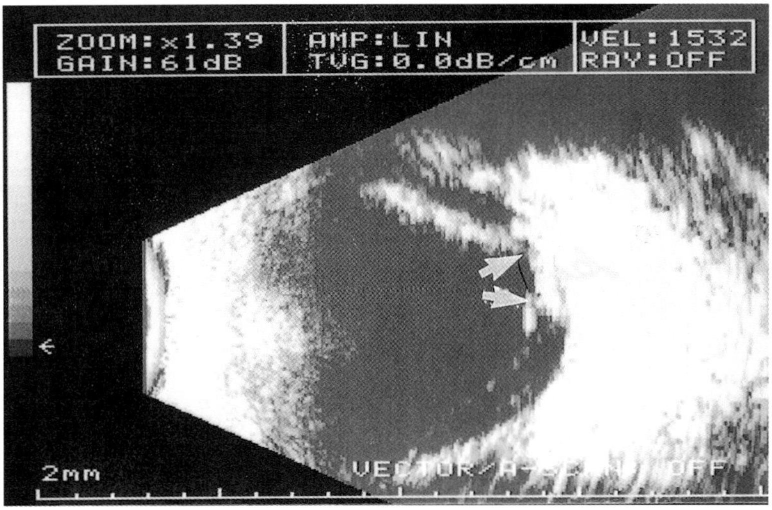

Figure 10.21
Tabletop retinal detachment, due to a broad vitreoretinal adherence.

of the foveal avascular zone and of the perifoveal intercapillary areas enlarged significantly with the retinopathy level.[40] No relationship could be found between decrease of capillary blood velocity and visual acuity, but such a relationship has been shown between vision and size of foveal avascular zone and perifoveal capillary area.[10] The decrease of capillary blood velocity in diabetic patients was comparable in patients with and without cystoid macular oedema.[41]

Blue field entoptic phenomenon

One own's leukocytes can be observed by looking at a uniform blue field. They appear as luminous dots, which move along curved paths and with a speed which is pulsatile and in phase with the heart cycle. The motion of the leukocytes is simulated on a screen and the speed of the simulated particles can be adjusted. The subject is then asked to match the speed of the particles on the screen with that of his/her own leukocytes. With such a technique Riva and Petrig[42] were able to calculate the speed of the leukocytes in the macular capillaries. The velocity was approximately 0.5 mm/second and the maximum velocity approximately 1 mm/second in various healthy subjects. With this method Fallon et al showed a significantly higher capillary flow velocity in patients with background retinopathy (0.74 mm ± 0.32 mm/second) as compared to normals (0.54 mm ± 0.19 mm/second) and diabetics without retinopathy (0.51 mm/second ± 0.29 mm/second). The blood flow decreased at the preproliferative stage.[43] Autoregulation could be demonstrated with the blue field entoptic technique in non-proliferative and in proliferative diabetic retinopathy using isocapnic hyperoxia and hyperoxia as stimuli.[44] Acute modification of plasma glucose level (either acute hyperglycaemia or reduction of the glycaemia by injection of insulin) did not significantly modify macular blood flow in patients with diabetic retinopathy or the autoregulatory changes induced by breathing 60% oxygen.[45,46] In patients with diabetic retinopathy the flow velocity diminished significantly over a follow-up period of 21–39 months.[45] This was observed both in patients with background retinopathy and those with preproliferative retinopathy, but not in the patients treated for proliferative retinopathy.[47] Increased macular circulation, assessed by blue field entoptic technique, may be associated with progression of retinopathy.[48]

Arend et al[49] compared the blue field entoptic technique in healthy subjects with velocity measurement using the scanning laser ophthalmoscope (SLO). They obtained significantly higher values with the SLO (2.68 ± 0.3 mm/second vs 0.89 ± 0.2 mm/second). Whereas with blue field entoptoscopy leukocyte flow is measured, with the SLO the velocity of erythrocyte rouleaux is quantified. The differences between the two techniques may also be due to different measuring sites.

Laser-Doppler velocitometry

Bidimensional laser velocimetry utilizes the shift in frequency produced when a monochromatic laser beam is reflected by moving red blood cells in the retinal vessels. This shift is proportional to the velocity of the red blood cells. To measure blood flow the calibre of the retinal vessel has to be taken into account. Usually, main superior or inferior temporal veins are chosen, avoiding sites close to venous junctions or to arteriovenous crossings.

With this technique it has been demonstrated that the retinal flow was slower in the nasal than in the temporal retina both in normals and in diabetics.[50,51] Whereas no difference was found between the superior and inferior retina in normals, in poorly controlled diabetic patients with diabetic retinopathy volumetric blood flow rate was higher in the superior than in the inferior hemiretina.[50]

Patients with early diabetes mellitus and patients with diabetic retinopathy have an increased volumetric blood flow rate,[50,52–54] although Feke et al[55] reported a 33% reduction in retinal arterial blood speed in diabetic patients with no or with background retinopathy and a duration of diabetes between 7 and 20 years. Hyperglycaemia increases retinal blood flow in experimental animals, but postprandial hyperglycaemia had little effect on retinal blood flow of type I diabetic and of non-diabetic subjects.[56]

Intravenous administration of insulin to obtain normoglycaemia in diabetics provoked a decrease in retinal blood flow. The decrease was larger in patients with shorter diabetes duration.[57] Retinal blood flow significantly increased in pregnant diabetic women, whose retinopathy worsened during pregnancy.[58]

The Doppler velocitometric findings can possibly help to identify patients at risk of progression of their retinopathy when metabolic control is improved. Grunwald et al[59] showed a correlation between the progression of the retinopathy and increased retinal venous blood flow, whereas those patients who on follow-up presented a stable retinopathy tended to have a decrease of retinal blood flow. The decrease in average volumetric blood flow can, however, also indicate progressive capillary closure.[60] As the diabetes duration becomes longer and the retinopathy becomes more severe, arterial blood flow may first decrease and later increase again, in the proliferative stage.[61] These modifications reflect the complexity of the changes occurring in the retina in diabetes.

Autoregulation, demonstrated by the change in vessel diameter and in red blood cell velocity after breathing of 60% oxygen, is variably affected in diabetes.[50,53,57,58]

Panretinal photocoagulation for proliferative diabetic retinopathy provokes a decrease of retinal volumetric blood flow rate and improves the autoregulatory reponse to hyperoxia.[62] Smoking, on the other hand, may even eliminate in diabetics the ability of retinal vessels to autoregulate to hyperoxia.[63]

FUNCTIONAL TESTS IN DIABETIC RETINOPATHY

Colour vision

Diabetic retinopathy is frequently associated with acquired colour vision deficiency.[64,65] This has its importance in the management of diabetes, as a number of patients still use colour-dependent urine or blood glucose tests for self-assessment.[12,66] Higher levels of illumination could, however, improve the correct interpretation of the strips.[67] The colour vision defects in diabetics characteristically follow a blue–yellow axis,[64,65,68–70] although Vassilou et al[71] most frequently found alterations in the red–green axis in young diabetics. Trick et al[72] noticed blue/yellow and red/green hue discrimination deficits with approximately equal frequency in diabetic patients with minimal or no retinopathy.

At least part of the blue/yellow defects could be caused by the absorption of blue light, due to premature yellowing of the lens.[73] When adjustments were made to correct for the effects of the yellowing of the lens, tritan deficits were no longer apparent.[74] Besides the lens and the retinopathy other pathologies may interfere with colour vision in diabetics, for example, glaucoma, optic neuropathy and vitreous haemorrhage.

Dean et al[75] reported on a small improvement in colour vision thresholds in diabetic patients with minimal or no retinopathy, who inhaled 100% oxygen for at least 5 minutes. This suggests that low retinal oxygenation may be one of the causes of retinal photoreceptor malfunctioning in diabetes.

Acquired defects in colour discrimination can be present in diabetics before diabetic retinopathy is clinically detected.[68,72,74,76–78] The Farnsworth–Munsell 100-Hue is, however, not sufficiently selective to be of value as a screening test for the detection of retinopathy.[77] Although for some authors duration of diabetes is a risk factor,[68,69,74] others did not find a significant association between presence or absence of colour vision deficits and deterioration of diabetes.[70,72,76,78]

Whereas Trick et al[72] obtained a correlation between hue discrimination deficits and metabolic control assessed by HbA_{1C} levels, such a correlation was not detected by others.[70,76] Peduzzi et al[79] noticed a moderately positive correlation between glycosylated haemoglobin and early loss of colour vision only in young insulin-dependent diabetics.

After a 6-year follow-up study of the colour vision in diabetic retinopathy, it was concluded that the Panel D-15, the desaturated panel or the Nagel I anomaloscope, had no predictive value for eyes at risk of developing retinopathy.[80]

The severity of diabetic maculopathy is correlated with progressive colour vision loss.[69,71,74] According to Bresnick et al[69] the Farnsworth–Munsell 100-Hue error score is more strongly related to macular fluorescein leakage than to macular non-perfusion. Colour vision after photocoagulation for diabetic retinopathy has not been extensively studied. Older studies, where blue–yellow argon laser was used, showed worsening of the blue defects.[81,82] Mäntyjärvi published a 5-year follow-up study on the colour vision of 60 diabetic patients treated with photocoagulation. Of the 32 eyes 22 (68.8%) had the same results in colour vision tests, 4 (12.5%) better results and 6 (18.8%) worse results. The groups with better or similar colour vision and the group with worse results differed significantly both in age and in visual acuity.[83]

The ETDRS showed that there was less loss of colour vision after 4 years in eyes with macular oedema and less severe retinopathy assessed with the Farnsworth–Munsell 100-Hue test assigned to immediate photocoagulation than in eyes assigned to deferral of photocoagulation. No significant difference was noted for eyes without

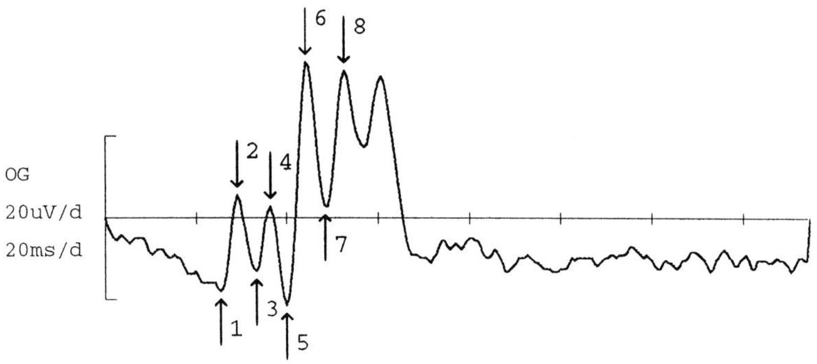

Figure 10.22
Normal oscillatory potentials in a 59-year-old person.

macular oedema and eyes with macular oedema and more severe retinopathy.[84]

Contrast sensitivity

Contrast sensitivity is of importance in daily activities and is not necessarily correlated with visual acuity obtained with standard optotypes.[85] Patients with reduced sensitivity at low contrast may have motility problems in rainy weather or in dim light. Contrast sensitivity can be measured with a video display of sinusoidal gratings of different spatial frequencies[12] or by using charts with standardized sinusoidal greys.[86]

Contrast sensitivity may be impaired in diabetics even with no or minimal retinopathy and with normal visual acuity.[87–90] Sokol et al[91] found normal contrast sensitivity in insulin-dependent diabetic patients with no retinopathy, abnormal contrast sensitivity only at 22.8 cpd in non-insulin-dependent diabetics with no retinopathy and an abnormal contrast sensitivity in all spatial frequencies tested in patients with background retinopathy. Contrast sensitivity worsens with advancing retinopathy.[78] Although some authors found a negative correlation between diabetic control expressed as HbA_{1C} levels and contrast sensitivity,[92] such a relationship was not detected by Trick et al,[72] who however noticed a significant correlation between sensitivity at 6.0 cpd and duration of diabetes in patients with little or no retinopathy In diabetics, smoking is associated with a further significant deterioration in contrast sensitivity.[88]

Contrast sensitivity thus appears as a sensitive test to detect early functional involvement in diabetes.[93] Still, the large variability in the scores limits its use as a clinical tool for screening diabetic patients.[87]

Electrophysiology

Electroretinography (ERG)

Early studies showed that conventional ERG does not exhibit significant changes in eyes with diabetic retinopathy untill a very advanced stage.[94,95]

Yonemura et al[96] were the first to describe deterioration of the oscillatory potentials in diabetic patients even with no obvious fundus changes. Oscillatory potentials (OPs) are low-amplitude wavelets superimposed on the b wave. They probably originate in the vicinity of the inner plexiform layer and could be generated by neural interactions[97] (*Fig. 10.22*). Oscillatory potentials can be used as an indicator of retinal ischaemia[98] (*Fig. 10.23*). A selective delay in the peak implicit time of the oscillatory potentials was found in non-insulin-dependent diabetic

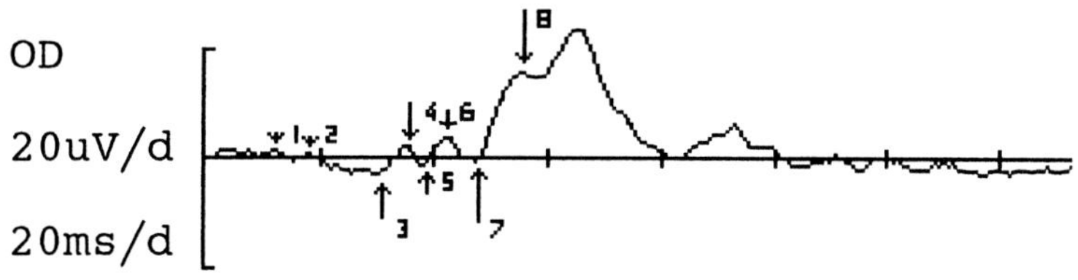

Figure 10.23
Markedly reduced oscillatory potentials in a 35-year-old diabetic patient with high-risk characteristics.

patients with no photographic and fluorescein angiographic evidence of diabetic retinopathy and who did not present increased permeability of the blood–retinal barrier.[99] In streptozotocin-induced diabetic rats significantly delayed OP peaks were found as early as 2 weeks after onset of diabetes, preceding by about 4 weeks the first ophthalmoscopic, angiographic or vitreous fluorophotometric changes,[100,101] suggesting a direct influence of hyperglycaemia in these OPs. However, short-time near normal blood glucose control by means of continuous subcutaneous insulin infusion did not influence OPs in diabetic patients with long-standing dysregulation.[102]

Although some authors considered mainly a selective delay of peak latency as an early sign of retinal dysfunction in diabetics without or with minimal retinopathy,[99,103,104] others also found a reduction in amplitude[105,106] Simonsen[107] even found OPs with amplitudes greater than normal in juvenile diabetics.[108] These disparities could be possibly explained by differences in methodology. The protocol of the International Society for Clinical Electrophysiology of Vision (ISCEV) recommends a considerably lower flash intensity than the protocol used by Bresnick in the study of diabetic retinopathy.[108] Most probably prolonged peak latency is the first sign, followed by reduction of the amplitude.[101] The attenuation or loss of OPs may be a distinctive feature of diabetic retinopathy.[109] It reflects the severity of retinal involvement[110,111] and may be of predictive value.[107,112] Bresnick and colleagues[113,114] showed that eyes with abnormal amplitudes had a 10-fold higher rate of progression to high-risk characteristics than eyes with normal OP amplitudes. Brinckmann-Hansen et al[115] did not identify an independent relation between changes in amplitude of the different OPs (OP1, OP2, OP3) or their sum and changes in glycaemic control but noted a significant reduction of OP2, OP3 or the sum of OPs when the retinopathy increased. In comparing the results between the start of the study and 7 years later, they obtained a negative correlation between all OPs and age and between OPs and the duration and microaneurysm counts.

Apart from the OPs the b wave amplitude and the scotopic threshold response may correlate with the severity of diabetic retinopathy.[116–118]

Pattern electroretinography (PERG)

Pattern electroretinography could reflect the activity of ganglion cells. It is abnormal in diseases of the optic nerve and ganglion cells. Arden et al[119] considered PERG more reliable than OPs in cases of fluoroangiographic evidence of capillary non-perfusion. Whereas Falsini et al[120] found a significant reduction in mean amplitude of the PERG in diabetics with no or minimal retinopathy, Coupland[109] measured normal PERG in diabetics without retinopathy who presented significantly reduced OPs. Others have observed a significant correlation between the reduction of the amplitude of the PERG and the severity of diabetic retinopathy.[121]

Electro-oculography (EOG)

The EOG measures the standing potential of the eye and reflects the functional status of the retinal pigment epithelium and the photoceptors. The light–dark or Arden ratio deteriorates with the duration of diabetes and the severity of the retinopathy.[122] Conventional EOG becomes abnormal only in advanced cases of retinopathy.[103,123] The standing potential can be influenced by hyperosmolarity, bicarbonate and acetazolamide.[101,103,124] The EOG amplitude is usually stabilized after about 30 minutes in the dark. Intravenous administration of a hypertonic solution or of acetazolamide provokes a decrease of the amplitude, which reaches its minimum after 8–20 minutes. The normal range of the response is 32.1–52.9% for acetazolamide. In diabetics even without retinopathy the mean amplitude of this response is significantly reduced. It further deteriorates as the retinopathy advances.[101]

Mori et al[125] obtained a slight reduction in the hyperosmolarity response with 50 ml mannitol 20% in background diabetic retinopathy, while the acetazolamide response and the light rise were normal. In the patients with proliferative retinopathy the hyperosmolarity response and light rise were markedly reduced while the acetazolamide response remained normal. This suggests that the retinal pigmented epithelium could be functionally affected early in diabetes and further suffer with the progression of the retinopathy. Still, in the light of the conflicting results, more studies are needed to establish the role of the EOG in diabetes.

Visual evoked potentials (VEPs)

A delay of the latency of the P100 component has been observed with pattern VEPs in some diabetics with no retinopathy and no visual complaints.[12, 126] In a study in diabetics, including patients with diabetic macular oedema, a correlation was found between the decrease of absolute amplitude of the pattern ERG and increasing VEP latencies.[127] Although optic nerve involvement cannot be dismissed, these results suggest that the retinopathy is mainly responsible for the VEP changes.

The increase in latency and the decrease in amplitude of the VEP responses after photostress is more important in diabetics even without retinopathy than in normals.

Magni et a[128] studied 12 diabetics with mild non-proliferative retinopathy and normal visual acuity and 14 normal controls. Whereas the VEPs, obtained by means of average were not significantly different between the groups, single-sweep VEPs showed a higher variability of the latency and more reduction of the amplitude in the diabetic group. The major problem of single-sweep VEPs is, however, the low signal to noise ratio. Flicker VEP could be useful in predicting visual outcome after vitrectomy in diabetic patients with vitreous haemorrhage.[129]

REFERENCES

1. Verougstraete C, Toussaint D, De Schepper J et al, First microangiographic abnormalities in childhood diabetes. Types of lesions, *Graefes Arch Clin Exp Ophthalmol* (1991) **229**:24–32.
2. Early Treatment Diabetic Retinopathy Study Research Group, Grading diabetic retinopathy from stereoscopic color fundus photographs. An extension of the modified Airlie House Classification, *Ophthalmology* (1991) **98**:786–806.
3. Hellstedt T, Vesti E, Immonen I, Identification of individual microaneurysms: a comparison

between fluorescein angiograms and red-free and colour photographs, *Graefe' Arch Clin Exp Ophthalmol* (1996) **234**:S13–S17.
4. Jalli PYI, Hellstedt TJ, Immonen IJR, Early versus late staining of microaneurysms in fluorescein angiography, *Retina* (1997) **17**:211–15.
5. Hellstedt T, Immonen I, Disappearance and formation rates of microaneurysms in early diabetic retinopathy, *Br J Ophthalmol* (1996) **80**:135–9.
6. Olk RJ, Lee CM, *Diabetic Retinopathy. Practical Management* (JB Lippincott: Philadelphia, 1993) 3–20.
7. Bresnick G.H, Condit R, Syrjala S et al, Abnormalities of the foveal avascular zone in diabetic retinopathy, *Arch Ophthalmol* (1984) **102**:1286–93.
8. Mansour AM, Schachat A, Bodiford G, Haymond R, Foveal avascular zone in diabetes mellitus, *Retina* (1993) **13**:125–8.
9. Arend O, Wolf S, Remky S et al, Perifoveal microcirculation with non-insulin dependent diabetes mellitus, *Graefes Arch Clin Exp Ophthalmol* (1994) **232**:225–31.
10. Arend O, Wolf S, Harris A, Reim M, The relationship of macular microcirculation to visual acuity in diabetic patients, *Arch Ophthalmol* (1995) **113**:610–14.
11. Early Treatment Diabetic Retinopathy Study Research Group, Classification of diabetic retinopathy from fluorescein angiography. EDTRS Report no. 91, *Ophthalmology* (1991) **98**:807–22.
12. Bresnick GH, Non-proliferative diabetic retinopathy. In: Ryan SJ, ed, *Retina,* 2nd edn (CV Mosby: St Louis, 1994) 1277–1318.
13. Shahidi M, Ogura Y, Blair MP et al, Retinal thickness analysis for quantitative assessment of diabetic macular oedema, *Arch Ophthalmol* (1991) **109**:1115–19.
14. Early Treatment Diabetic Retinopathy Study Research Group, Fluorescein angiographic risk factors for progression of diabetic retinopathy. ETDRS Report no. 13, *Ophthalmology* (1991) **98**:834–40.
15. Shimizu K, Kobayashi Y, Muraoka K, Midperipheral fundus involvement in diabetic retinopathy, *Ophthalmology* (1981) **88**:601–12.
16. Niki T, Muraoka K, Shimizu K, Distribution of capillary non-perfusion in early stage diabetic retinopathy, *Ophthalmology* (1984) **91**:1431–9.
17. Saracco JB, Gastaud P, Ridings A, Ubaud CA, La choroïdopathie diabétique, *J Fr Ophtalmol* (1982) **5**:231–6.
18. Morone G, Tazzi A, Carella G et al, L'uvéopathie diabétique, *Bull Mém Soc Fr Ophtalmol* (1984) **85**:343–7.
19. Fryczkowski AW, Hoder BL, Walker J, Diabetic and iris vasculature scanning electron microscopy findings, *Int Ophthalmol* (1989) **13**:269–79.
20. Ho AC, Retina and retinal vascular lesions. In: Yannuzzi LA, Flower RW, Slakter JS, eds, *Indocyanine-green Angiography* (CV Mosby: St Louis, 1997) 340–7.
21. Bisschoff P, Flower RA, Ten years experience with choroidal angiography using ICG dye: a new routine examination or an epilogue, *Doc Ophthalmol* (1985) **60**:235–91.
22. Shimizu K, The plasticity of the choroidal circulation. Presented at the Symposium on ICG angiography at the International Congress of Ophthalmology, Amsterdam, June 1998.
23. Algvere P, Kornacki B, Fluorescein angiography of the iris: a correlation of microangiopathy in the iris and retina, *Acta Ophthalmol* (1978) **56**: 803–16.
24. Bandello F, Brancato R, Lattanzio R et al, Relation between iridopathy and retinopathy in diabetes, *Br J Ophthalmol* (1994) **78**:542–5.
25. Maruyama Y, Kishi S, Kamei Y et al, Infrared angiography of the anterior ocular segment, *Surv Ophthalmol* (1995) **39**:S40–S48.
26. Pavese T, Insler MS, Effects of extracapsular cataract extraction with posterior chamber lens implantation on the development of neovascular glaucoma in diabetics, *J Cataract Refract Surg* (1987) **13**:197–201.
27. Basad P, Setna PH, Dunne JA, Accelerated ocular neovascularization in diabetics following posterior

chamber lens implantation on the development of neovascular glaucoma in diabetics, *Br J Ophthalmol* (1990) 74:313–14.
28. Klein R, Klein BEK, Moss SE, Visual impairment in diabetes, *Ophthalmology* (1984) **91**:1–8.
29. Zeimer RC, Shahidi M, Mori MT, Benhamou E, In vivo evaluation of a non-invasive method to measure the retinal thickness in primates, *Arch Ophthalmol* (1989) **107**:1006–9.
30. Shahidi M, Ogura Y, Blair H et al, Retinal thickness analysis for quantitative assessment of diabetic macular edema, *Arch Ophthalmol* (1991) **109**:1115–19.
31. Hee MR, Izatt JA, Swanson E et al, Optical coherence tomography of the human retina, *Arch Ophthalmol* (1995) **113**:325–32.
32. Hee MR, Puliafito CA, Wong C et al, Quantitative assessment of macular oedema with optical coherence tomography, *Arch Ophthalmol* (1995) **113**:1019–29.
33. Hee MR, Puliafito RA, Duker JS et al, Topography of diabetic macular edema with optical coherence tomography, *Ophthalmology* (1998) **105**:360–70.
34. Ossoinig KC, Standardized echography: basic principles, clinical applications and results, *Int Ophthalmol Clin* (1979) **19**:127–210.
35. Green RL, Byrne SF, Diagnostic ophthalmic ultrasound. In: Ryan SJ, ed, *Retina* (CV Mosby: St Louis, 1994) 217–309.
36. McLeod D, Restori M, Ultrasonic examination in severe diabetic eye disease, *Br J Ophthalmol* (1979) **63**:533–8.
37. Poujol J, *Echography in Ophthalmology* (Masson: New York, 1985) 36–9.
38. Chu TG, Lopez PF, Cano MR et al, Posterior vitreoschisis. An echographic finding in proliferative diabetic retinopathy, *Ophthalmology* (1996) **103**:315–22.
39. Wolf S, Arend O, Toonen H et al, Retinal capillary bloodflow measurement with a scanning laser ophthalmoscope, *Ophthalmology* (1991) **98**:996–1000.
40. Arend O, Wolf S, Jung F et al, Microcirculation in patients with diabetes mellitus: dynamic and morphological analysis of perifoveal capillary network, *Br J Ophthalmol* (1991) **75**:514–18.
41. Arend O, Remky A, Harris A et al, Macular microcirculation in cystoid maculopathy of diabetic patients, *Br J Ophthalmol* (1995) **79**:628–38.
42. Riva CE, Petrig B, Blue field entoptic phenomenon and blood velocity in the retinal capillaries, *J Opt Soc Am* (1980) **70**:1234–8.
43. Fallon TJ, Chourincyzk P, Kohner EM, Measurement of retinal bloodflow in diabetes by the blue light entoptic phenomenon, *Br J Ophthalmol* (1986) **70**:43–6.
44. Fallon TJ, Maxwell DL, Kohner EM, Autoregulation of retinal bloodflow in diabetic retinopathy, measured by the bluelight entoptic technique, *Ophthalmology* (1987) **94**:1410–15.
45. Fallon TJ, Sleightholm MA, Merrick C et al, The effect of acute hyperglycemia or flow velocity in the macular capillaries, *Invest Ophthalmol Vis Sci* (1987) **28**:1027–30.
46. Davies EG, Hyer SL, Kohner EM et al, Macular blood flow response to acute reduction of plasma glucose in diabetic patients, measured by the blue field light entoptic technique, *Ophthalmology* (1990) **97**:160–4.
47. Rimmer T, Fallon TJ, Kohner EM, Long-term follow-up of retinal bloodflow in diabetes using the blue light entoptic phenomenon, *Br J Ophthalmol* (1989) **73**:1–5.
48. Grunwald JE, Riva CE, Petrig BL et al, Strict control of glycaemia: effects on bloodflow in the large retinal vessels and in the macular microcirculation, *Br J Ophthalmol* (1995) **79**:735–41.
49. Arend O, Harris A, Sponsel WE et al, Macular capillary particle velocities: a blue field and scanning laser comparison, *Graefes Arch Clin Exp Ophthalmol* (1995) **233**:244–9.
50. Grunwald JE, Riva CE, Baine J, Brucker AJ, Total retinal volumetric bloodflow in diabetic patients with poor glycemia control, *Invest Ophthalmol Vis Sci* (1992) **33**:356–63.
51. Rassam SMB, Patel V, Chen HC, Kohner EM, Regional retinal blood flow and vascular autoregulation, *Eye* (1996) **10**:331–7.
52. Grunwald JE, Riva CE, Sinclair H et al, Laser

doppler velocimetry study of retinal circulation in diabetes mellitus, *Arch Ophthalmol* (1986) **104**:991–6.
53. Patel V, Rassam S, Newsom R et al, Retinal blood flow in diabetic retinopathy, *Br Med J* (1992) **305**:678–83.
54. Grunwald JE, Dupont J, Riva CE, Retinal haemodynamics in patients with early diabetes mellitus, *Br J Ophthalmol* (1996) **80**:327–31.
55. Feke GT, Burney SM, Ogasawa H et al, Retinal circulatory abnormalities in type 1 diabetes, *Invest Ophthalmol Vis Sci* (1994) **35**:2968–75.
56. Sullivan PM, Perfitt VJ, Jagae R et al, Effect of meal on retinal bloodflow in IDDM patients, *Diabetes Care* (1991) **14**:756–8.
57. Grunwald JE, Riva CE, Martin DB et al, Effect of an insulin-induced decrease in blood glucose on the human diabetic retinal circulation, *Ophthalmology* (1987) **94**:1614–20.
58. Chen HC, Newsom RSB, Patel V et al, Retinal blood flow change during pregnancy in women with diabetes, *Invest Ophthalmol Vis Sci* (1994) **35**:3199–3208.
59. Grunwald JE, Brucker AJ, Braunstein SN et al, Strict metabolic control and retinal bloodflow in diabetes mellitus, *Br J Ophthalmol* (1994) **78**:598–604.
60. Grunwald JE, Brucker AJ, Grunwald SE, Riva CE, Retinal haemodynamics in proliferative diabetic retinopathy. A laser doppler velocimetry study, *Invest Ophthalmol Vis Sci* (1993) **34**:66–71.
61. Konno S, Feke GT, Yoshida A et al, Retinal bloodflow changes in type I diabetes. A long term follow-up study, *Invest Ophthalmol Vis Sci* (1996) **37**:1140–8.
62. Grunwald JE, Brucker AJ, Petrig BL, Riva CE, Retinal bloodflow regulation and the clinical response to panretinal photocoagulation in proliferative diabetic retinopathy, *Ophthalmology* (1989) **96**:1518–22.
63. Morgado PB, Chen HC, Patel V et al, The acute effect of smoking on retinal bloodflow in subjects with and without diabetes, *Ophthalmology* (1994) **101**:1220–6.
64. Verriest G, Further studies on acquired deficiency of color discrimination, *J Opt Soc Am* (1963) **53**:185–96.
65. Pokorny J, Smith VC, Verriest G, Pinckers AJLG, *Congenital and Acquired Color Vision Defects* (Grune & Stratton: New York, 1979) 282–4.
66. Mäntyjärvi M, Screening of diabetics who read incorrectly colour-dependent glucose test-strips, *Doc Ophthalmol* (1992) **80**:323–8.
67. Bresnick GH, Crawford J, Groo A, Urine testing inaccuracies among diabetic patients with color vision deficiency. In: Verriest G, ed, *Colour Vision Deficiencies VII. Doc. Ophthalmol. Proc. Series*, (1984) **39**:393–405.
68. Kinnear PR, Aspinall PA, Lakowski R, The diabetic eye and colour vision, *Trans Ophthalmol Soc UK* (1972) **92**:62–78.
69. Bresnick GH, Condit RS, Palta M et al, Association of Hue discrimination loss and diabetic retinopathy, *Arch Ophthalmol* (1985) **103**:1317–24.
70. Roy MS, Gunkel RD, Podgor MJ, Color vision defects in early diabetic retinopathy, *Arch Ophthalmol* (1986) **104**:225–8.
71. Vassilou G, Simonetas G, Kasnantas A, Colour vision deficiencies in young diabetics, *Mod Probl Ophthalmol* (1975) **17**:299–311.
72. Trick GL, Burde RM, Gordon MO et al, The relationship between Hue discrimination and contrast sensitivity deficits in patients with diabetes mellitus, *Ophthalmology* (1988) **95**:693–8.
73. Hardy KJ, Scardello JHB, Foster DH, Moreland JD, Effect of diabetes associated increases in lens optical density on colour discrimination in insulin-dependent diabetes, *Br J Ophthalmol* (1994) **78**:754–6.
74. Tregear SJ, Knowles PJ, Ripley LG, Coswell AG, Chromatic contrast threshold impairment in diabetes, *Eye* (1997) **11**:537–46.
75. Dean FM, Arden GB, Dornhorst A, Partial reversal of protan and tritan colour defects with inhaled oxygen in insulin-dependent diabetes subjects, *Br J Ophthalmol* (1997) **81**:27–30.
76. Kurtenbach A, Wagner V, Heer A et al, Brightness matching and colour discrimination in young diabetics without retinopathy, *Vision Res* (1994) **34**:115–22.

77. Green FD, Ghafour IM, Allan D et al, Colour vision of diabetics, *Br J Ophthalmol* (1985) **69**:533–6.
78. Brinckmann-Hansen O, Bangstad HJ, Hultgren S et al, Psychophysical visual function, retinopathy and glycemic control in insulin-dependent diabetics with normal visual acuity, *Acta Ophthalmol* (1993) **71**:230–57.
79. Peduzzi M, Longanesi L, Ascari A et al, Dépistage des altérations précoces de la vision des couleurs chez les patients diabétiques, *J Fr Ophtalmol* (1989) **12**:791–6.
80. Mäntyjärvi M, Tuppurainen K, Could colour vision tests predict or find retinopathy in diabetic school children? *Br J Ophthalmol* (1995) **79**:711–12.
81. Birch-Cox J, Defective colour vision in diabetic retinopathy before and after laser photocoagulation, *Mod Probl Ophthalmol* (1978) **19**:326–9.
82. Cambie E, Functional results following argon laser photocoagulation for diabetic retinopathy. In: Little H, Jack RL, Patz A, Forsham PH, eds, *Diabetic Retinopathy* (Thieme-Stratton: New York, 1983) 274–84.
83. Mäntyjärvi M, Colour vision in diabetics after photocoagulation treatment. A five-year follow-up, *Acta Ophthalmol* (1993) **71**:514–18.
84. Early Treatment Diabetic Retinopathy Study Research Group, ETDRS Report no. 9, Early photocoagulation for diabetic retinopathy, *Ophthalmology* (1991) **98**:766–85.
85. Arden GB, Visual loss in patients with normal visual acuity, *Trans Ophthalmol Soc UK* (1978) **98**:219–31.
86. Arden GB, The importance of measuring contrast sensitivity in cases of visual disturbance, *Br J Ophthalmol* (1978) **62**:198–209.
87. Ghafour IM, Foulds WS, Allan D, McClure F, Contrast sensitivity in diabetic subjects with and without retinopathy, *Br J Ophthalmol* (1982) **66**:492–5.
88. Moloney J, Drury MI, Retinopathy and retinal function in insulin-dependent diabetes mellitus, *Br J Ophthalmol* (1982) **66**:759–61.
89. Hyvärinen L, Laurinen P, Rovamo J, Contrast sensitivity in evaluation of visual impairment due to diabetes, *Acta Ophthalmol* (1983) **61**:94–101.
90. Della Sala S, Bertoni G, Somazzi C et al, Impaired contrast sensitivity in diabetic patients with or without retinopathy: a new technique for rapid assessment, *Br J Ophthalmol* (1985) **69**:136–42.
91. Sokol S, Moskowitz A, Skarf B et al, Contrast sensitivity in diabetics with and without background retinopathy, *Arch Ophthalmol* (1985) **103**:51–4.
92. Banford D, North RM, Dolben J et al, Longitudinal study of visual functions in young insulin-dependent diabetics, *Ophthalm Physiol Opt* (1994) **14**:339–46.
93. Bresnick GH, Diabetic retinopathy viewed as a neurosensory disorder, *Arch Ophthalmol* (1986) **104**:989–90.
94. Fracçois J, De Rouck A, ERG dans la rétinopathie diabétique et dans la rétinopathie hypertensive, *Acta Ophthalmol* (1954) **32**:391–4.
95. Karpe G, Kornerup T, Wulfing B, The clinical ERG, *Acta Ophthalmol* (1958) **36**:281–91.
96. Yonemura D, Aoki T, Tsuzuki K, Electroretinogram in diabetic retinopathy, *Arch Ophthalmol* (1962) **68**:19–24.
97. Karwoski C, Kawasaki K, Oscillatory potentials. In: Heckenlively JR, Arden GR, eds, *Principles and Practice of Clinical Electrophysiology of Vision* (CV Mosby: St Louis, 1991) 125–8.
98. Speros P, Price J, Oscillatory potentials. History, techniques and potential use in the evaluation of disturbances of the retinal circulation, *Surv Ophthalmol* (1981) **25**:237–52.
99. Yoshida A, Kohima M, Ogasawa H, Ishiko S, Oscillatory potentials and permeability of the blood retinal barrier in non-insulin-dependent diabetic patients without retinopathy, *Ophthalmology* (1991) **98**:1266–71.
100. Sakai H, Tani Y, Shirasawa E et al, Development of electroretinographic alterations in streptozotocin-induced diabetes in rats, *Ophthalmic Res* (1995) **27**:57–63.
101. Shirao Y, Kawasaki K, Electrical responses from diabetic retina, *Progr Retin Eye Res* (1998) **17**:59–76.

102. Frost-Larsen K, Christiaensen JS, Lauritzen T, Parving HH, The effect of short-term near normal blood glucose control on oscillatory potential and macular recovery time in insulin-dependent diabetic patients with longstanding dysregulation, *Acta Ophthalmol* (1989) **67**:405–8.
103. Yonemura D, Kawasaki K, New approaches to ophthalmic electrodiagnosis by retinal oscillatory potential, drug-induced responses from retinal pigment epithelium and cone potential, *Doc Ophthalmol* (1979) **48**:163–222.
104. Bresnick GH, Palta M, Temporal aspects of the electroretinogram in diabetic retinopathy, *Arch Ophthalmol* (1987) **105**:660–4.
105. Vander Torren K, Van Lith G, Oscillatory potentials in early diabetic retinopathy, *Doc Ophthalmol* (1989) **71**:375–9.
106. Juen S, Kieselbach G, Electrophysiological changes in juvenile diabetics without retinopathy, *Arch Ophthalmol* (1990) **108**:372–5.
107. Simonsen SE, Prognostic value of ERG (oscillatory potential) in juvenile diabetics, *Acta Ophthalmol* (1974) **123** (Suppl):223–4.
108. Severns ML, Johnson MA, Bresnick GH, Methodologic dependence of electroretinogram oscillatory potential amplitudes, *Doc Ophthalmol* (1994) **86**:23–31.
109. Coupland SG, A comparison of oscillatory potential and pattern electroretinogram measures in diabetic retinopathy, *Doc Ophthalmol* (1987) **66**:207–18.
110. Algvere P, Gjöttenberg M, The diagnostic value of the oscillatory potentials of the ERG and fluorescein angiography in diabetic proliferative retinopathy, *Ophthalmologica* (1974) **168**:97–108.
111. Bresnick GH, Palta M, Oscillatory potential amplitudes: relation to severity of diabetic retinopathy, *Arch Ophthalmol* (1987) **105**:929–33.
112. Simonsen SE, The value of the oscillatory potential in selecting juvenile diabetics at risk of developing proliferative retinopathy, *Acta Ophthalmol* (1980) **58**:865–78.
113. Bresnick GH, Korth K, Groo A, Palta M, Electroretinographic oscillatory potentials predict progression of diabetic retinopathy: preliminary report, *Arch ophthalmol* (1984) **102**:1307–11.
114. Bresnick GH, Palta M, Predicting progression to severe proliferative diabetic retinopathy, *Arch. Ophthalmol* (1987) **105**:810–14.
115. Brinkmann-Hansen O, Dahl-Jaegersen K, Hanssen KF, Sandvik L, Oscillatory potentials, retinopathy and long-term glucose control in insulin-dependent diabetes, *Acta Ophthalmol* (1992) **70**:705–12.
116. Roecker EB, Pulos E, Bresnick GH, Severns M, Characterization of the electroretinographic scotopic b-wave amplitude in diabetic and normal subjects, *Invest Ophthalmol Vis Sci* (1992) **33**:1575–83.
117. Aylward G, The scotopic threshold response in diabetic retinopathy, *Eye* (1989) **3**:626–37.
118. Holopigian K, Seiple W, Lorenzo M, Carr R, A comparison of photopic and scotopic electroretinographic changes in early diabetic retinopathy, *Invest Ophthalmol Vis Sci* (1992) **33**:2773–80.
119. Arden GB, Hamilton AMP, Wilson-Holt J et al, Pattern electroretinograms become abnormal when background diabetic retinopathy deteriorates to a preproliferative stage: possible use as a screening test, *Br J Ophthalmol* (1986) **70**:330–5.
120. Falsini B, Porciatti V, Scalia G et al, Steady-state pattern electroretinogram in insulin-dependent diabetics with no or minimal retinopathy, *Doc Ophthalmol* (1989) **73**:193–200.
121. Pragger T, Garcia C, Mincker D et al, The pattern electroretinogram in diabetes, *Am J Ophthalmol* (1990) **109**:279–84.
122. Henkes HE, Houtsmuller AJ, Fundus diabeticus: an evaluation of the preretinopathic stage, *Am J Ophthalmol* (1965) **60**:662–70.
123. François J, De Rouck A, Cambie E, Cartenheira-Dimin A, Electrophysiological studies before and after argon laser photocoagulation in diabetic retinopathy, *Ophthalmologica* (1978) **176**:133–44.
124. Kawasaki K, Tanabe J, Wakabayashi K, Nonphotic standing potential responses: hyperosmolarity, bicarbonate and Diamox response. In: Heckenlively JR, Arden GB, eds, *Principles and*

Practice of Clinical Electrophysiology of Vision (CV Mosby: St Louis, 1991) 163–6.

125. Mori T, Marmor MF, Miyoshi K, Tazawa Y, Combined photic and non-photic electro-oculographic responses in the clinical evaluation of the retinal pigment epithelium, *Doc Ophthalmol* (1991) **76**:315–22.

126. Parisi V, Uccioli L, Monticone G et al, Visual evoked potentials after photostress in insulin dependent diabetic patients with or without retinopathy, *Graefes Arch Clin Exp Ophthalmol* (1994) **232**:193–8.

127. Ryan S, Arden GL, Weinstein GW, Electrophysiological discrimination between retinal and optic nerve disorders, *Metabol Ped Syst Ophthalmol* (1989) **12**:69–73.

128. Magni R, Giunti S, Bianchi A et al, Single-sweep analysis using an auto-regressive with exogenous input (ARX) model, *Doc Ophthalmol* (1994) **86**:95–104.

129. Schönfeld CL, Schneider R, Körner U et al, Prognostic factors in vitreous surgery for proliferative diabetic retinopathy, *Ger J Ophthalmol* (1994) **3**:137–43.

11 Epidemiology of diabetic retinopathy

Michael W Ulbig and Jan P Hoops

CLASSIFICATION

Today's classification of diabetic retinopathy is a modified Airlie House Classification.[1] Diabetic retinopathy is subdivided into non-proliferative diabetic retinopathy and proliferative diabetic retinopathy. Non-proliferative diabetic retinopathy is graded as mild, moderate or severe depending on the number of microaneurysms, intraretinal haemorrhages, venous beading and intraretinal microvascular abnormalities (IRMAs). Cotton wool spots are also a sign of diabetic retinopathy but may indicate coexisting hypertensive retinopathy (*Fig. 11.1*). Proliferative diabetic retinopathy is characterized by epiretinal outgrowth of new vessels and finally fibrous membrane formation. The severity is graded using low-risk and high-risk criteria (*Fig. 11.2*). The high-risk criteria are as follows:

(a) Neovascularization at the disc (NVD) that is at least one-fourth to one-third of the disc area in extent.

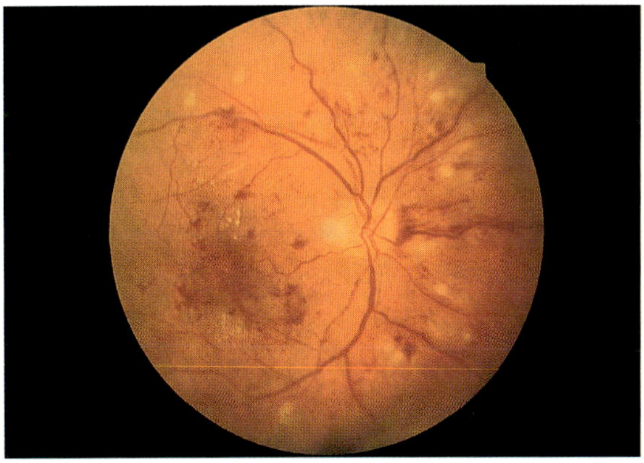

Figure 11.1
Right fundus of a 68-year-old male patient with combined hypertensive retinopathy and severe non-proliferative diabetic retinopathy. Note the multiple cotton wool spots located around the optic nerve head, especially on the nasal side, indicating coexisting arterial hypertension in a type II diabetic patient.

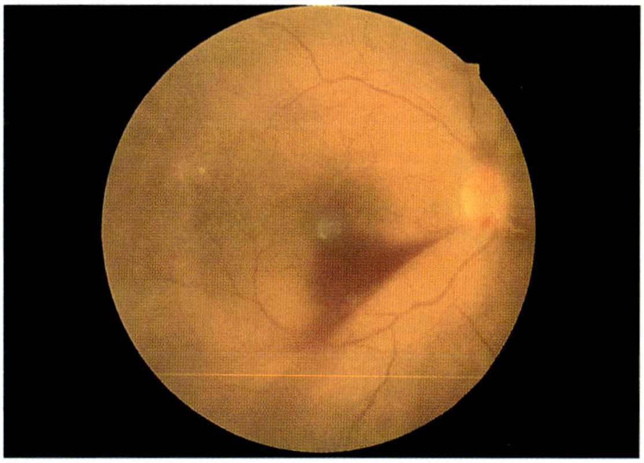

Figure 11.2
Right fundus of a 41-year-old female type I diabetic patient with high-risk proliferative diabetic retinopathy. Neovascularization at the disc (NVD) and preretinal haemorrhage are present.

(b) NVD that is associated with preretinal or vitreous haemorrhage.
(c) Neovascularization elsewhere that is at least one-half of the disc area in extent and is associated with preretinal or vitreous haemorrhage.

Diabetic macular oedema can be associated either with non-proliferative or proliferative diabetic retinopathy. The most common classification of diabetic macular oedema is based on the Early Treatment Diabetic Retinopathy Study (ETDRS) definition of clinically significant macular oedema.[2] Clinically significant macular oedema is defined as the presence of any one of the following: (a) retinal thickening at or within 500 μm of the macular centre; (b) hard exudates at or within 500 μm of the macular centre, if associated with thickening of the adjacent retina; or (c) retinal thickening of at least one disc area in extent, any part of which is within one disc diameter of the macular centre.

PREVALENCE

The Framingham Eye Study reported a 3.1% prevalence of diabetic retinopathy within a population of 2477 people aged 52–85 years.[3] In the Beaver Dam Eye Study only diabetic patients aged 43–84 years were included. The prevalence of any diabetic retinopathy was 10% for cases with newly discovered non-insulin-dependent diabetes and 37% for the entire group of 435 patients.[4] The United Kingdom Prospective Diabetes Study found 39% of men and 35% of women to have retinopathy out of 2964 patients with newly diagnosed non-insulin-dependent diabetes mellitus.[5]

The most renowned data available are from the Wisconsin Epidemiologic Study of Diabetic Retinopathy which is a population-based study of diabetic patients in southern Wisconsin, USA[6,7] (*Table 11.1*) The patients were subdivided into two groups according to their age at diagnosis of diabetes (below 30 years of age or beyond 30 years).

Data from 996 insulin-dependent younger-onset diabetics were obtained[6] (*Table 11.1*) No retinopathy was detected in 29%, non-proliferative retinopathy in 47%, and proliferative retinopathy in 23%. Seventeen per cent of patients with diabetes mellitus of less than 5 years' duration showed diabetic retinopathy in contrast to 98% after at least 15 years' duration. Non-proliferative diabetic retinopathy was found in 17% after less than 5 years', in 71% after 10 years', in 69% after 15 years', and in 42% after

Table 11.1 Prevalence of diabetic retinopathy in the Wisconsin Epidemiologic Study.

Stage of retinopathy		Prevalence (%)	
	Younger-onset insulin-dependent	Older-onset insulin-dependent	Older-onset non-insulin-dependent
None	29	30	61
Non-proliferative	47	56	36
Proliferative	23	14	3
Macular oedema	11	15	4

30 years' duration of diabetes mellitus. Proliferative diabetic retinopathy developed in none of the patients with less than 5 years of duration, in 1% after 10 years, in 25% after 15 years, and in 57% after at least 30 years. The prevalence rate of macular oedema,[8] which was defined as thickening of the retina within one disc diameter from the centre of the macula, was 11% and varied from 0% in those who had had diabetes for less than 5 years to 29% in those whose duration of diabetes was 20 or more years.

In the second group prevalence data from 696 patients with non-insulin-dependent and from 674 with insulin-dependent older-onset diabetes were evaluated[7] (*Table 11.1*). No retinopathy occurred in 30% of insulin-dependent patients, vs 61% of non-insulin-dependent subjects. Data for non-proliferative diabetic retinopathy were 56% and 36%, respectively, for proliferative retinopathy 14% and 3%. After less than 5 years' duration of diabetes, retinopathy was diagnosed in 25% of non-insulin-dependent vs 40% of insulin-dependent patients. After more than 15 years 58% vs 85% had diabetic retinopathy.

Proliferative diabetic retinopathy occurred early after diagnosis of the disease. Three per cent of non-insulin-dependent patients with diabetes for 2 years or less and 4% of insulin-dependent patients with diabetes for 3–4 years had proliferative retinopathy. After more than 15 years' duration of diabetes 4% vs 20% had proliferative diabetic retinopathy.

The prevalence rate of macular oedema[8] was 8% and varied from 3% in those who had had diabetes for less than 5 years to 28% in those whose duration of diabetes was 20 or more years. Amongst insulin-dependent diabetics, 15% had macular oedema in contrast to 4% of the non-insulin-dependent diabetics.

INCIDENCE

Again, the most renowned data available are derived from the Wisconsin Epidemiologic Study assessing the fundus changes in a diabetic population after 4 years of follow-up[9,10] (*Table 11.2*) and 10 years of follow-up[11] (*Table 11.3*).

Of the younger-onset diabetics (30 years of age or less at diagnosis of insulin-dependent diabetes mellitus) 59% of patients without retinopathy at study entrance developed it after 4 years of follow-up. Forty-one per cent of

Table 11.2 Incidence of diabetic retinopathy in the Wisconsin Epidemiologic Study after 4-year follow-up.

Initial status	Status after 4 years	Incidence of fundus changes (%)		
		Younger-onset insulin-dependent	Older-onset insulin-dependent	Older-onset non-insulin-dependent
No retinopathy	Any retinopathy	59	47	34
Any retinopathy	Deterioration	41	34	25
Any	New prolif. retinopathy	11	7	2
No macular oedema	Macular oedema	8	8	3

Table 11.3 Incidence of diabetic retinopathy in the Wisconsin Epidemiologic Study after 10-year follow-up.

Initial status	Status after 10 years	Incidence of fundus changes (%)		
		Younger-onset insulin-dependent	Older-onset insulin-dependent	Older-onset non-insulin-dependent
No retinopathy	Any retinopathy	89	79	67
Any retinopathy	Deterioration	76	69	53
Any	New prolif. retinopathy	30	24	10

subjects with diabetic retinopathy showed progression, but only 7% improvement. Eleven per cent of patients initially free of proliferative diabetic retinopathy finally developed it during the period of review.[9]

After 4 years of follow-up the data for the older-onset group (insulin-dependent group over 30) were the following: 47% development of any retinopathy, 34% deterioration of retinopathy and 7% with progression to proliferative retinopathy. The data for non-insulin-dependent patients were 34%, 25% and 2%, respectively.

The overall incidence of macular oedema (defined as thickening of the retina within one disc diameter from the centre of the macula) after a 4-year follow-up was 8% (50/610) in the younger-onset group.[12] The data for the older-onset persons using insulin were 8% (23/273) and 3% (11/379) in the group of those not using insulin.

The 10-year results[11] of the Wisconsin Epidemiologic Study were calculated for three groups (age at diagnosis of insulin-dependent diabetes less than 30 years, age at diagnosis 30 years or more (insulin-dependent or non-insulin-dependent). The 10-year incidence of retinopathy (89%, 79% and 67%), progression of retinopathy (76%, 69% and 53%), and progression to proliferative retinopathy (30%, 24% and 10%) were highest in the group diagnosed before the age of 30 years, intermediate in the insulin-dependent group diagnosed at the age of 30 years or older, and lowest in the non-insulin-dependent group, respectively.

NATURAL HISTORY

These days, the natural history of diabetic retinopathy is difficult to assess since effective laser treatment is available. Furthermore, control of diabetes mellitus has much improved in the past 20 years.

The natural history of diabetic retinopathy can be assessed in terms of the type of diabetes mellitus, change in fundus appearance and effect of retinopathy on visual outcome.[13]

Concerning the type of diabetes mellitus, insulin-dependent diabetics (type I) are more likely to have proliferative diabetic retinopathy, whereas non-insulin-dependent patients (type II) predominantly have macular oedema. Fifty per cent of all the patients with proliferative retinopathy experienced onset of diabetes before the

Table 11.4 Ten-year incidence of visual loss in diabetic subjects in the Wisconsin Study.

Group	Blindness (%) (vision ≤ 20/200)	Visual impairment (%) (vision ≤ 20/40)
Younger-onset	1.8	9.4
Older-onset taking insulin	4.0	37.2
Older-onset without insulin	4.8	23.9

age of 20, while 75% of those with diabetic macular oedema experienced onset of diabetes after the age of 40.[14]

The change in retinopathic appearance was also studied by Kohner.[14] Fifty-eight per cent of cases of mild non-proliferative retinopathy were unchanged after 4 years of follow-up, whereas 42% had progressed. Amongst the cases of severe non-proliferative diabetic retinopathy followed up for 4 years, 35% remained unchanged, 65% progressed and 14% developed proliferative retinopathy. Once macular oedema is present and remains untreated, it will increase in most cases.

Table 11.4 shows the 10-year incidence of visual loss in diabetic subjects in the Wisconsin Study.[15]

FACTORS INFLUENCING THE NATURAL COURSE

Factors that may interfere with the natural history of diabetic retinopathy are discussed below. These factors can be subdivided into systemic and ocular factors and may be listed as follows:

Systemic factors
Age
Duration of diabetes
Diabetic control
Smoking habits
Alcohol consumption
Aspirin
Arterial hypertension
Serum lipids
Renal disease
Anaemia
Contraceptive pill
Pregnancy

Ocular factors
Myopia
Glaucoma
Posterior vitreous detachment
Old chorioretinopathy
Cataract surgery
Rubeosis iridis

Systemic factors

Age

Age dictates to a very large extent the development and progression of diabetic retinopathy. Younger-onset diabetics are usually insulin-dependent and are prone to develop proliferative retinopathy, whereas late-onset patients with non-insulin-dependent diabetes are more likely to have macular oedema. In the Wisconsin Epidemiologic Study, in younger-onset patients prevalence of retinopathy was positively correlated with age.[6] It seems, however, that the correlation with age is likely to be due to development and progression of retinopathy with the duration of diabetes mellitus.

Duration of diabetes

General agreement has evolved that the duration of diabetes mellitus and severity of hyperglycaemia are fundamental risk factors for the development of diabetic retinopathy. Almost all studies of prevalence of diabetic retinopathy have proved that the duration of diabetes mellitus is a most important characteristic associated with increased risk. Once retinopathy is present, duration of diabetes appears to be a less important factor for the progression from earlier to advanced stages of retinopathy, but the degree of hyperglycaemia remains important as a risk factor for progression.[16]

In the Wisconsin Epidemiologic Study, diabetic retinopathy was uncommon before the age of 13. Those who were older than 13 years at diagnosis of diabetes mellitus were more likely to have retinopathy than those who were younger even when the duration of diabetes was considered.

Diabetic control

The metabolic control measured by the glycosylated haemoglobin level seems to be a most important prognostic factor for the incidence and progression of diabetic retinopathy. The Wisconsin Epidemiologic Study data demonstrate that there is a correlation between glycosylated haemoglobin levels and severity of retinopathy in all groups at baseline.[6–8] After a follow-up of 4 years in the younger-onset group, comparing the highest with the lowest quartile of glycosylated haemoglobin, the relative risk for developing any diabetic retinopathy was 1.9, for proliferative retinopathy 21.8 and for progression 4.0. Among older-onset insulin-dependent patients, the corresponding relative risks were 1.9, 4.0 and 2.1. Among older-onset non-insulin-dependent patients, relative risks were 4.0 for any retinopathy and 6.2 for progression. A positive correlation between incidence and progression of retinopathy and glycosylated haemoglobin was found after correction for duration of diabetes, age, sex and baseline retinopathy.[17] Furthermore, hyperglycaemia is a risk factor for diabetic macular oedema after 4-year and 10-year follow-up.[12,18]

The KROC study followed up insulin-dependent patients with non-proliferative diabetic retinopathy assigned to continuous subcutaneous insulin infusion or unchanged conventional injection treatment.[19] After 8 months of follow-up the level of glycosylated haemoglobin had profoundly improved in the continuous subcutaneous insulin infusion group but remained unchanged in the conventional treatment group. The level of retinopathy, assessed from standard photographs, progressed in both groups. Continuous subcutaneous insulin infusion was associated with slightly more deterioration. At 2 years the degree of retinopathy in the two treatment groups was indistinguishable, with a tendency to lesser overall deterioration with continuous insulin infusion.[20] It was concluded that, in diabetics with mild to moderate non-proliferative retinopathy, the acceleration of progression associated with tightened control was not sustained and did not initiate vasoproliferative deterioration in retinopathy. Another study following up type II diabetics could not find any deterioration of retinopathy associated with tightened control of blood glucose levels.[21]

The Stockholm study compared insulin-dependent diabetics with non-proliferative retinopathy and unsatisfactory blood glucose control randomized to either intensified conventional treatment (ICT) or regular treatment (RT). After 18 months the glycosylated haemoglobin (HbA_{1c}) was reduced in both groups, but significantly more in the ICT group. Thirty of the RT patients and 16 from the ICT group deteriorated with respect retinopathy.[22] After 5 years retinopathy increased in both groups, but it was worse in the RT group. The increase in retinopathy was related to the mean HbA_{1c} value during the study.[23] Similar results were published after 10-year follow-up.[24]

The Oslo study enrolled insulin-dependent diabetic patients to study possible changes in the non-proliferative retinopathy in these patients and its relation to glycaemic control.[25] After 7 years it was stated that secondary intervention by long-term lowering of $HgbA_{1C}$ had a beneficial impact on non-proliferative retinopathy.

The Diabetes Control and Complications Trial Research Group (DCCT) assessed the effect of intensive treatment of diabetes on the development and progression of long-term complications in insulin-dependent diabetes mellitus.[26] In the primary prevention cohort (726 patients without any retinopathy at baseline), intensified control reduced the adjusted mean risk for the development of retinopathy by 76%, as compared with conventional therapy. In the secondary intervention cohort (715 patients with mild retinopathy at baseline), intensive therapy slowed the progression of retinopathy down by 54% and reduced the development of proliferative or severe non-proliferative retinopathy by 47%. Overall reduction for need of photocoagulation was 56%. There seems to be a point of no return once more severe diabetic retinopathy has become established. In the presence of large areas of non-perfused retina, even perfect normoglycaemia as achieved by pancreatic transplantation is unable to protect against the development of proliferative diabetic retinopathy.[27]

In general, sudden tight diabetic control can cause a temporary progression of non-proliferative retinopathy. In the long term, however, improved control appears to delay the onset and slow down the progression of diabetic retinopathy, including diabetic macular oedema and proliferative disease.

Smoking habits

Previous studies of the association between cigarette smoking and the incidence or progression of diabetic retinopathy have produced inconsistent results. Some studies found a positive correlation[23] whereas others found none.[18,28–30]

In the Stockholm study smoking habits had an influence on the progression of retinopathy,[23] while in the same study smoking habits did not correlate with the angiographically demonstrated capillary loss and leakage.[30]

The association between cigarette smoking and the incidence of diabetic retinopathy was examined in the Wisconsin Epidemiologic Study at baseline and after 4 and 10 years of follow-up. Cigarette smoking was neither a risk factor for the long-term incidence of retinopathy[29,31] nor for the long-term incidence of macular oedema.[18]

Alcohol consumption

Few studies have examined the effect of alcohol intake on diabetic retinopathy. The Wisconsin Epidemiologic Study of diabetic retinopathy showed no significant association with incidence or progression of retinopathy,[32] although there was a hint that moderate alcohol intake could diminish the prevalence of proliferative diabetic retinopathy in the younger-onset group.[33] A study from the Veneto region in Italy found no correlation between retinopathy and alcohol intake.[34] In contrast, Young et al showed heavy alcohol consumption to be a risk factor for the development of diabetic retinopathy in patients without retinopathy at baseline.[35]

Aspirin

The ETDRS examined the influence of aspirin use on the formation and advancement of existing diabetic retinopathy and could not find any

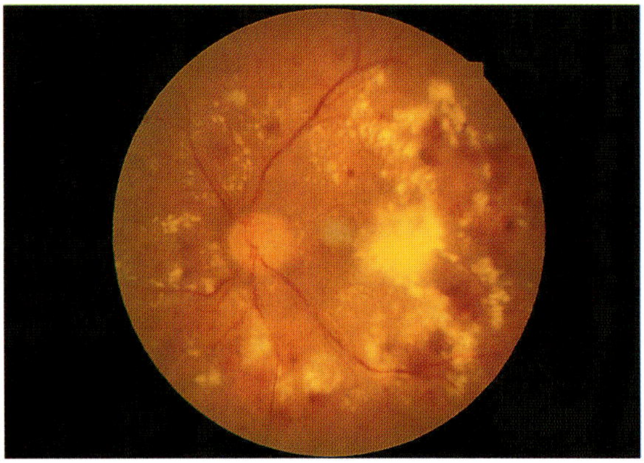

Figure 11.3
Left fundus of a 66-year-old male patient with hypertensive and diabetic retinopathy. Foveal plaque exudates are present due to long-standing uncontrolled arterial hypertension and diabetic macular oedema non-responding to focal and grid laser coagulation. Note the exudates nasally of the optic nerve head, which are a sign for coexisting arterial hypertension.

beneficial effect.[36] On the other hand 650 mg aspirin per day had no clinically important harmful effects for diabetic patients with retinopathy. The severity and duration of vitreous or preretinal haemorrhages were not significantly affected by the use of aspirin. These findings suggest that there are no ocular contraindications to aspirin when required for cardiovascular disease or any other medical indications.[37]

Arterial hypertension

The Wisconsin Epidemiologic Study demonstrated a modest correlation between hypertension and progression to proliferative retinopathy in the younger-onset group.[38] No consistent association of blood pressure and retinopathy in subjects with older-onset diabetes was observed. Mortality did not affect the correlation of blood pressure and diabetic retinopathy. Diastolic blood pressure was a risk factor for the 10-year incidence of macular oedema in the older-onset group[18] (*Fig. 11.3*).

Knowler et al stated that control of blood pressure might reduce the incidence of retinal exudates in diabetics not treated with insulin.[39] In an Italian study, the prevalence of retinopathy was significantly related to both systolic and diastolic blood pressure.[34] Bodansky et al found an association between hypertension and proliferative retinopathy.[40]

Serum lipids

Several investigators have reported on the relation of cholesterol or triglycerides and diabetic retinopathy, but the results were not consistent. The ETDRS demonstrated that elevated serum lipid levels are associated with an increased risk of retinal hard exudate formation in persons with diabetic retinopathy.[41] In the Wisconsin Epidemiologic Study, cholesterol was not a significant factor with the respect to the severity of retinopathy in any group examined, but was a significant factor with respect to the severity of retinal hard exudates.[42] Diastolic blood pressure added significantly to explaining the severity of hard exudates in older-onset insulin users. These data support the current management strategies for diabetes, which include control of level of glycaemia, blood pressure and blood lipids.

Renal disease

Diabetic nephropathy aggravates retinopathy too, an effect that may be mediated through an increase in blood pressure, fibrinogen levels and lipoproteins.[43] The preferred mode of treatment to control renal failure in respect to visual acuity is renal transplantation and peritoneal dialysis as compared to haemodialysis.[27]

Anaemia

There are single case reports on the association of severe anaemia and diabetic retinopathy.[44,45] Recent data support the view that treating anaemia slows down the progression of diabetic retinopathy.[16]

Contraceptive pill

Progression of diabetic retinopathy is known to occur with the use of high-dose progesterone pills.[13] The use of modern low-level hormone pills among young women with insulin-dependent diabetes mellitus does not seem to pose an additional risk for the development of early diabetic retinopathy.[46] The effect of hormone replacement therapy in the elderly female diabetic is as yet uncertain.

Pregnancy

Pregnancy may accelerate the development or advancement of diabetic retinopathy.[47,48] Risk factors are pregnancy per se, hypertension, hyperglycaemia, rapid normalization of blood glucose levels, duration of diabetes and stage of retinopathy at baseline.[47,49] Therefore, blood glucose levels should be normalized slowly over a period of 6–8 months prior to conception.

Patients without any retinopathy or with mild non-proliferative retinopathy when pregnant are at low risk for progression of retinopathy.[47,50] In contrast, an untreated proliferative diabetic retinopathy will progress in 58% of cases during pregnancy.[50] If proliferative diabetic retinopathy is treated before pregnancy, progression rate is reduced to 26%.

Ocular factors

Myopia, glaucoma, old chorioretinopathy

High myopia with choroidal degeneration, glaucoma, and extensive old chorioretinopathy all protect against diabetic retinopathy and are believed to act in the same way as panretinal photocoagulation by reducing the metabolic needs of the retina.[51,52]

Posterior vitreous detachment

A complete posterior vitreous detachment may prevent the development of proliferative diabetic retinopathy because the hyaloid is needed as a scaffold for retinal neovascularization.[53] An attached posterior hyaloid has also been associated with an increased risk of macular oedema.[54,55]

Cataract surgery, rubeosis iridis

Removal of a cataract may aggravate both existing macular oedema and non-proliferative or proliferative retinopathy and may hasten the onset of rubeosis.[56,57] After extracapsular cataract surgery or phacoemulsification with implantation of a posterior chamber lens, progression of mild diabetic retinopathy is reported in up to 18% of cases.[58–60] An intracapsular operation with implantation of an anterior chamber lens is associated with a higher rate of progression of retinopathy. In cases of active proliferative retinopathy, progression occurs in up to 65% after cataract surgery. No major studies are available concerning the influence of intraocular lens implantation, but clinical experience gives the impression that intraocular lens implantation itself is not a risk factor for progression of diabetic retinopathy.[61] After uncomplicated cataract surgery in diabetic eyes, anterior hyaloidal fibrovascular proliferation, which is common in vitrectomized phacic diabetic eyes,[62] can occur as shown by Ulbig et al.[63] Therefore, retinopathy should be treated prior to cataract surgery provided the cataract is not too dense and allows access for photocoagulation.

REFERENCES

1. Early Treatment Diabetic Retinopathy Study Research Group, Grading diabetic retinopathy from stereoscopic colour fundus photographs – an extension of the modified Airlie House Clas-

sification: ETDRS report No 10, *Ophthalmology* (1991) **98**(Suppl 5):786–806.
2. Early Treatment Diabetic Retinopathy Study Research Group, Photocoagulation for diabetic macular edema: Early Treatment Diabetic Retinopathy Study Report no. 1, *Arch Ophthalmol* (1985) **103**:1796–806.
3. Kini MM, Leibowitz HM, Colton T et al, Prevalence of senile cataract, diabetic retinopathy, senile macular degeneration, and open-angle glaucoma in the Framingham eye study, *Am J Ophthalmol* (1978) **85**:28–34.
4. Klein R, Klein BEK, Moss SE, Linton KLP, The Beaver Dam Eye Study. Retinopathy in adults with newly discovered and previously diagnosed diabetes mellitus, *Ophthalmology* (1992) **99**: 58–62.
5. Kohner EM, Aldington SJ, Stratton IM et al, United Kingdom Prospective Diabetes Study, 30: diabetic retinopathy at diagnosis of non-insulin-dependent diabetes mellitus and associated risk factors, *Arch Ophthalmol* (1998) **116**:297–303.
6. Klein R, Klein BEK, Moss SE et al, The Wisconsin Epidemiologic Study of Diabetic Retinopathy. II. Prevalence and risk of diabetic retinopathy when age at diagnosis is less than 30 years, *Arch Ophthalmol* (1984) **102**:520–6.
7. Klein R, Klein BEK, Moss SE et al, The Wisconsin Epidemiologic Study of Diabetic Retinopathy. III. Prevalence and risk of diabetic retinopathy when age at diagnosis is 30 or more years, *Arch Ophthalmol* (1984) **102**:527–32.
8. Klein R, Klein BEK, Moss SE et al, The Wisconsin Epidemiologic Study of Diabetic Retinopathy. IV. Diabetic macular edema, *Ophthalmology* (1984) **91**:1464–74.
9. Klein R, Klein BEK, Moss SE et al, The Wisconsin Epidemiologic Study of Diabetic Retinopathy. IX. Four-year incidence and progression of diabetic retinopathy when age at diagnosis is less than 30 years, *Arch Ophthalmol* (1989) **107**:237–43.
10. Klein R, Klein BE, Moss SE et al, The Wisconsin Epidemiologic Study of Diabetic Retinopathy. X. Four-year incidence and progression of diabetic retinopathy when age at diagnosis is 30 years or more, *Arch Ophthalmol* (1989) **107**:244–9.
11. Klein R, Klein BEK, Moss SE, Cruickshanks KJ, The Wisconsin Epidemiologic Study of Diabetic Retinopathy. XIV. Ten-year incidence and progression of diabetic retinopathy, *Arch Ophthalmol* (1994) **112**:1217–28.
12. Klein R, Moss SE, Klein BEK et al, The Wisconsin Epidemiologic Study of Diabetic Retinopathy. XI. The incidence of macular edema, *Ophthalmology* (1989) **96**:1501–10.
13. Ulbig MRW, Hamilton AMP, Factors influencing the natural history of diabetic retinopathy, *Eye* (1993) **7**:242–9.
14. Kohner EM, The evolution and natural history of diabetic retinopathy, *Int Ophthalmol Clin* (1978) **18**:1–16.
15. Moss SE, Klein R, Klein BEK, Ten-year incidence of visual loss in a diabetic population, *Ophthalmology* (1994) **101**:1061–70.
16. Davis MD, Fisher MR, Gangnon RE et al, Risk factors for high-proliferative diabetic retinopathy and severe visual loss: Early Treatment Diabetic Retinopathy Study Report no. 18, *Invest Ophthalmol Vis Sci* (1998) **39**:233–52.
17. Klein R, Klein BEK, Moss SE et al, Glycosylated hemoglobin predicts the incidence and progression of diabetic retinopathy, *JAMA* (1988) **260**:2864–71.
18. Klein R, Klein BEK, Moss SE, Cruickshanks KJ, The Wisconsin Epidemiologic Study of Diabetic Retinopathy. XV. The long-term incidence of macular edema, *Ophthalmology* (1995) **102**: 7–16.
19. KROC Collaborative Study Group, Blood glucose control and the evolution of diabetic retinopathy and albuminuria. A preliminary multicenter trial, *N Engl J Med* (1984) **311**:365–72.
20. KROC Collaborative Study Group, Diabetic retinopathy after two years of intensified insulin treatment. Follow-up of the KROC Collaborative Study, *JAMA* (1988) **260**:37–41.
21. Emanuele N, Klein R, Abraira C et al, Evaluations of retinopathy in the VA Cooperative Study on Glycemic Control and Complications in Type II Diabetes (VA CSDM). A feasibility study, *Diabetes Care* (1996) **19**:1375–81.

22. Reichard P, Britz A, Cars I et al, The Stockholm Diabetes Intervention Study (SDIS): 18 months' results, *Acta Med Scand* (1988) **224**:115–22.
23. Reichard P, Berglund B, Britz A et al, Intensified conventional insulin treatment retards the microvascular complications of insulin-dependent diabetes mellitus (IDDM): the Stockholm Diabetes Intervention Study (SDIS) after 5 years, *J Intern Med* (1991) **230**:101–8.
24. Reichard P, Pihl M, Rosenqvist U, Sule J, Complications in IDDM are caused by elevated blood glucose level: the Stockholm Diabetes Intervention Study (SDIS) at 10-year follow up, *Diabetologia* (1996) **39**:1483–8.
25. Brinchmann-Hansen O, Dahl-Jorgensen K, Sandvik L, Hanssen KF, Blood glucose concentrations and progression of diabetic retinopathy: the seven year results of the Oslo study, *BMJ* (1992) **304**:19–22.
26. The Diabetes Control and Complications Trial Research Group, The effect of intensive treatment of diabetes on the development and progression of long-term complications in insulin-dependent diabetes mellitus, *N Engl J Med* (1993) **329**:977–86.
27. Ulbig M, Kampik A, Thurau S et al, Long-term follow-up of diabetic retinopathy for up to 71 months after combined renal and pancreatic transplantation, *Graefes Arch Clin Exp Ophthalmol* (1991) **229**:242–5.
28. Chase HP, Garg SK, Marshall G et al, Cigarette smoking increases the risk of albuminuria among subjects with type I diabetes, *JAMA* (1991) **265**:614–17.
29. Moss SE, Klein R, Klein BEK, Cigarette smoking and ten-year progression of diabetic retinopathy, *Ophthalmology* (1996) **103**:1438–42.
30. Reichard P, Sule J, Rosenqvist U, Capillary loss and leakage after five years of intensified insulin treatment in patients with insulin-dependent diabetes mellitus, *Ophthalmology* (1991) **98**: 1587–93.
31. Moss SE, Klein R, Klein BEK, Association of cigarette smoking with diabetic retinopathy, *Diabetes Care* (1991) **14**:119–26.
32. Moss SE, Klein R, Klein BEK, The association of alcohol consumption with the incidence and progression of diabetic retinopathy, *Ophthalmology* (1994) **101**:1962–8.
33. Moss SE, Klein R, Klein BEK, Alcohol consumption and the prevalence of diabetic retinopathy, *Ophthalmology* (1992) **99**:926–32.
34. Segato T, Midena E, Grigoletto F et al, The epidemiology and prevalence of diabetic retinopathy in the Veneto region of north east Italy. Veneto Group for Diabetic Retinopathy, *Diabet Med* (1991) **8**:S11–6.
35. Young RJ, McCulloch DK, Prescott RJ, Clarke BF, Alcohol: another risk factor for diabetic retinopathy? *Br Med J Clin Res Ed* (1984) **288**:1035–7.
36. Early Treatment Diabetic Retinopathy Study Research Group, Effects of aspirin treatment on diabetic retinopathy. ETDRS Report no. 8, *Ophthalmology* (1991) **98**(Suppl 5):757–65.
37. Chew EY, Klein ML, Murphy RP et al, Effects of aspirin on vitreous/preretinal hemorrhage in patients with diabetes mellitus. Early Treatment Diabetic Retinopathy Study Report No. 20, *Arch Ophthalmol* (1995) **113**:52–5.
38. Klein BEK, Klein R, Moss SE, Palta M, A cohort study of the relationship of diabetic retinopathy to blood pressure [published erratum appears in *Arch Ophthalmol* (1996) **114**:109]. *Arch Ophthalmol* (1995) **113**:601–6.
39. Knowler WC, Bennett PH, Ballintine EJ, Increased incidence of retinopathy in diabetics with elevated blood pressure. A six-year follow-up study in Pima Indians, *N Engl J Med* (1980) **302**:645–50.
40. Bodansky HJ, Cudworth AG, Drury PL, Kohner EM, Risk factors associated with severe proliferative retinopathy in insulin-dependent diabetes mellitus, *Diabetes Care* (1982) **5**:97–100.
41. Chew EY, Klein ML, Ferris III FL et al, Association of elevated serum lipid levels with retinal hard exudate in diabetic retinopathy. Early Treatment Diabetic Retinopathy Study (ETDRS) Report no. 22, *Arch Ophthalmol* (1996) **114**:1079–84.

42. Klein BEK, Moss SE, Klein R, Surawicz TS, The Wisconsin Epidemiologic Study of Diabetic Retinopathy. XIII. Relationship of serum cholesterol to retinopathy and hard exudate, *Ophthalmology* (1991) **98**:1261–5.
43. Kostraba JN, Klein R, Dorman JS et al, The epidemiology of diabetes complications study. IV. Correlates of diabetic background and proliferative retinopathy, *Am J Epidemiol* (1991) **133**:381–91.
44. Berman DH, Friedman EA, Partial absorption of hard exudates in patients with diabetic end-stage renal disease and severe anemia after treatment with erythropoietin, *Retina* (1994) **14**:1–5.
45. Shorb SR, Anemia and diabetic retinopathy, *Am J Ophthalmol* (1985) **100**:434–6.
46. Garg SK, Chase HP, Marshall G et al, Oral contraceptives and renal and retinal complications in young women with insulin-dependent diabetes mellitus, *JAMA* (1994) **271**:1099–102.
47. Axer-Siegel R, Hod M, Fink-Cohen S et al, Diabetic retinopathy during pregnancy, *Ophthalmology* (1996) **103**:1815–19.
48. Moloney JB, Drury MI, The effect of pregnancy on the natural course of diabetic retinopathy, *Am J Ophthalmol* (1982) **93**:745–56.
49. Jovanovic-Peterson L, Peterson CM, Diabetic retinopathy, *Clin Obstet Gynecol* (1991) **34**:516–25.
50. Sunnes JS, The pregnant woman's eye, *Surv Ophthalmol* (1988) **32**:219–38.
51. Boulton M, Patel B, Khaliq A et al, Modulators and milieu in preretinal neovascularisation, *Eye* (1992) **6**:650–5.
52. Moss SE, Klein R, Klein BEK, Ocular factors in the incidence and progression of diabetic retinopathy, *Ophthalmology* (1994) **101**:77–83.
53. Akiba J, Arzabe CW, Trempe CL, Posterior vitreous detachment and neovascularization in diabetic retinopathy, *Ophthalmology* (1990) **97**:889–91.
54. Nasrallah FP, Jalkh AE, van Coppenolle F et al, The role of the vitreous in diabetic macular edema, *Ophthalmology* (1988) **95**:1335–9.
55. Lewis H, Abrams GW, Blumenkranz MS, Campo RV, Vitrectomy for diabetic macular traction and edema associated with posterior hyaloidal traction, *Ophthalmology* (1992) **99**:753–9.
56. Benson WE, Brown GC, Tasman W et al, Extracapsular cataract extraction with placement of a posterior chamber lens in patients with diabetic retinopathy, *Ophthalmology* (1993) **100**:730–8.
57. Schatz H, Atienza D, McDonald HR, Johnson RN, Severe diabetic retinopathy after cataract surgery, *Am J Ophthalmol* (1994) **117**:314–21.
58. Fung WE, Phacoemulsification and implantation of posterior chamber intraocular lens in eyes with quiescent proliferative diabetic retinopathy, *Graefes Arch Clin Exp Ophthalmol* (1987) **225**:251–3.
59. Pollack A, Leiba H, Bukelman A et al, The course of diabetic retinopathy following cataract surgery in eyes previously treated by laser photocoagulation, *Br J Ophthalmol* (1992) **76**:228–31.
60. Sebestyen JG, Intraocular lenses and diabetes mellitus, *Am J Ophthalmol* (1986) **101**:425–8.
61. Cunliffe IA, Flanagan DW, George ND et al, Extracapsular cataract surgery with lens implantation in diabetics with and without proliferative retinopathy, *Br J Ophthalmol* (1991) **75**:9–12.
62. Lewis H, Abrams GW, Williams GA, Anterior hyaloidal fibrovascular proliferation after diabetic vitrectomy, *Am J Ophthalmol* (1987) **104**:607–13.
63. Ulbig MRW, Hykin PG, Foss AJE et al, Anterior hyaloidal fibrovascular proliferation after extracapsular cataract extraction in diabetic eyes, *Am J Ophthalmol* (1993) **115**:321–6.

12 The blood–retinal barrier in diabetes

José G Cunha-Vaz

THE BLOOD–RETINAL BARRIER

The most important function of the blood–retinal barrier (BRB) is maintenance of the homeostasis of the retinal environment by separating the retina from the blood circulation. The organization of the BRB is such that the retina is protected from blood-borne compounds, since a strict homeostasis of the neuronal environment and intact barrier is essential for optimal retinal functioning.

The BRB is formed by a complex cellular system of endothelial cells, retinal glial cells and retinal pigmented epithelial cells. The retina does have two sites of direct relationship with the blood, namely, at the level of the retinal vessels and at the chorioretinal interface – the inner and outer BRB, respectively.

In the inner BRB, the lumen of the retinal capillaries is covered by endothelial cells which are the first structure in the frontier separating the blood and the retinal tissue (*Fig. 12.1*). The retinal endothelial cells (RECs) have various functional and morphological differences in comparison with endothelial cells derived from peripheral organs. The RECs possess narrow

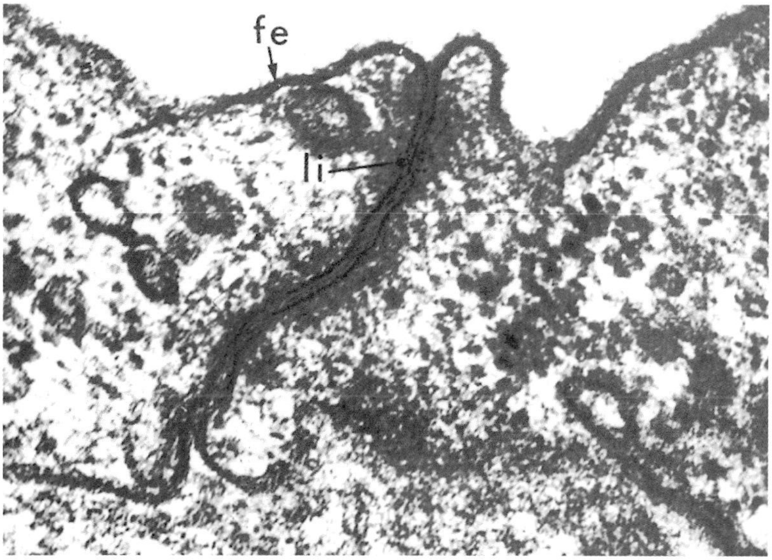

Figure 12.1
Small retinal vessel of a rabbit showing a junction between two endothelial cells. An extensive zonula occludens is visible all along the junction. The outer leaflets (fe) of the lateral cell membranes of two adjoining cells fuse into an intermediate line (li). Specimen fixed in osmium tetroxide stained in block with KMn 04 and embedded in Epon. Uranyl acetate and lead citrate stained section. ×124 000.

intercellular tight junctional structures.[1] The tight junctions are composed of a complex of belt-like zonula occludens. These narrow tight junctions hinder paracellular transport of hydrophilic compounds across the endothelium. The absence of fenestrae in the endothelial plasma membrane and little pinocytotic vesicular activity together with high densities of mitochondria are other prominent morphological features of the RECs.

Accessory roles are played by the astrocytes, which project their endfeet to the vessel walls, influencing the barrier function of these cells and the pericytes.

In the outer BRB, the retinal pigmented epithelium (RPE) is the main structure to be crossed or opposed by any substance originating from the blood and making its way into the retina. Adjacent epithelial cells are united by extensive zonulae occludentes very similar to the ones described between the RECs. The RPE is formed by highly polarized cells which play a fundamental role in the visual process. These cells are characterized by numerous folds in their basal and apical membranes and high mitochondrial density.

Certain enzymes residing selectively in the RECs and RPE constitute a metabolic barrier contributing to the protective function of the BRB. Rather high activities of barrier-selective enzymes have been detected in these cells, such as angiotensin-converting enzyme, dopa decarboxylase, γ-glutamyl transpeptidase (γ-GTP), pseudocholinesterase, monoaminoxidases and alkaline phosphatase. Most of these enzymes are involved in the degradation of neurotransmitters released in the retina and also compounds that have entered the BRB cells can be degraded into metabolites. Na^+ K^+ ATPase is localized predominantly in the abluminal membrane of the RECs, catalysing active transport of K^+ and Na^+ between blood and the retinal extracellular fluid.

Astrocytes and Müller cells surround the retinal vessels and appear to play an important role in the development and maintenance of the BRB characteristics. Astrocytic processes are not joined together and therefore allow substances that have crossed the endothelial barrier to diffuse into the retina. However, the presence of astrocytes is apparently required to differentiate a tight BRB.[2]

Transport across the BRB

The presence of the BRB has major implications for the passage of relatively large and hydrophilic compounds into the retina. As a result, essential nutrients must be transported by means of selective carrier mechanisms. Several transport systems have been characterized, varying from passive transport (like diffusion) to active and energy-requiring processes.

Bleeker and Maas[3] showed a good correlation between diffusion across the BRB and penetration into the vitreous, and lipid solubility of compounds. Lipid-soluble substances penetrated according to their oil/water partition coefficient, the more fat-soluble substances penetrating more easily.

A review of the molecular size and penetration rate of a variety of substances across the BRB shows that substances like inulin (r-14 Å) and sucrose (r-5.3 Å) do not penetrate easily into the vitreous, whereas smaller molecules, like glycerol (r-3 Å) and sodium (r-2.5 Å), were described as penetrating very slowly.

Personal studies in collaboration with David Maurice[4] produced the first approximate value for the permeability coefficient of a substance at the level of the BRB. The results obtained showed that fluorescein, which has a molecular radius of approximately 5.5 Å, has a permeability coefficient at the BRB in the order of 0.14×10^{-5} cm/second comparable to the value for the BRB for fructose, 0.16×10^{-5} cm/second. It is particularly interesting to compare the value obtained for the permeability of the BRB to fluorescein with the value found by Darson and Danielli[5] for the permeability of a cell to sucrose (5.3 Å). The passive transfer at the level of the BRB appears, therefore, to be extremely restricted, being similar to that considered for cellular permeability in general.

Specific carrier systems mediating active transport of certain compounds into the retina have been identified. A selective glucose carrier system has been characterized, transporting 2–deoxyglucose, mannose, galactose and glucose with a high capacity. In the brain vessels Glut-1 (55 kDa) is expressed asymetrically both at the abluminal and luminal membrane of the endothelial cell.

An active transport for organic anions has also been demonstrated at both the inner and outer BRBs. Fluorescein has the characteristics of an organic anion. Using fluorophotometry techniques it was possible to characterize this active transport in a situation of 'uphill' gradient and using various inhibitors, competitive and metabolic. This transport showed a clear analogy with other transport systems for organic anions existing in the body, indicating that all ions with similar characteristics are actively transported by the BRB.

The function of this active transport process, at the level of the BRB, appears to be to block the penetration of organic anions from the blood into the retinal tissue and to pump them out whenever they are present. This pumping process may therefore be considered as an important part of the barrier mechanism especially for the removal of toxic agents from the retina.

In the brain, three high-affinity amino acid carrier systems have been described for large neutral amino acids, for basic amino acids and for acidic amino acids, respectively. Furthermore, carrier systems for purine, thiamine, monocarboxylic acid and thyroid hormones have been identified.

Finally, proteins can be transported through the barrier endothelial cells into the retina by means of receptor-mediated transcytosis. The initial step in this process is the specific interaction of a ligand with its receptor on the luminal side of the endothelial cell. After association, the complex of receptor and ligand is endocytosed and endosomes cross the cell cytoplasm by means of diffusion without interaction with lysosomic vesicles. Receptor-mediated exocytosis at the abluminal side of the endothelial cell releases the peptide into the brain interstitial space. One of the proteins that can cross the BRB in this manner is transferrin, for which the retinal endothelial cell possesses a relatively high density of receptors.

The insulin-like growth factors I and II (IGF) and insulin can also be transported through the endothelium by means of transcytosis.

Assessment of BRB

Tracer particles in experimental studies and the clinical use of fluorescein angiography were the first methods used to assess the BRB. During the past decades the emphasis of BRB research has changed from qualitative studies demonstrating alterations of the BRB using fluorescein angiography (*Fig. 12.2*) to quantitative investigation using vitreous fluorometry (*Fig. 12.3*). It is important to realize that present knowledge on the permeability of the BRB refers generally to the BRB as a whole, including both outer and inner barriers, because information on differences in the permeability rates between these parts of the BRB is very scant and has been obtained only in experimental situations.

Measurement of in vivo transport

The presence of concentration gradients within the intraocular fluids and between intraocular fluids and blood represents the best physiological criterion for the existence and direction of

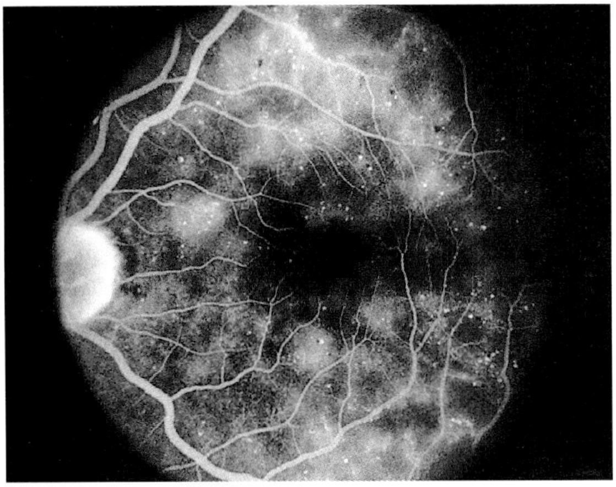

Figure 12.2
Fluorescein angiography of a diabetic eye showing multiple microaneurysms and leakage, demonstrating well the alteration of the blood–retinal barrier.

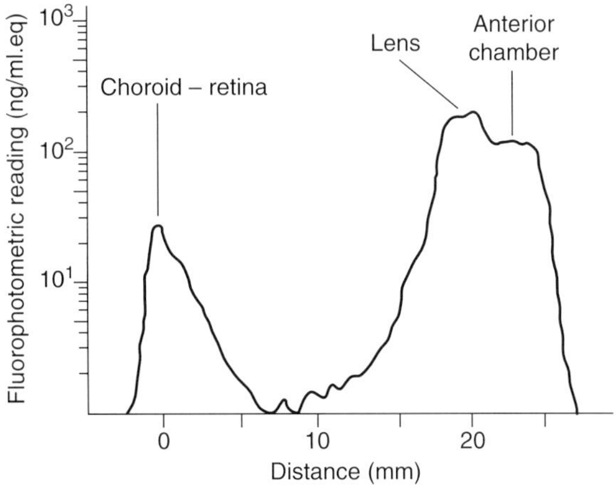

Figure 12.3
Diagram of the ocular fluorometry recording demonstrating the positioning of the choroid–retina interface and the lens posterior and anterior peaks. The presence of fluorescence in the vitreous and anterior chamber is due to penetration of fluorescein into the eye after its intravenous injection.

transport processes across the BRB. It requires detailed knowledge on the concentrations of the substances within all regions of the intraocular fluids.

During the last two decades, a method has been extensively used in clinical and experimental ophthalmology to measure the permeability of fluorescein in the BRB: vitreous fluorophotometry (VF). Fluorescein, the tracer used, has a small molecular size and is actively transported by the retinal vessels and the retinal pigmented epithelium, making this method a highly sensitive probe to study the barrier function.

Vitreous fluorophotometry, originally introduced by Cunha-Vaz et al,[6] reflects the behaviour of fluorescein as it penetrates into the chambers of the eye, allowing the examination of the dynamics of the intraocular fluids, and traverses the blood–ocular barriers demonstrating their properties of permeability to fluorescein.

After systemic administration, the distribution of fluorescein in the vitreous of the normal eye follows a well-defined pattern which constitutes the fluorometric recording and gives much information regarding the retina–vitreous interface and other intraocular compartments (*Fig. 12.4*).

The fluorescein concentration contours in the vitreous, recorded at 1, 2, 3, 4 and 5 hours following a single intravenous administration of fluorescein (14 mg/kg), show clearly that fluorescein penetrates into the vitreous of the normal eye from two main sources. Anteriorly, from the ciliary body and aqueous humor, and posteriorly, from the retinal and choroid vessels through the BRB.

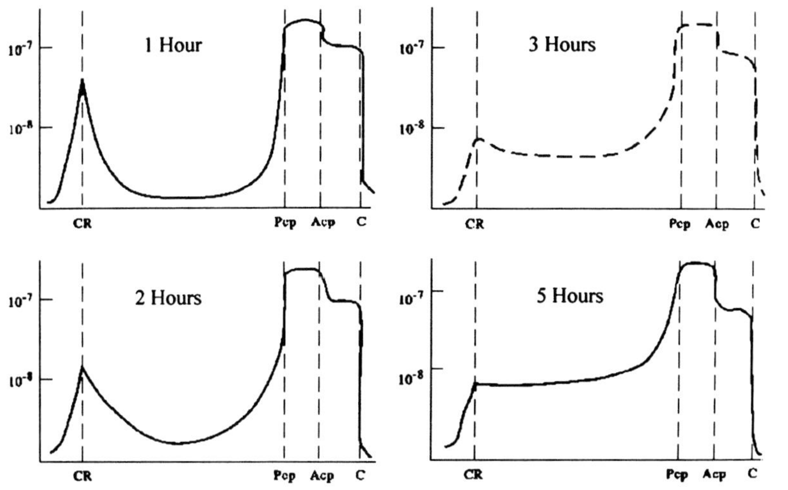

Figure 12.4
Diagram showing fluorescein contours in the normal eye at various time intervals after an intravenous fluorescein injection. CR, Choroid–retina; Pcp and Acp, posterior and anterior limits of the lens; C, cornea.

The inward permeability across the BRB can be estimated by calculating the mass of fluorescein that penetrated posteriously into the vitreous and the integral over time of the free plasma fluorescein concentration.

A formula representing these values is:

$$Pin = Cv(r) \times \mathrm{dv} \,/\, Cp\ (t) \times \mathrm{dt}$$

where *Pin* is the inward permeability; *Cv (r)* is the concentration in the vitreous at location r; dv is a volume element; *Cp (t)* is the time element. The movements of fluorescein should be measured within the first hours after systemic administration when transport may still be ignored.[7]

Values for BRB permeability coefficient obtained by different authors have shown good agreement. The European Clinical Network of Ocular Fluorometry, using a dedicated software, and the Fluorotron Master, found a mean value of $1.97 \pm 0.93 \times 10^{-7}$ cm/second on data collected from six centres for a total of 81 healthy volunteers.[8]

When performing VF, important information is obtained not only from the value of inward permeability of the BRB, which quantifies its function in health and disease, but also from the configuration of the recording. It is also possible to calculate the outward transport of the BRB (*Pout*).

The major advantage of the determination of BRB *Pout* is the information given on BRB function, because of its probable reversibility in the early stages of disease and the fact that further development of these measurements may dispense with blood sampling.

VF remains the only available method that can quantify an alteration of the BRB. It appears also to be particularly suited for the early detection of functional changes of the BRB, before lesions are visible in the retina on ophthalmoscopy or fluorescein angiography,[6,9] because the vitreous must not be detached in order for the method to give reliable results.

Recently, a retinal leakage analyser was developed to measure localized alterations of the BRB while simultaneously imaging the retina.[10,11] The instrument is based on a prototype Zeiss confocal scanning laser ophthalmoscope that was

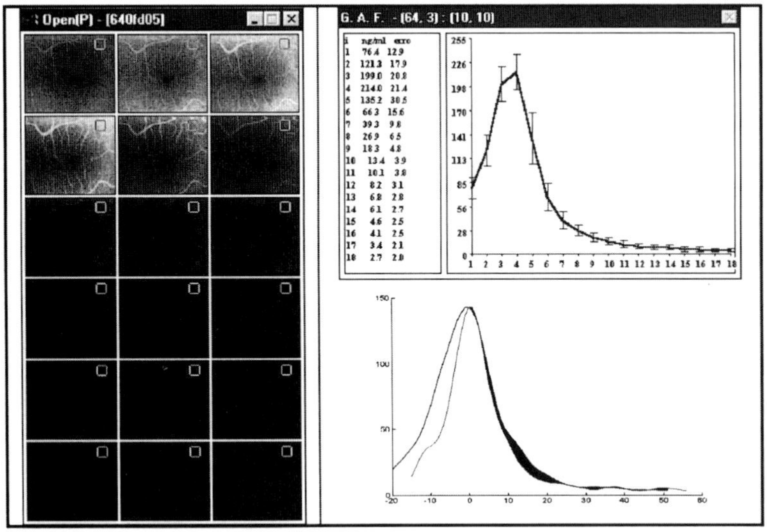

Figure 12.5
Retinal leakage analyser. Left: scan obtained 5 minutes after injection showing the 18 images. Top right: fluorometric profile of the 18 images. Bottom right: subtraction of two profiles (e.g. 30 and 5 minutes). The shaded area represents the fluorescein that penetrated into the vitreous.

modified into a confocal scanning laser fluorometer (*Fig. 12.5*).

Measurement of in vitro BRB transport

A major limitation of in vivo models is the difficulty of determining the relative contribution of the two components of the BRB. One approach to this problem is to study in vitro the transport processes in isolated preparations of retinal pigmented epithelium and retinal capillaries.

Different methodologies have been developed.

In vitro utilization of the Ussing–Zerahn chamber methodology, in which accurate transmembrane tracer flux measurements under short-circuited conditions are performed, has been another alternative. This technique has been widely and successfully used in studies involving the choroid-retina interface.[12] In contrast with an increasing number of studies in isolated retinal pigmented epithelium, the study of the permeability characteristics in the retinal vasculature was limited mainly owing to the difficulty in dissecting and isolating these structures.

In vitro studies have been performed in isolated retinal vessel[13] and in primary cultures of microvascular endothelial cells.[14]

However, transport studies using the methods mentioned are very limited because of the difficulties involved in maintaining polarity of the cells involved.

We have developed an experimental model which is suitable for the study in vitro of the permeability of normal and diabetic retinal vessels using microperfusion techniques adapted from kidney tubule studies.[15,16] Segments of retinal arterioles are isolated with forceps by freehand dissection and mounted on a microperfusion apparatus (*Fig. 12.6*). The retinal vessels of the rabbit are uniquely appropriate for these studies because of their location, lying free on the surface of the retina in the vitreous, thus permitting easy isolation (*Fig. 12.7*).

Finally, a variety of tracer particles have been used to study the permeability of the BRB in experimental situations. Carbon particles, horseradish peroxidase, natural albumin identification and lanthanum are only a few of the tracers used,

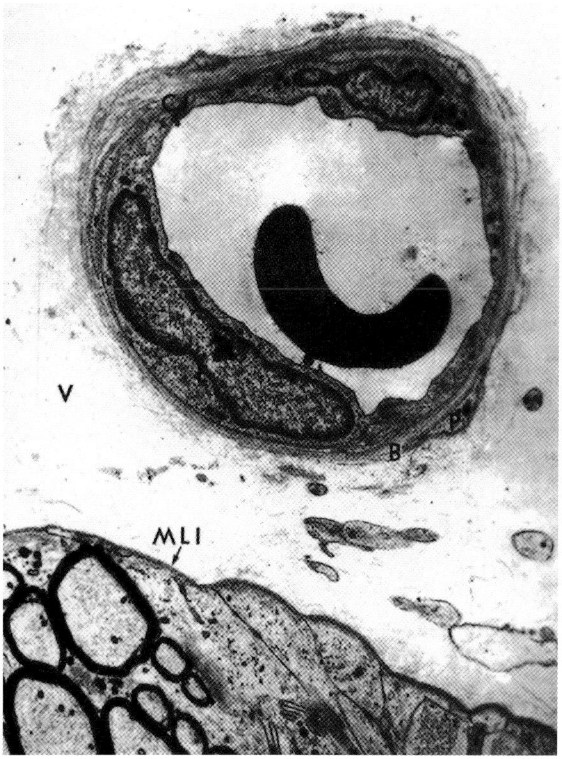

Figure 12.6
Section of a rabbit retinal vessel seen in the electron microscope. The direct contact of the vitreous humour with the endothelial cells and the tight cellular junctions should be noted. Osmium tetroxide fixed, embedded in araldite. Section stained with uranyl acetate and lead citrate. MLI = Internal limiting membrane; V = vitreous.

generally associated with histochemical methods or using electron microscopy.

BLOOD–RETINAL BARRIERS IN DIABETES MELLITUS

Since the early 1950s, two research groups have contributed significantly to our understanding of the pathological picture of diabetic retinopathy: Ashton and his group[17] and Cogan and his co-workers[18] in Boston. Injection and digestion techniques allowed the observation and characterization of the initial vascular changes occurring in diabetic retinal disease. The first changes are limited to the cellular constituents of the retinal vessels, involving both the endothelial cells and pericytes. Microaneurysms appear associated with endothelial proliferation, being localized predominantly on the venous side of the retinal circulation. With progression of the disease the capillaries on the arterial side show increased cell loss and capillary closure.

From these observations the endothelial cells were seen to be affected from the earlier stages of diabetic retinopathy. When the BRB was found to be located primarily at the level of the endothelial membrane of the retinal vessels it was only natural to assume that an alteration of the endothelial

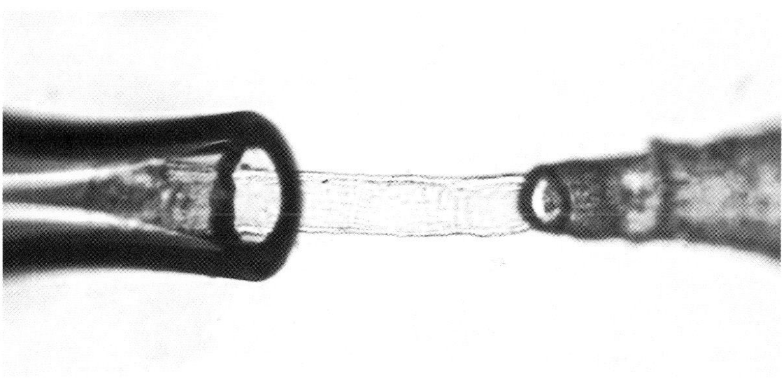

Figure 12.7
Cannulated rabbit retinal arteriole in the microperfusion system.

cells could play a major role in diabetic retinal disease. Ashton, in his 1965 Bowman Lecture, stated that early lesions of diabetic retinopathy are 'focal breakdowns of the BRB'.[19]

The advent of fluorescein angiography confirmed most of what was known about the initial pathological picture of diabetic retinopathy and showed in the initial stages of the disease focal leaks of fluorescein, demonstrating well, in a clinical setting, the existence of focal breakdowns of the BRB.

In 1975, vitreous fluorometry, a clinical quantitative method for the study of the BRB, was introduced by our group, showing that an alteration of the BRB could be detected and measured in diabetic eyes with apparently normal fundi.[6] The disturbance of the BRB, as evidenced by vitreous fluorometry, appeared before microaneurysms or capillary closure could be demonstrated by fluorescein angiography. These results were soon confirmed by Waltman et al.[20]

Thereafter, many experimental and clinical studies have examined the alteration of the BRB in diabetes with conflicting results at times, but showing in general that an alteration of the BRB is present in the diabetic retina and may have an important role in its development and progression.

Garner,[21] when reviewing the pathology of diabetic retinopathy, combined available clinical and histological information and described a 'functional' or prepathological stage followed by the development of permament pathological changes. He described the following characteristics of the functional stage:

1. Diffuse dilatation of retinal veins.
2. Breakdown of the BRB, due to abnormalitites in the endothelial layer and the retinal pigmented epithelium. Vitreous fluorometry documents this leakage very well.
3. Increased blood flow in the diabetic circulation either from hyperglycaemia or as a result of an autoregulatory response to tissue hypoxia.

Pathological changes occur primarily in the inner half of the retina, important findings being related to morphological changes in the arterioles, venules and capillaries. These morphological changes consist of alterations in vascular structure and they are different from those which are associated with simple ageing. The main changes are:

- thickening of basement membranes
- endothelial cell proliferation
- hyalinization
- loss of intramural pericytes.

Thickening of the basement membranes leads to closure of capillaries, whereas loss of pericytes leads to weakening of the capillary walls. Both changes may result from abnormal vessel permeability and contribute to eventual formation of microaneurysms, hence the presence of retinal microaneurysms as a usual initial presenting sign at the posterior pole of diabetic fundi.

The damaged capillaries leak contents intraretinally, resulting in the formation of hard yellow exudates (confluents of lipids and lipoproteins) in the nerve fibre layer and oedema. A haemorrhage is also possible in the presence of excessive porosity. If present, haemorrhages take the form of dots and blots, this appearance being attributable to sequestration of blood in an anatomically compact retina.

Closure of the capillaries produces swelling or death in the retinal nerve fibre layer supplied by these capillaries. These manifest as cotton wool spots or soft exudates.

Breakdown of the BRB appears, therefore, to play a major initiating role in the development of the pathological picture of diabetic retinopathy.

Experimental studies

An alteration of the BRB has, indeed, been observed in a variety of studies using different models of experimental diabetes. These studies, initiated by Waltman and co-workers,[22] showed an alteration of the BRB in rats with streptozotocin-induced diabetes, well demonstrated by vitreous fluorometry, soon after the induction of chronic hyperglycaemia. Furthermore, this alteration of the BRB was reversed by the administration of insulin and regularization of the glycaemia.

Other studies have confirmed the alteration of the BRB in the rat in streptozotocin-induced diabetes, only 1 week after the administration of streptozotocin. There were, however, contradicting observations regarding the site of the BRB breakdown. Studies using horseradish peroxidase as a tracer for electron microscopic investigation, pointed to the retinal pigmented epithelium as the main structure affected.[23] However, studies using histochemical localization of naturally occurring albumin, performed by Murata et al[24] and Viñores et al[25] have clearly shown that the main site of increased permeability of the BRB is located at the level of the inner BRB involving the retinal vessels. More recently, our group in Coimbra[26] have demonstrated using confocal microscopy that the breakdown of the BRB occurring in rats 1 week after onset of streptozotocin-induced diabetes is localized preferentially in the inner BRB.

In alloxan-induced diabetes, Engerman[27] was able to demonstrate in the dog the development of a retinopathy presenting many of the features seen in man. Ultrastructural studies, using horseradish peroxidase, a relatively large protein, demonstrated the breakdown of the BRB in eyes showing microaneurysms and focal capillary closure. The breakdown of the inner BRB was manifested by the presence of the tracer in the cytoplasm of the endothelial cells and in ruptured junctions. It is noteworthy that the breakdown of the BRB was observed preferentially in vessels showing signs of endothelial proliferation.

An alteration of the transport of glucose has also been demonstrated in the retinal vessels of rabbits with alloxan-induced diabetes, using a model of microperfusion.[28] These studies may offer an explanation for the differences in retinal and brain involvement in diabetes. In the alloxan-diabetic rabbit, the transport of glucose increases significantly increasing its Tm and promoting increased access of glucose to the retina, in contrast to the brain where the transport of glucose has been shown to be decreased, maintaining a low Tm in diabetic animals.

Clinical studies

Our clinical studies on the application of vitreous fluorophotometry to diabetes were reported for the first time in 1975.[6] The examination of a series of predominantly adult-onset diabetics with apparently normal fundi revealed the presence of a significant alteration of the BRB. The disturbance of the BRB appeared before microaneurysms or capillary closure could be demonstrated by fundus fluorescein angiography. The fluorescein concentration curves in the vitreous in the diabetic patients followed a typical pattern, the gradient indicating penetration of fluorescein across the BRB (*Fig. 12.8*).

Our results were confirmed by Waltman and co-workers,[20] in St Louis, who reported on the vitreous fluorometry examination of a series of juvenile-onset, insulin-dependent diabetics.

Initial studies suggested a direct association between an increase in vitreous fluorometry values and development of the retinal lesions. Higher fluorescein concentrations in the vitreous were observed in eyes showing more pathology. Another aspect of much interest was the observation of a relation between breakdown of the BRB, as shown by vitreous fluorometry, and metabolic control.[29]

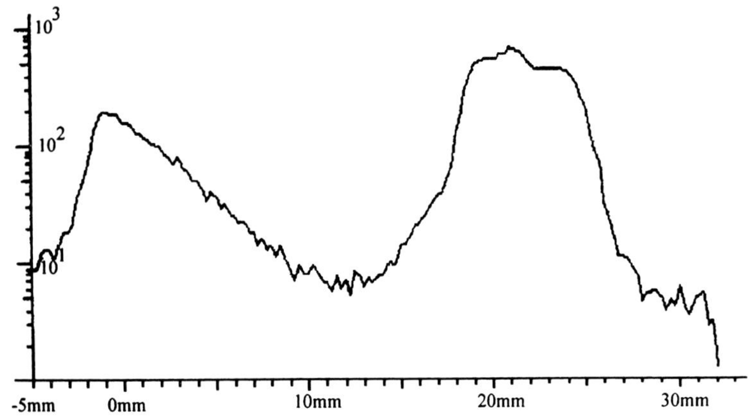

Figure 12.8
Vitreous fluorometry recording in a diabetic eye with minimal retinopathy, 60 minutes after the intravenous injection of fluorescein. Note the increased fluorescence in the posterior vitreous demonstrating an abnormal blood–retinal barrier to fluorescein.

A series of subsequent studies have examined diabetic patients with different degrees of retinopathy with conflicting results. Increased vitreous fluorometry results have generally been observed when retinopathy is present, but there is still controversy regarding the percentage of diabetic patients who show an alteration of the BRB without visible retinopathy.

During the following years many of the research efforts were directed at improving the instrumentation and standardization of the method.[7,30,31] An ocular fluorometer described by Zeimer et al[30] finally became available commercially, thus making it possible to repeat studies at different centres and avoiding much of the variability in instrumentation that characterized some of the earlier studies.

More recently, in 1997, the results of a European multicentre study involving six different research groups showed that vitreous fluorometry, performed using the Fluorotron Master and following a well-defined protocol, is a highly sensitive and reliable method for measuring the permeability of the BRB.[8]

A general review of the many studies performed using vitreous fluorometry, in both type I and type II diabetes, show that there is, in both types of diabetes, an alteration of the BRB which is always present after development of ophthalmoscopically visible retinopathy and sometimes present even before the development of clinically visible retinopathy. This breakdown of the BRB increases with duration of the disease and is associated with poor metabolic control.

Prognostic value of vitreous fluorometry

Waltman[32] and Krupin et al[33] published for the first time a 5-year follow-up study involving 59 type I diabetic patients, examining the correlation between vitreous fluorometry values and the deterioration of the retinopathy. They found that increasing vitreous fluorometry values were harbingers of more rapid progression of diabetic retinopathy.

We have recently published a 7-year prospective follow-up study of a group a 40 patients with adult-onset diabetes mellitus, with retinopathy no greater than level 3 of the modified Airlie House Classification of diabetic retinopathy at the commencement of the study.[34] They were examined by fundus photography, fluorescein angiography and vitreous fluorometry, at entry into the study and 1, 4, 5 and 7 years after the initial examination. After 7 years of follow-up a total of 22 of the 40 eyes had received photocoagulation. The eyes that needed photocoagulation were those that had higher vitreous fluorometry values at entry to the study and showed higher rates of deterioration. The eyes that did not need photocoagulation during the 7 years follow-up showed stable vitreous fluorometry readings. Abnormally high vitreous fluorometry values and their rapid increase over time were shown to be good indicators of progression and worsening of the retinopathy in diabetes type II.

Similar findings have been reported by Engler et al[35] in an 8-year follow-up study of 50 type I diabetic patients. Initially, the patients were submitted to fundus photography and vitreous fluorometry for determination of the BRB permeability. After 8 years the patients were re-examined. A positive correlation between a high initial permeability value and an unfavourable clinical course, using photocoagulation as the outcome parameter, was found. In summary, in patients showing the same retinal morphology, high permeability of the BRB indicates an unfavourable disease course.

It appears, therefore, that the alteration of the BRB, measured by vitreous fluorometry, is an early finding in diabetic retinal disease and correlates well with progression and worsening of the retinopathy, both in type I and in type II diabetics. The quantitative nature of vitreous fluorometry and the demonstration of its clinical significance makes it the preferred outcome variable when evaluating drug therapy directed at the earliest stages of diabetic retinopathy.

Randomized studies using fundus photography as the main outcome have consistently produced negative results, particularly when studying initial stages of the retinopathy. Clinical studies using the alteration of the BRB as the outcome variable have shown that the progressive deterioration of the BRB that occurs in the diabetic patients may be decreased and possibly stabilized by drug administration.[36] A favourable effect on the BRB has been observed in pilot studies using aldose reductase inhibitors, such as sorbinil, sulindac and calcium dobesilate[37] antioxidants and antihistamine drugs. Angiotensin-converting enzyme (ACE) inhibitors have also been shown to stabilize the BRB in type I diabetics. A prospective, randomized study of 20

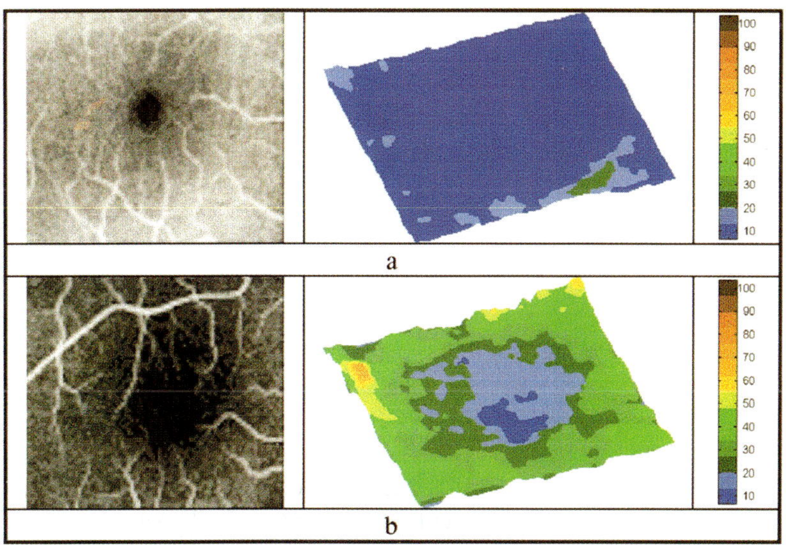

Figure 12.9
(a) Retinal leakage analyser examination of a normal eye. Left: fundus image obtained less than 5 minutes after the fluorescein injection. Right: Retinal leakage map obtained 30 minutes after fluorescein injection. (b) Retinal leakage analyser examination of a diabetic eye with minimal retinopathy. Left: fundus image obtained less than 5 minutes after the fluorescein injection. Right: retinal leakage map obtained 30 minutes after the fluorescein injection.

normotensive insulin-dependent diabetic patients showed that the alteration of the BRB, measured by vitreous fluorometry, was stabilized by captopril administration.[38]

Permeability of the BRB, measured by vitreous fluorometry, appears to be particularly valuable in the early stages of retinal disease as a quantifiable outcome variable of clinical significance.

The development of a retinal leakage analyser, with the ability to map retinal fluorescein leakage while simultaneously imaging the retina, is expected to improve in the near future our understanting of the role of breakdown of the BRB in diabetic retinal disease. It is now possible to follow the natural history of the main morphological changes occurring in the diabetic retina, such as microaneurysms, capillary closure and retinal oedema, and study their association with localized alterations of the BRB identified and measured by the retinal leakage analyser (*Fig. 12.9*).

SUMMARY

The BRB plays a fundamental role in the regulation of the homeostasis of the retinal environment. The BRB has specific morphological characteristics and is involved in a variety of transport mechanisms.

Alteration of the BRB has been proposed as one of the earliest changes in diabetes. Early lesions of diabetic retinopathy appear to be focal breakdowns of the BRB. This breakdown of the BRB may be identified and quantified by measuring fluorescein leakage into the vitreous using a technique called vitreous fluorometry. This technique has shown that abnormal leakage may occur before retinopathy could be demonstrated angiographically. It has also shown a close correlation between the degree of the alteration of the BRB and the severity of the vascular lesions that characterize the pathological picture of diabetic retinopathy.

A number of studies have suggested a relationship between increased fluorescein leakage in diabetics and the ultimate deterioration into frank retinopathy and need for photocoagulation treatment. The alteration of the BRB may, indeed, be a marker for evaluating the activity of diabetic retinopathy and for predicting its progression.

REFERENCES

1. Shakib M, Cunha-Vaz JG, Studies on the permeability of the blood–retinal barrier. IV. Junctional complexes of the retinal vessels and their role in the permeability of the blood–retinal barrier, *Exp Eye Res* (1966) **5**:229–34.
2. Chan-Ling T, Stone J, Degeneration of astrocytes in feline retinopathy of prematurity causes failure of the blood–retinal barrier, *Invest Ophthalmol Vis Sci* (1992) **33**:2148–59.
3. Bleeker GM, Maas EH, Penetration of penethamate penicillin esther into the tissue of the eye, *Arch Ophthalmol* (1958) **60**:1013–20.
4. Cunha-Vaz JG, Maurice DM, The active transport of fluorescein by the retinal vessels and retina, *J Physiol (Lond)* (1967) **191**:467–86.
5. Darson H, Danielli JF, *The Permeability of Natural Membranes* (Cambridge University Press: London, 1952).
6. Cunha-Vaz JG, Faria de Abreu JR, Campos AJ, Figo G, Early breakdown of the blood–retinal barrier in diabetes, *Br J Ophthalmol* (1975) **59**:649–56.
7. Zeimer RC, Blair NP, Cunha-Vaz JG, Vitreous fluorophotometry for clinical research. II Methodology of data acquisition and processing, *Arch Ophthalmol* (1983) **11**:1757–61.
8. van Schaik HJ, Heintz B, Larsen M et al, Permeability of the blood–retinal barrier in healthy humans, *Graefes Arch Clin Exp Ophthalmol* (1997) **235**:639–46.
9. Gieser DJ, Fishamn GA, Cunha-Vaz JG, X-linked

recessive retinitis pigmentosa and vitreous fluorophotometry. A study of female heterozygotes, *Arch Ophthalmol* (1980) **98**:307–10.

10. Bernardes R, Santos F, Lobo C, Cunha-Vaz JG, Mapping fluorescein leakage across the BRB using a modified confocal scanning laser ophthalmoscope, *Invest Ophthalmol Vis Sci* (1998) **39**(suppl): S596.
11. Lobo C, Bernardes R, Santos F, Cunha-Vaz JG, Clinical validation of the retinal leakage analyser, *Invest Ophthalmol Vis Sci* (1998) **39**(Suppl): S595.
12. Zadunaisky JA, Degnam KJ, Passage of sugars and urea across the isolated retina pigment epithelium of the frog, *Exp Eye Res* (1976) **23**:191–6.
13. Betz AL, Golstein GW, Transport of hexoses, potassium and neutral amino acids into capillaries isolated from bovine retina, *Exp Eye Res* (1980) **30**:593–605.
14. Betz AL, Bowman PD, Goldstein GW, Hexoses transport in microvascular endothelial cells cultured from bovine retina, *Exp Eye Res* (1983) **36**:269–77.
15. Murta JN, Cunha-Vaz JG, Sabo CA, Laski ME, Microperfusion studies of retinal vessels. I. A new model demonstrating organic anion transport and reabsorptive fluid flux, *Invest Ophthalmol Vis Sci* (1990) **31**:471–80.
16. Murta JN, Serra A, Cunha-Vaz JG, Organic anion transport and reabsorptive fluid flux in diabetic retinal vessels: a microperfusion study, *Exp Eye Res* (1994) **58**:567–72.
17. Ashton N, Studies of retinal capillaries in relation to diabetic and other retinopathies, *Br J Ophthalmol* (1963) **47**:521–38.
18. Cogan DG, Kwabara T, Capillary shunts in the pathogenesis of diabetic retinopathy, *Diabetes* (1963) **12**:293–300.
19. Ashton N, The blood–retinal barrier and vasoglial relationships in retinal disease, *Trans Ophthalmol Soc UK* (1965) **85**:199–229.
20. Waltman SR, Oestrich C, Krupin T et al, Quantitative vitreous fluorometry: a sensitive technique for measuring early breakdown of the blood–retinal barrier in young diabetic patients, *Diabetes* (1978) **27**:85–7.
21. Garner A, Pathogemesis of diabetic retinopathy, *Semin Ophthalmol* (1987) **2**:4–11.
22. Waltman SR, Krupin T, Hanish S et al, Alteration of the blood–retinal barrier in experimental diabetes mellitus, *Arch Ophthalmol* (1978) **96**:878–9.
23. Tso MOM, Cunha-Vaz JG, Shih CY et al, Clinical pathologic study of blood–retinal barrier in experimental diabetes mellitus, *Arch Ophthalmol* (1980) **98**:2032–40.
24. Murata T, Ishibashi T, Inomata H, Immunohistochemical detection of blood–retinal barrier breakdown in streptozotocin-diabetic rats, *Graefes Arch Clin Exp Ophthalmol* (1993) **231**:175–7.
25. Viñores SA, McGree R, Lee A et al, Ultrastructural localization of blood–retinal barrier breakdown in diabetic and galactosemic rats, *J Histochem Cytochem* (1990) **38**:1341–52.
26. Do carmo A, Ramos P, Reis A et al, Breakdown of the inner and outer blood–retinal barriers in streptozotocin-induced diabetes, *Exp Eye Res* (1998) **67**:569–75.
27. Engerman RL, Animal models of diabetic retinopathy, *Trans Am Acad Ophthalmol Otolaryngol* (1976) **81**:710–15.
28. Murta JN, Serra A, Cunha-Vaz JG, Characterization of D-glucose transport across diabetic retinal vessels, *Invest Ophthalmol Vis Sci* (1996) **38**(suppl):S979
29. Cunha-Vaz JG, Fonseca JR, Faria de Abreu JR, Ruas MA, A follow-up study by vitreous fluorophotometry of early involvement in diabetes, *Am J Ophthalmol* (1978) **86**:467–73.
30. Zeimer RC, Blair NP, Cunha-Vaz JG, Vitreous fluorophotometry for clinical research. I. Description and evaluation of a new fluorophotometer, *Arch Ophthalmol* (1983) **101**:1753–1756.
31. Lund-Andersen H, Krogsaa B, LaCour M, Larsen J, Quantitative vitreous fluorofotometry applying a mathematical model of the eye, *Invest Ophthalmol Vis Sci* (1985) **26**:698–710.
32. Waltman SR, Sequential vitreous fluorophotometry in diabetes mellitus: a five-year prospective study, *Trans Am Ophthalmol Soc* (1989) **82**:827–940.

33. Krupin T, Waltman SR, Fluorophotometry in juvenile-onset diabetes: long-term follow-up, *Jpn J Ophthalmol* (1985) **29**:139–45.
34. Cunha-Vaz JG, Lobo C, Castro Sousa JP et al, Progression of retinopathy and alteration of the blood–retinal barrier in patients with type 2 diabetes: a 7-year prospective follow-up study, *Graefes Arch Clin Exp Ophthalmol* (1998) **236**:264–8.
35. Engler C, Krogsaa B, Lund-Andersen H, Blood-retinal barrier permeability and its relation to the progression of diabetic retinopathy in type 1 diabetes, *Graefes Arch Clin Exp Ophthalmol* (1991) **229**:442–6.
36. Cunha-Vaz JG, Perspectives in the treatment of diabetic retinopathy, *Diabetes Metab Rev* (1992) **8**:105–16.
37. Leite E, Mota MC, Faria de Abreu JR, Cunha-Vaz JH, Effect of calcium dobesilate on the blood–retinal barrier in early diabetic retinopathy, *Int Ophthalmol* (1990) **14**:81–8.
38. Larsen M, Hammel E, Parving HE, Lund-Andersen H, Protective effect of captopril on the blood-retina barrier in normotensive insulin-dependent diabetic patients with nephropathy and background retinopathy, *Graefes Arch Clin Exp Ophthalmol* (1990) **228**:505–9.

13 Histopathology and pathophysiology of diabetic retinopathy

Toke Bek

INTRODUCTION

Over the past 50 years huge resources have been invested in elucidating the pathophysiology of diabetic retinopathy. The motives for this are both clinical and general scientific.

From a clinical point of view it is important that diabetic retinopathy is the most frequent cause of blindness among young adults in the Western world, even when measures are taken to ensure optimal prevention with tight control of blood glucose and blood pressure, early detection of vision-threatening changes and efficient treatment with photocoagulation and vitrectomy. A basic precondition for introducing new preventive, diagnostic and therapeutic measures for diabetic retinopathy on a rational basis is knowledge of the pathophysiology of the disease.

From a general scientific point of view it is important that the morphological and functional changes characteristic of diabetic retinopathy can also be seen in a number of other retinal diseases. Knowledge of the pathophysiology of diabetic retinopathy may therefore potentially provide knowledge about the pathological reaction potential of the retina in general. This may be used for detecting, diagnosing and treating retinal diseases other than diabetic retinopathy.

In spite of considerable research activity using a large number of theoretical and experimental approaches, only little light has so far been shed on the pathophysiology of diabetic retinopathy. The purpose of the this chapter is to present current knowledge of the pathophysiology of the disease viewed from one approach, that is the histopathological one. In order to limit this topic and come as close as possible to a description of clinical diabetic retinopathy, I will mainly focus on histopathological studies made on human diabetic retinas. References to animal studies will only be made when necessary to confirm, clarify or support the findings in humans. Furthermore, the histopathological findings will be supplemented with evidence gained from other experimental approaches when necessary to clarify the text of the presentation. As compared to other experimental approaches, histopathological examinations have both advantages and limitations (*Table 13.1*). The main advantage of the histopathological approach is the opportunity to study the consequences of diabetic retinopathy directly on the retina, whereas it is a limitation that the complications can only be studied after they have developed so that no direct evidence is obtained as to how this happened. Finally, a significant limitation for the design of histopathological studies is that selection of tissue with particular lesions or lesion patterns of interest is difficult, so that researchers have to make do with what tissue is made available by chance.

Table 13.1 Experimental approaches to the study of the pathophysiology of diabetic retinopathy at different stages of the disease.

Stage in disease development	Experimental methods
Before	Genetics Epidemiology
During	Natural history Clinical intervention Experimental diabetes
After	Histopathology

HISTOPATHOLOGY OF DIABETIC RETINOPATHY

Techniques

The earliest histopathological studies of diabetic retinopathy were done using general histological staining techniques on paraffin-embedded sections.[1,2] These investigations mainly confirmed the ophthalmoscopical impression indicating that diabetic retinopathy is a disease involving changes in the retinal blood vessels. Therefore, a breakthrough in the study of diabetic retinopathy came with the introduction of new techniques for examining the retinal vascular system. In his classical work on the retinal vascular system in man and animals, Michaelson[3] used a technique he had developed some years earlier. He injected ink into the systemic circulation postmortem, and after the optics of the eye were removed, the ink-stained black retinal vessels could be observed by direct inspection. Ashton worked with similar ideas, and he described a modification of the technique suitable for studying human postmortem retinas.[4] However, it was a disadvantage of the ink injection technique that observation of the deeper-lying retinal vessels was difficult due to a blurred view through the overlying layers of the retina. Consequently, during the 1950s different attempts at isolating the retinal vascular tree from the surrounding tissue were made, either by mechanical shaking or by alkali corrosion of neoprene casts of the vascular tree.[5] A few years later an elegant method was described to solve the problem.[6] It took advantage of the fact that the neuroglial components of the retina are much more loosely joined than is its vascular tree. By exposing the retina to a brief controlled digestion with trypsin a complete resolution of the neuroglial parts of the retina was achieved, exposing the vascular tree for observation. This accomplishment became the beginning of a very profitable period for the study of vascular pathology in diabetic retinopathy, and trypsin digestion is still used as a basis for studies of new aspects of retinal vascular pathology.[7,8] The disadvantage of the enzyme digestion technique was that it did not allow an examination of the interaction between pathological vascular changes and changes in the surrounding retinal tissue. In a series of comprehensive histopathological studies during the 1960s the types of retinal damage in diabetic retinopathy were studied structurally and ultrastructurally[9,10] but lacking the gross overview of the pathological vascular structure that could be obtained with ink injection combined with trypsin digestion. The histopathological examinations have later been supplemented with immunohistochemistry, enzyme histochemistry,[11] and in situ hybridization.[12] In the 1990s methods have been developed for casting the retinal vascular system that allow for subsequent histopathological, immunohistochemical and in situ hybridization studies of areas with well-defined vascular pathology, as seen on the cast.[13,14] These new methodological approaches have contributed further knowledge about the pathophysiology of diabetic retinopathy.[15,16]

Limitations

Histopathological studies on human eyes can be carried out on fresh tissue obtained during vitrectomy or from eyes enucleated because of other ocular diseases such as malignancies, or the examinations can be carried out as part of routine autopsy. Retinal tissue has a comparatively higher postmortal stability than for example, brain tissue. This is probably a consequence of metabolic buffering of the vitreous body combined with a high content of glycogen in retinal Müller cells that may serve as an energy reservoir for anaerobic glycolysis during the first postmortem hours.[17] In spite of this fact, postmortal degradation implies that retinas obtained by autopsy are less suited for ultrastructural studies and for studies of easily degradable compounds such as neurotransmitters and nucleic acids. On the other hand, autopsy tissue is highly suitable for histopathological and immunohistochemical determination of structural proteins and other compounds with high postmortal stability.

CYTOPATHOLOGICAL CHANGES

Changes in the vascular walls

Retinal capillaries are composed of an endothelial cell layer anchored to a basement membrane which has vascular pericytes embedded.

Endothelial cells

Remarkably few studies have been done on the cytopathology of retinal vascular endothelial cells in diabetic retinopathy. When studied on trypsin digests retinal vascular endothelial cells are the last cell type to disappear when or before the capillary bed is obliterated.[18] Furthermore, proliferation of endothelial cells has been shown in the smaller retinal vessels in diabetic retinopathy, possibly owing to a shortened cell cycle and/or as an adaptive mechanism to ensure endothelial cell covering of the lumen of the distended vessels. A recent study using DNA labelling of apoptotic cells in the diabetic retina has also shown increased degradation of vascular endothelial cells.[7] Finally, endothelial cell proliferation is a prominent feature of neovascularization in proliferative diabetic retinopathy.[5]

Altogether this evidence suggests that vascular endothelial cells in diabetic retinopathy proliferate for the formation of new vessels, when it is necessary to cover a larger vascular lumen, and because of increased turnover of this cell type.

Basement membranes

A basement membrane is a layer of extracellular matrix composed of type IV collagen, glycoproteins and acid mucopolysaccharides in a composition specialized for the purpose of anchoring cells to underlying loose connective tissue.[19] Under normal conditions the basement membrane of retinal capillaries is thicker than that of capillaries elsewhere in the body.[20] In diabetes mellitus a generalized thickening of vascular basement membranes develops, which can be evidenced by increased periodic acid-Schiff (PAS) staining of their glycoproteins.[21] In the retinal vessels this increased PAS staining has been shown to correlate with the glycoproteins laminin and fibronectin (*Fig. 13.1*), but not with vitronectin and type VI collagen.[22] The basement membrane thickening is more pronounced in arterial than in venous environments and more pronounced in the inner than the other retinal vascular layers.[23,24] By electron microscopy the thickened basement membrane in the retinal vessels from diabetic patients is seen to be irregular, in some places only encompassing parts of the vascular circumference, and often smaller basement membrane processes are seen to

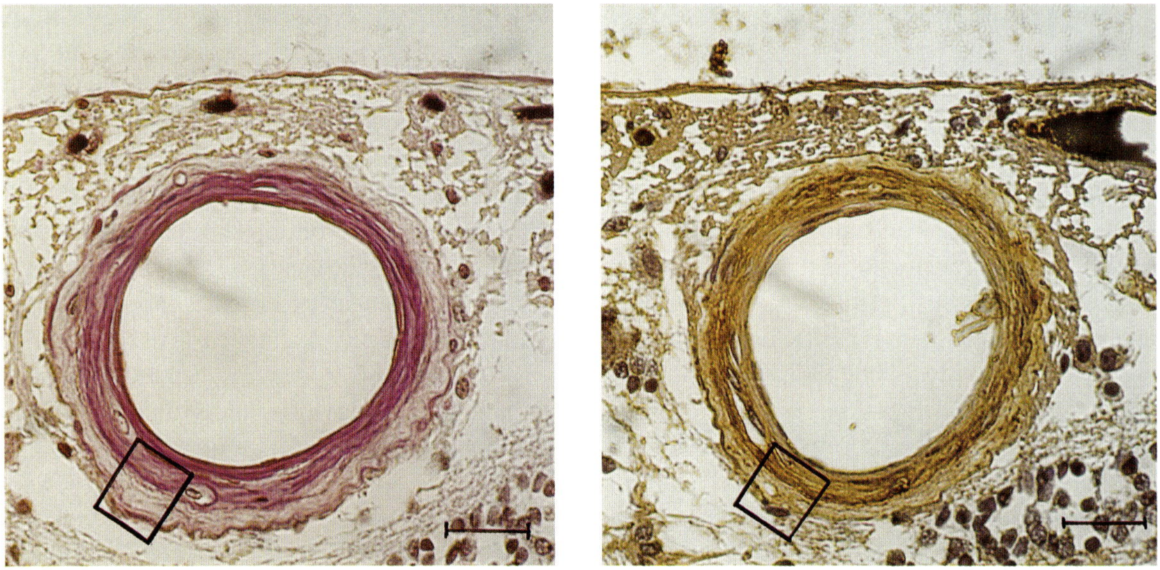

(a) (b)

Figure 13.1
Closely adjacent sections through a retinal arteriole from a diabetic patient. Apart from the endothelial cell lining there is identical distribution of staining with periodic acid-Schiff (a) and immunoreactivity to fibronectin (b) in the arteriolar wall (compare staining pattern in boxes). The black material inside some of the smaller vessels represents casting material. Haematoxylin. Bars = 25 μm. Reproduced with permission from Ref 22.

extend between neurons and glial cells.[9,10,25,26] The retinal vascular basement membrane is very resistant to disease changes, and it is the only structure that is left when the vessels are occluded and the cells of the vascular walls disappear.[27]

Many speculations have been raised as to whether thickening of retinal vascular basement membranes is simply part of the generalized basement membrane thickening in diabetes mellitus, or whether it plays a specific role for the development of diabetic retinopathy. However, there is so far no certain evidence that thickening of basement membranes has any significance for the development of diabetic retinopathy.

Pericytes

Pericytes are multipotent cells situated inside or in close association with the vascular basement membrane, for which reason they have also been termed mural cells. Pericytes are developed from the same stem cell as the vascular endothelial cells, but they are differentiated to have other morphological and functional characteristics.[28] The exact function of vascular pericytes is unknown, but it is assumed that they are important for maintaining the structural and functional integrity of the retinal vascular walls. It has been shown, however, that the pericytes have potential contractile capacity, and on the venolar side of microcirculatory units transition forms may occur with features in common with smooth muscle cells.[20] Under normal conditions the ratio between retinal vascular pericytes and endothelial cells is 1:1, but it is larger in other organs.[18,20] This has led to speculations about whether reduced spare capacity of pericytes in the retinal vessels might confer a special vulnerability to retinal vessels in response to loss of this cell type. The interest for retinal vascular pericytes in diabetes mellitus is harboured by a selective loss of this cell in the early stages of the disease.[7,29] On trypsin digests the pericyte loss is seen as an increased endothelial cell/pericyte ratio, and histologically the degenerated pericytes are seen as eosinophilic ghost cells lacking nuclear staining.[30] It has been proposed that pericyte loss is the primary pathophysiological change in the retina leading to diabetic retinopathy. Thus, it has been suggested that the weakening of the vascular wall secondary to pericyte loss could be the cause of the extension of the capillary lumen leading to the formation of microaneurysms, and that the lack of support from the pericytes might lead to death and occlusion of the vessel. A primary role of the pericytes in the pathophysiology of diabetic retinopathy is supported by the fact that this cell type contains large amounts of aldose reductase, which mediates degradation of glucose by an alternative metabolic pathway when exposed to hyperglycaemia, leading to toxic cell damage.[31] However, this hypothesis has been difficult to verify in practice because of difficulties in establishing the temporal relation between pericyte loss and other pathological changes in diabetic retinopathy.

Changes in retinal neuroglial components

Glial cells

The retina contains a number of glial cell types, of which the Müller cell and the perivascular glial cell[32] have been shown to display histopathological changes in diabetic retinopathy.[16] A possible role of astrocytes and the microglia for the pathophysiology of this disease has not yet been established.[16,33]

The Müller cell is the radial glia of the retina. This cell type has received much attention as being involved in the pathophysiology of diabetic retinopathy, partly stimulated by the fact that the b wave of the ERG, which is assumed to be generated in the retinal Müller cells,[34] is changed early in the course of diabetic retinopathy. In the retina from diabetic patients the Müller cells can be seen to be activated to display increasing immunoreactivity to the intermediary filament glial fibrillary acid protein,[35] and there is evidence that the Müller cells may be involved in retinal capillary occlusion in diabetic patients.[15,16] Finally, extensive Müller cell proliferation is seen to accompany the healing response in the outer retina secondary to retinal photocoagulation. However, an understanding of the precise relation between these histopathological findings and the pathophysiology of diabetic retinopathy is still lacking.

The perivascular glial cells were originally identified by the silver carbonate staining method of Rio Hortega and were shown to display pathological activation in a number of retinal diseases, including diabetic retinopathy.[33,36] As studied by immunohistochemistry these cells are seen to display increased immunoreactivity to S-100 protein;[16] however, the significance of pathological changes in the perivascular glial cells for the pathophysiology of diabetic retinopathy is still unknown.

Neurons

Loss of the neuronal components of the retina leads to permanent reduction of vision. Histologically, this cell loss displays three different forms. When an arteriole belonging to the central retinal vascular system is occluded, neurons in the supplied area from the inner retinal layers down to the outer plexiform layer atrophy,[37] while laser treatment leads to loss of the photoreceptor layer, perhaps including some of the inner retinal layers.[38] Finally, diffuse loss of retinal neurons is seen in areas with retinal oedema. It has been proposed that diabetic retinopathy might be a primary neurosensory disorder,[39] but the general notion is that the observed loss of retinal neurons is secondary to the vascular changes.

HISTOPATHOLOGICAL CHANGES IN THE POSTERIOR POLE OF THE EYE

The cytopathological changes in the retina secondary to diabetes mellitus together form the lesions that can be seen by ophthalmoscopy as clinical diabetic retinopathy. However, the different ophthalmoscopic lesions display a different distribution in the ocular background, with some lesions predominating in the posterior pole of the eye, and other lesions predominating in the retinal periphery. The changes predominating in the posterior pole, designated *background retinopathy* or *simple retinopathy*, can be attributed to pathological changes in the integrity of the retinal capillary walls and disturbances of axoplasmic flow in retinal nerve fibres.

Changes in the integrity of capillary walls

The pathological changes in the cellular and extracellular constituents of the capillary walls in background retinopathy lead to localized dilation of the capillary lumen and breakdown of the barrier function of the capillaries to the formed and unformed constituents of the blood.

Microaneurysms

Microaneurysms are localized dilations of the retinal capillaries, and together with small retinal haemorrhages in the posterior pole of the eye they are the first ophthalmoscopically visible sign of diabetic retinopathy. The size of microaneurysms varies from 10 to 100 μm, and according to their shape they are described as sacculate, fusiform or as having shapes in between (*Fig. 13.2*).

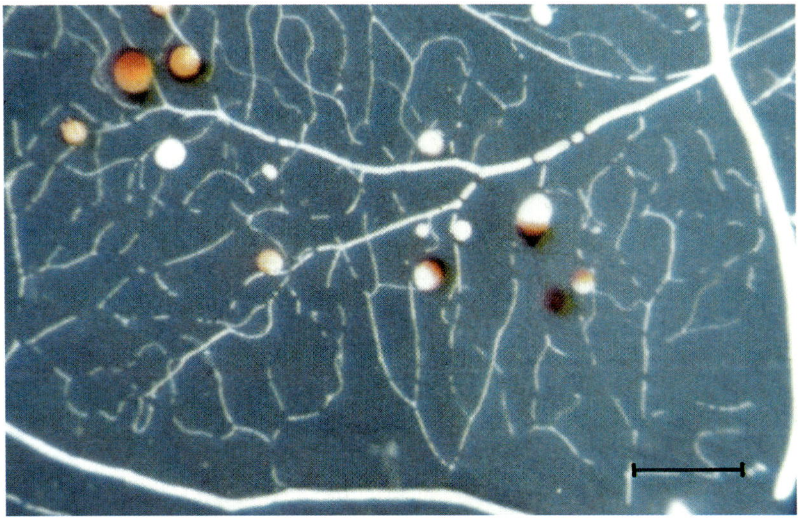

Figure 13.2
Cast of retinal vessels showing sacculate microaneurysms on capillaries in the venous part of a microcirculatory unit. The red caps represent erythrocytes adhering to the internal surface of the microaneurysms. The casting of the retinal vessels is fragmented, but there is no capillary occlusion. Bar = 250 μm.

Histologically, several types of microaneurysm can be differentiated, which are assumed to represent different stages in the cycle of the lesions: (1) small hypercellular aneurysms, (2) large thin-walled aneurysms, (3) thick-walled aneurysms, (4) hyalinized aneurysms with obliterated lumen.[9,40,41] In addition to this, when the aneurysms are included in areas of capillary occlusion, they may have an occluded lumen because of ingrowth of retinal Müller cells (Bek, unpublished). Ultrastructurally the wall of microaneurysms consists of endothelial cells with normal tight junctions but with an increased lipid content. The basement membrane of microaneurysms has the same thickness as the capillaries they emerge from, but the vascular pericytes have disappeared or are visible as debris in the aneurysmal wall.[10,25,41] The mechanism underlying the formation of microaneurysms is unknown. A previous hypothesis suggesting that microaneurysms represent the initial stages of retinal neovascularization has been abandoned,[5,42] and it is now the general impression that the formation of microaneurysms is due to weakening of the vascular wall caused by changes in their structure, loss of pericytes, etc. combined with increased hydrostatic pressure in the capillaries because of changes in the retinal blood flow.

Haemorrhages

Retinal haemorrhages are erythrocytes extravasated from the retinal vascular bed because of breaks in the vascular wall. The mechanism underlying these breaks is unknown, but as with microaneurysms their formation is probably influenced by decreased structural integrity of the vascular walls combined with increased hydrostatic pressure in the vascular lumens. Pathologically gross haemorrhages are easily seen on unfixated tissue because of the red colour of the extravasated haemoglobin (*Fig. 13.3*). The lesions often become less visible after histological preparation because of bleaching of the haemoglobin during fixation and dehydration. By microscopy haemorrhages can be identified as localized assemblances of erythrocytes not surrounded by a basement membrane (*Fig. 13.4*).[9] Retinal haemorrhages are resolved by disintegration and phagocytosis of the

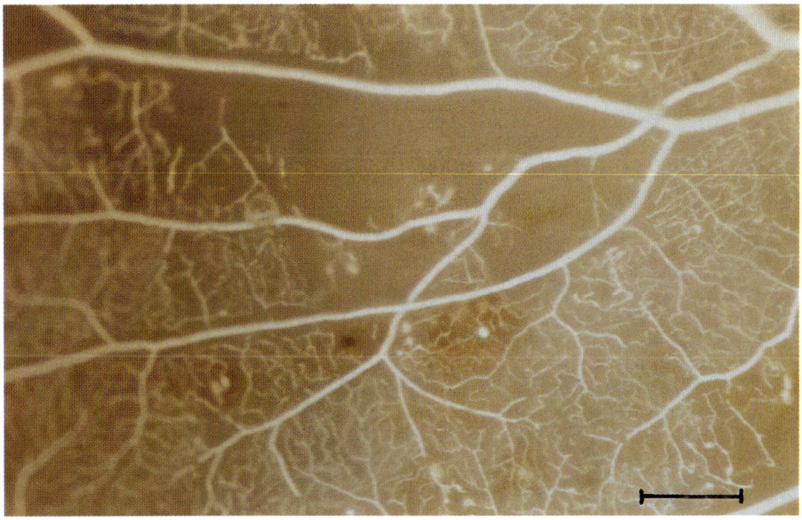

Figure 13.3
Cast of retinal vessels with an area of capillary occlusion. Microaneurysms (white dots) are seen dispersed in the capillary bed. The reddish areas represent extravasated blood. Bar = 1000 μm.

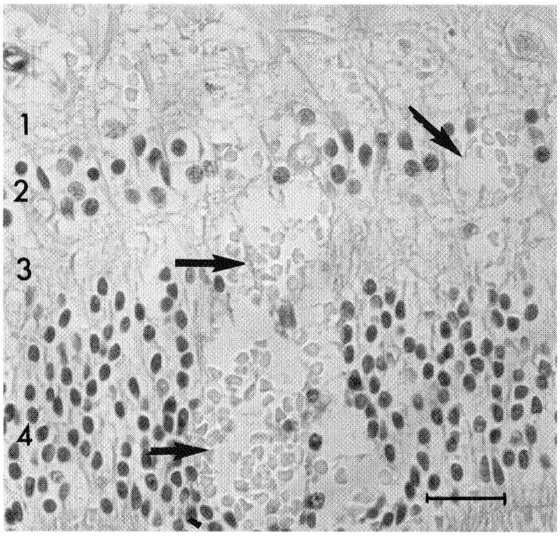

Figure 13.4
Section through intraretinal haemorrhage. Haemorrhages are seen as clusters of erythrocytes (arrows) not surrounded by basement membrane. Inner plexiform layer (1), inner nuclear layer (2), outer plexiform layer (3), outer nuclear layer (4). Haematoxylin. Bar = 25 μm.

extravasated erythrocytes in the tissue. Haemorrhages often disappear without any trace, but they may leave behind neuronal damage due to the pressure exerted on the surrounding tissue, and larger haemorrhages may result in the formation of fibrotic scars.[2]

Breakdown of the blood–retina barrier

Similarly to the brain, the retinal tissue is protected from the bloodstream by a tight barrier. Due to the dual blood supply there is both an anterior blood–retina barrier towards the retinal circulation, and a posterior barrier towards the choroidal circulation. Experiments using peroxidase diffusion[43–45] have suggested that the anatomical basis for the blood–retina barrier is tight junctions between the pigment epithelial cells (the posterior blood–retina barrier) and between the retinal vascular endothelial cells (the anterior blood–retina barrier). Clinically, breakdown of the blood–retina barrier is seen by leakage of intravenously administered fluorescein. The anatomical background for this leakage has not yet been finally settled, but the fact that fenestrated endothelial cells in new vessels without tight junctions display fluorescein leakage,[46,48] supports the notion that these tight junctions hold the barrier properties of the vessels. However, other suggestions as to the structural basis of the blood–retina barrier have also been made, for example, the retinal Müller cells and the vascular basement membrane. The Müller cells are involved in the development and maintenance of the blood–retina barrier,[48] but this fact can hardly be used to conclude that they represent the barrier itself. The fact that microaneurysms with thickened basement membrane leak fluorescein while microaneurysms without basement membrane thickening do not[40] argues against the idea that the barrier properties should be due to the basement membrane. Barrier leakage in itself as seen by fluorescein angiography does not lead to visual loss.[49]

Exudates

Hard exudates are whitish extravascular precipitates of lipoprotein in the retinal tissue.[50] Histologically, hard exudates appear as periodic acid-Schiff-positive sudanophilic conglomerates in the retina (*Fig. 13.5*), predominating in the outer plexiform layer.[9,51] It has been shown by immunohistochemistry that hard exudates contain fibrinogen and thus probably represent plasma proteins that have exuded from the bloodstream.[52] This is supported by the fact that hard exudates are often arranged in circular precipitation lines around a point with leakage as seen by fluorescein angiography. The presence of hard exudates is an indication of disturbances in the balance between formation and removal of plasma proteins in the

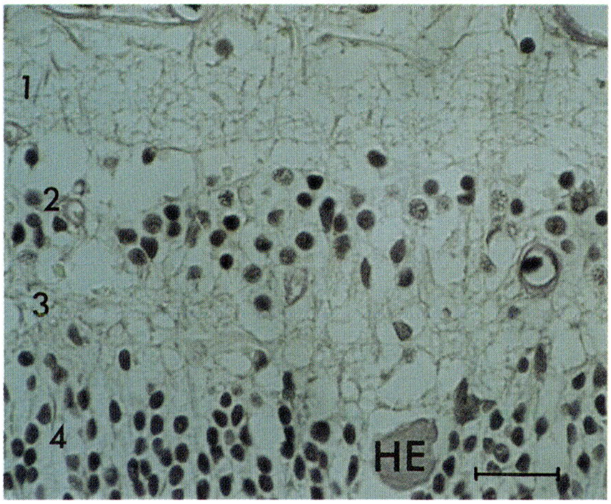

Figure 13.5
Section through retinal area with hard exudate (HE) in the outer nuclear layer. The exudates and the vascular walls stain weakly with periodic acid-Schiff (PAS). Inner plexiform layer (1), inner nuclear layer (2), outer plexiform layer (3), outer nuclear layer (4). Haematoxylin. Bar = 25 μm.

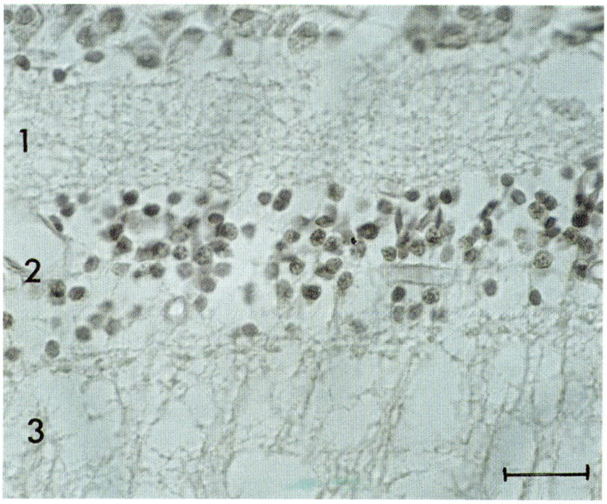

Figure 13.6
Section through area with retinal oedema. The numbering is similar to that in *Fig. 13.5*. The outer plexiform layer (3) is much thicker than on the section without oedema in *Fig. 13.5*. Haematoxylin. Bar = 25 μm.

retinal tissue. However, the removal of plasma proteins from the retinal tissue is probably very limited since the retina contains no lymphatic vessels, leaving increased leakage of plasma proteins from the bloodstream as the probable predominant contributor to the exudates. Hard exudates can accumulate into large conglomerates that give localized defects in retinal function, partly because of compression of the surrounding retinal tissue and partly because they prohibit light from reaching the photoreceptors located underneath the lesion.[49] Hard exudates are dynamic,[53] and their resolution is probably due to altered perfusion in the retina and an active removal by the reticuloendothelial system.[54] Larger exudate areas may after resolution result in fibrous scars with permanent retinal damage.[55]

Retinal oedema

Diabetic background retinopathy complicated by retinal oedema in the posterior pole of the eye is termed 'diabetic maculopathy'. The oedema is the result of disturbances in the retinal fluid haemostasis that may involve increased leakage of fluid from the blood vessels, reduced removal of fluid or local production of fluid. In exudative maculopathy the oedema is extracellular and most frequently is combined with hard exudates, while a more diffusely extended oedema is often accompanied by few or no exudates.[56] By histological examination an enlargement of the extracellular space is seen in the early stages of retinal oedema, combined with a thickening of the outer plexiform layer of the retina (*Fig. 13.6*). If the oedema progresses it may become confluent into cysts located in the outer plexiform layer and confined by retinal Müller cells bridging the inner and the other retinal layers.[51,57,58] In ischaemic maculopathy the oedema is intracellular and is caused by osmotic drag secondary to acidosis. Histologically, the retinal cells are seen to be swollen with vacuolized cytoplasm and disintegration of the nuclei resulting in cell death. Diabetic retinal oedema is often accompanied by visual loss because of the damage caused to the neuroglial elements in the retina.

Cotton wool spots

Retinal cotton wool spots are white fluffy lesions in the posterior pole of the eye, approximately the size of one-third disc diameter. Cotton wool spots have been known since the middle of the nineteenth century[59] and since that time the lesion has been given many names, of which the most misleading alludes to exudation as its cause. The lesion can be seen in a number of retinal and systemic diseases of which diabetic retinopathy is the most prominent.[60] In the earliest histopathological studies of cotton wool spots it was established that the lesion is a result of swelling of the retinal nerve fibres.[50,61,62] It was observed that the retinal nerve fibres contained small accumulations of cell-like elements which motivated the term ‘cytoid bodies’.[63] In clinical studies cotton wool spots were found to be dynamic with a cycle depending on the underlying disease, in diabetes this being approximately 1 year.[64]

The pathophysiology of cotton wool spots was established in an elegant histopathological study by McLeod and co-workers.[65] They studied the incorporation of radioactively labelled leucin into retinal ganglion cells of pigs after experimental occlusion of smaller retinal arterioles leading to the formation of cotton wool spots. They found that radioactive leucin administered a few days before the occlusion accumulated in the retinal nerve fibres, corresponding to a cotton wool spot on each side of the site of occlusion, whereas radioactive leucin taken up after the occlusion only was accumulated in the nerve fibres corresponding to the cotton wool spot on the peripheral aspect of the lesions. The conclusion was that cotton wool spots develop because of accumulation of cytoplasmic material in the retinal nerve fibres secondary to disturbances in the anterograde and/or retrograde axoplasmic transport. Clinically, cotton wool spots are often seen adjacent to a retinal area supplied by a retinal end arteriole, suggesting that the aetiology is similar to what was observed in experimentally produced lesions in pigs. However, cotton wool spots in diabetic retinopathy also occur in areas that are not related to an end arterial supply. Therefore, it can be assumed that mechanisms other than ischaemia may also result in the formation of cotton wool spots. One such mechanism might be metabolic disturbances that could, for example, account for the fact that the number of cotton wool spots may increase considerably in periods with large fluctuations in the regulation of blood glucose.[66] The swollen nerve fibres in retinal cotton wool spots diffuse and block light illuminating the retina, leading to localized scotomas in the visual field.[67] However, these scotomas often persist when the lesions have resolved, indicating that the damage caused to the tissue at the site of the lesion has led to permanent damage of retinal neurons. The function of the swollen nerve fibres themselves seems to be rather robust since it is unusual to find arcuate scotomas in the visual field corresponding to the nerve fibres traversing the lesion.[68] Retinal cotton wool spots normally do not lead to clinically significant changes in visual function since they are not located near the foveal area.

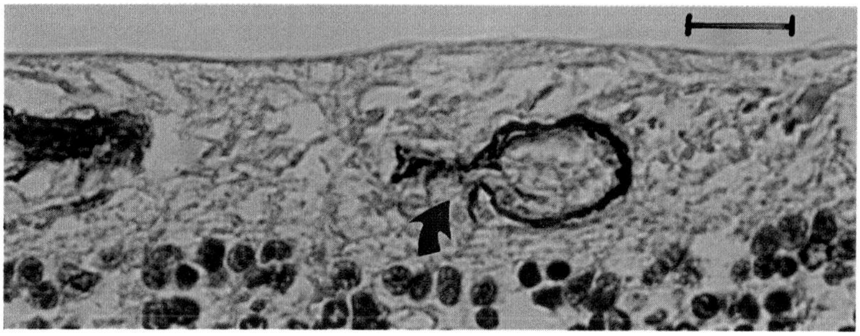

(a)

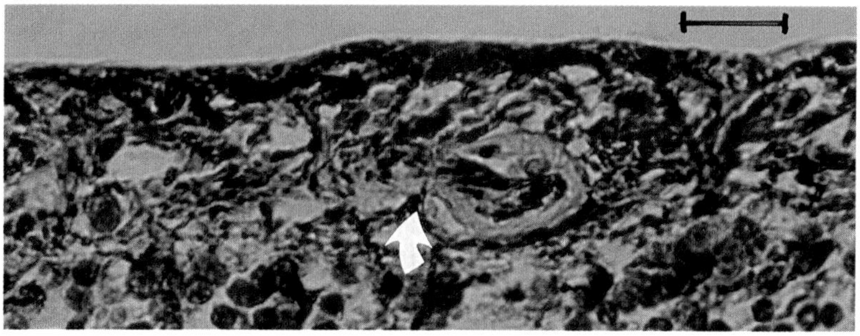

(b)

Figure 13.7
Adjacent sections through a retinal arteriole supplying an occluded retinal microcirculatory unit. (a) Immunoreactivity to type IV collagen (the vascular basement membrane) displays a continuity break (arrow). (b) Communication between intravascular glial fibrillary acidic protein immunoreactivity and extravascular glial cells through the break in the wall (arrows). Haematoxylin. Bars = 25 μm. Reproduced with permission from Ref 36.

HISTOPATHOLOGICAL CHANGES OF THE LARGE VESSELS AND THE RETINAL PERIPHERY

Capillary occlusion

Occlusion of the retinal capillaries secondary to diabetic retinopathy often starts in the retinal midperiphery and extends to the retinal periphery while the macular area is included last. Using the trypsin digestion technique Ashton showed that the occlusion is predominantly located on the arteriolar part of the capillary bed,[69] from which it extends to include the whole capillary bed in the affected microcirculatory units. A later clinicopathological study showed that the histopathological signs of capillary occlusion as seen in a trypsin-digested retina were related to clinical angiographic findings of retinal capillary non-perfusion.[70] On retinal casts areas of capillary occlusion can be recognized by their lack of filling with casting material and the lack of nuclear staining in the ghosts of former vascular endothelial cells and pericytes.[29] In cross-section the capillary is seen to have a preserved basement membrane but an obliterated lumen.[27,37] Immunohistochemically, this accumulated material can be seen to represent retinal Müller cells that have invaded the vessel and extended inside its lumen until its obliteration[10,15,16] (*Fig. 13.7*). On the arteriolar side of microcirculatory units the occluded vessels are totally obliterated with Müller cell processes, while the venules are seen to be partially collapsed with Müller cell processes filling out the residual lumen. Such a collapse can be expected as a consequence of the low hydrostatic pressure in the retinal venules when the vascular bed is occluded from the arteriolar side of microvascular units. In the areas with inner retinal vascular occlusion an amorphous material can be seen to be accumulated between the photoreceptor outer segments and the pigment epithelium.[37] The cause of this accumulation is unknown, but its shadowing of the choroidal background fluorescence may explain the uniformly black appearance of retinal non-perfusion as seen by fluorescein angiography[71] (*Fig. 13.8*).

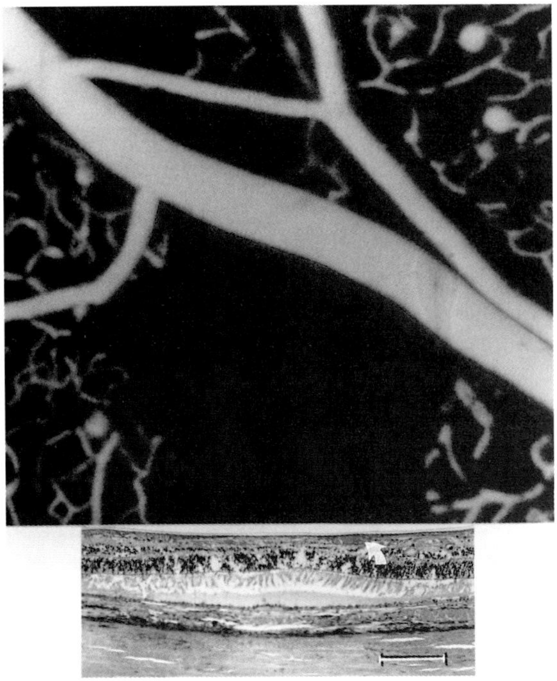

Figure 13.8
A composite photograph of a vascular cast and a histological section. The photograph of the cast has been cut so that its lower edge corresponds to the histological sectioning plane. Corresponding to the capillary-free area on the cast the histological section shows pronounced inner retinal tissue loss, and an eosinophilic substance accumulated between the photoreceptor outer segments and the pigment epithelium. The arrow points to an occluded arteriole. Bar = 200 μm. Reproduced with permission from Ref 15.

Several hypotheses have been proposed to account for the initial changes leading to capillary occlusion in diabetic retinopathy, that is, abnormalities of vascular flow regulation, thickening of retinal vascular basement membranes, microthrombosis or the Müller cell ingrowth that is seen to obliterate the retinal vessels when studied at autopsy. Several findings argue against basement membrane thickening or microthrombosis being the aetiological factor. Thus, these elements are not found corresponding to the former lumen of the occluded vessels at autopsy, and there are no differences in the thickness of basement membranes in areas of capillary occlusion and in adjacent areas without occlusion[22]. Some observations speak in favour of the Müller cell ingrowth being the causative factor. For instance, the ingrown Müller cells seen at autopsy fill out the lumen corresponding to the whole occluded vascular bed from open arteriole to open venule, and abortive or incipient ingrowth of Müller cells is seen in otherwise open and perfused vessels.[15] However, it should be emphasized that histopathological findings cannot exclude the possibility that other structural or functional disturbances may have preceded the Müller cell ingrowth[72] and be the initiating factor. The occlusion of retinal vessels leads to localized scotomas in the visual field[71] that may lead to reduction in central vision if it extends to the foveal area (ischaemic maculopathy).

Venous abnormalities

Retinal venous abnormalities in diabetic retinopathy comprise a heterogenous group of changes including venous beading, venous loops, venous reduplications and some intraretinal microvascular abnormalities (IRMAs) and arteriovenous communications. Only few histopathological studies have been done on these abnormalities in diabetic retinopathy,[73] and they

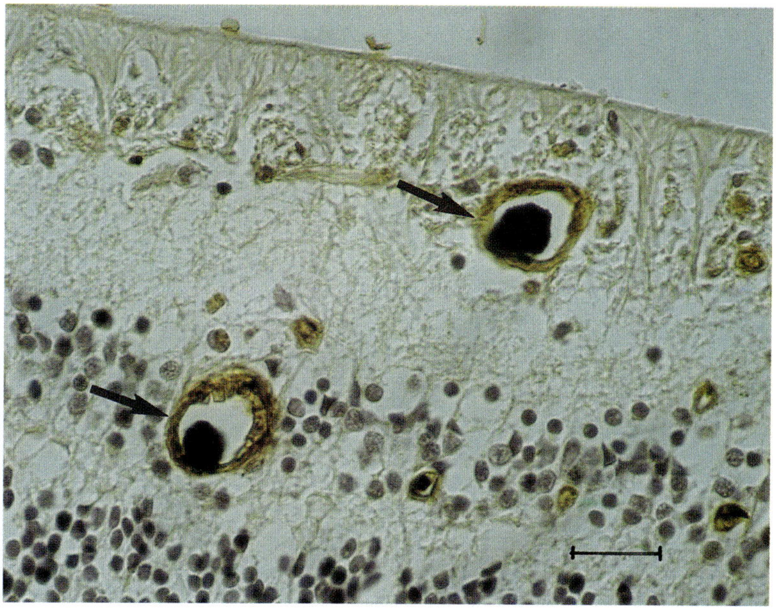

Figure 13.9
Section through two larger retinal vessels (arrows). The upper right vessel is located normally in the ganglion cell layer. The lower left vessel has too large a calibre for its location in the inner nuclear layer. The black areas inside the vessels represent casting material. Bar = 25 μm.

have mainly confirmed what can be inferred from the ophthalmoscopic appearance, that is that there is uneven thickening of the vessel walls, and endothelial cell proliferation in areas of dilation and evidence of venous thrombosis.[74] Histopathologically, arteriovenous communications can be seen as large thin-walled vessels with an aberrant localization in the outer retinal layers, presumably representing pre-existing smaller vessels that have adapted to the increased flow (*Fig. 13.9*). However, the exact histopathological characteristics of and differences between different types of venous abnormalities in diabetic retinopathy still remain to be fully elucidated.[75]

Retinal neovascularization

In proliferative diabetic retinopathy new retinal vessels develop from the large venules at the optic disc or in the retina, often starting at the edge of ischaemic retinal areas. The growth of new vessels is assumed to be stimulated with the purpose of replacing the occluded capillaries in the retinal periphery. However, the growth pattern is abnormal. The new vessels grow preretinally along the posterior hyaloid membrane in front of the tissue it is intended to supply (*Fig. 13.10*). This growth pattern forms the basis for the morphological characteristics of new retinal vessels:

1. They are not connected with the arterial side of the retinal vascular system.
2. They grow preretinally.
3. They loop back to their venous origin.
4. They may be seen to cross their feeder vessel.

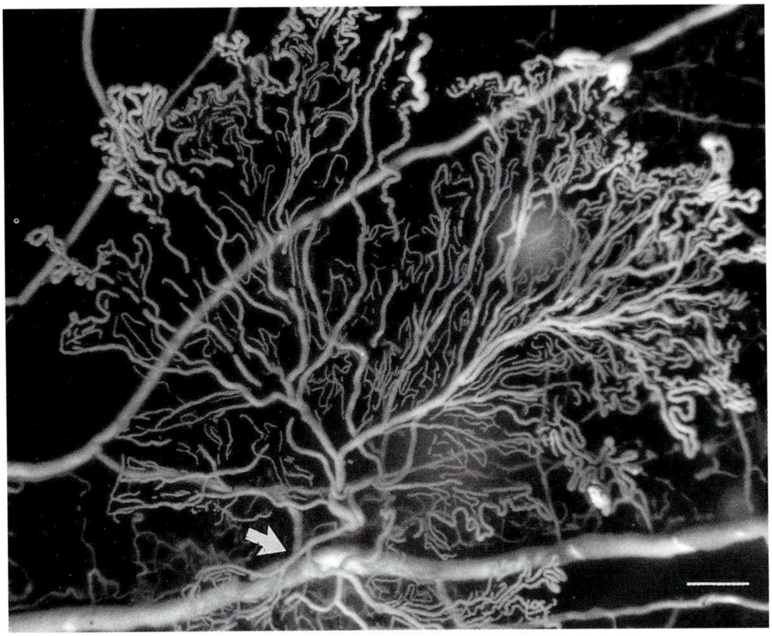

Figure 13.10
Cast of retinal neovascularization in proliferative diabetic retinopathy. The tuft of new vessels is seen to originate from a larger retinal venule (arrow) and crosses preretinally over this feeder vessel. Bar = 400 μm.

Histologically the preretinal new vessels consist of proliferating endothelial cells with a basement membrane and embedded vascular pericytes (*Fig. 13.11*). In newly formed vessels the endothelial cells are fenestrated so that they lack the normal barrier properties of retinal vessels that prevent the leakage of intravenously administered fluorescein.[46,47] The new vessels are surrounded by a collagenous amorphous ground substance that may be transformed into more or less pronounced fibrosis. A significant characteristic of preretinal new vessels, however, is that they are not surrounded by glial cells as are normal retinal vessels. This fact may in some way be related to their pathological growth pattern.

In recent years much effort has been invested in identifying the possible cytokines that may be responsible for the development of retinal new vessels in proliferative diabetic retinopathy. Several candidates have been suggested, including insulin-like growth factor and fibroblast growth factor.[76] However, most attention has been

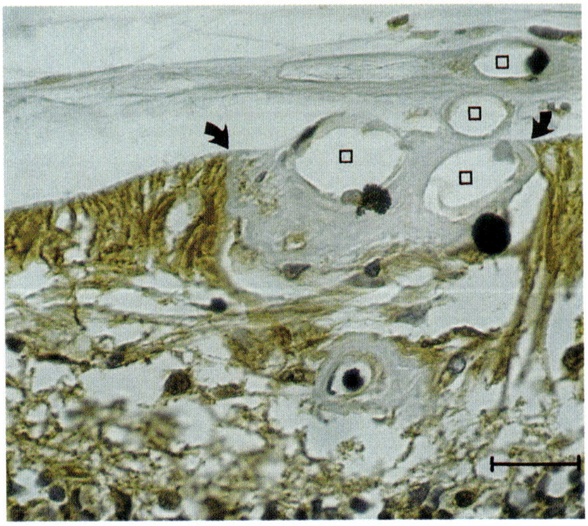

Figure 13.11
Section of preretinal neovascularization (boxes) at the site of outgrowth from the retina through the inner limiting membrane (arrows). Immunoreactivity to the vascular endothelial growth factor receptor KDR is seen corresponding to vascular pericytes and retinal Müller cells. Haematoxylin. Bar = 25 μm.

given to vascular endothelial growth factor (VEGF), which has been shown to be synthesized in the retina secondary to hypoxia and which is present in increased amounts in the retina and in ocular fluids in diabetic retinopathy.[77,78] Furthermore, it has been shown that VEGF stimulates neovascularization when synthesized in the photoreceptors of transgenic mice. Finally, intraocular administration of VEGF can stimulate neovascularization in experimental animals, while inhibition of the VEGF action can suppress this neovascularization.[79] Therefore, there are good arguments for believing that VEGF is involved in retinal neovascularization, but a final determination of the role of VEGF in the pathogenesis of proliferative diabetic retinopathy is awaited.

Retinal neovascularizations by themselves do not lead to reduced visual acuity, but may indirectly lead to visual loss when complicated by vitreous haemorrhage or tractional retinal detachment.

RETINAL PHOTOCOAGULATION

Diabetic retinopathy is treated by retinal photocoagulation. The light energy is absorbed in the pigmented epithelium and leads to coagulation necrosis in the outer retinal layers. Histologically, retinal photocoagulation can be seen to result in destruction of the choriocapillaris, the pigmented epithelium and the photoreceptors, sometimes including the inner retinal layers if the treatment is intense. A photocoagulation lesion heals by proliferation of the pigmented epithelium in the border zone to bridge over the lesion, whereby the outer blood–retina barrier is reformed. Corresponding to the destroyed parts of the neuroretina the retinal Müller cells will transform to fibroblast-like cells that form fibrotic scars. Several hypotheses have been proposed to account for the positive effect of photocoagulation treatment in diabetic retinopathy. Thus, it has been suggested that the effect could be due to altered properties of the outer blood–retina barrier, such as better oxygen supply and increased outward transport of oedema fluid through the newly proliferated pigment epithelium, and it has been suggested that the effect is due to destruction of the energy-demanding photoreceptors with a consequent elimination of retinal hypoxia.[80] However, the exact background for the positive effect of retinal photocoagulation in diabetic retinopathy remains unknown.

CONCLUSION

From the previous account it appears that histopathological studies have played a crucial role for acquiring the current knowledge of the pathophysiology of diabetic retinopathy. However, it also appears that many aspects of the disease process are still largely unknown and the histopathological approach has inherent limitations as to what information about the pathophysiology of diabetic retinopathy can be acquired. From an immediate consideration, histopathology might be regarded as an outlived examination technique of the past. However, several potentially fruitful experimental approaches can be expected to further extend the knowledge of the pathophysiology of diabetic retinopathy in future:

1. Some of the more rarely studied lesions, for example, venous abnormalities, may become available for study on autopsy material.
2. New advances in molecular biology, for example, in situ hybridization, may introduce new experimental possibilites for exploiting the information available in the retinal tissue with changes secondary to diabetic retinopathy.

3. The development of new experimental animal models of diabetic retinopathy may generate a need for histopathological examinations.
4. The formulation of a new working hypothesis for the pathophysiology of diabetic retinopathy may generate a need for reconsidering available histopathological evidence of the disease.

It is hoped that, in combination with other techniques, the histopathological approach will in the near future give a better understanding of the pathophysiology of diabetic retinopathy that may ultimately lead to a better prevention, diagnosis and treatment of its vision-threatening consequences.

REFERENCES

1. Ballantyne AJ, Loewenstein A, The pathology of diabetic retinopathy, *Trans Ophthalmol Soc UK* (1943) **63**:95–115.
2. Gartner S, Ocular pathology of diabetes, *Am J Ophthalmol* (1950) **33**:727–41.
3. Michaelson JC, *Retinal Circulation in Man and Animals* (Thomas: Springfield, Illinois, 1954) 1–146.
4. Ashton N, Injection of the retinal vascular system in the enucleated eye in diabetic retinopathy, *Br J Ophthalmol* (1949) **33**:38–41.
5. Ashton N, Studies of the retinal capillaries in relation to diabetic and other retinopathies, *Br J Ophthalmol* (1963) **47**:521–38.
6. Kuwabara T, Cogan DG, Studies of retinal vascular patterns: part I. Normal architechture, *Arch Ophthalmol* (1960) **64**:904–11.
7. Mizutani M, Kern TS, Lorenzi M, Accelerated cell death of retinal microvascular cells in human and experimental diabetic retinopathy, *J Clin Invest* (1996) **97**:2883–90.
8. Foreman DM, Bagley S, Moore J et al, Three dimensional analysis of the retinal vasculature using immunofluorescent staining and confocal laser scanning microscopy, *Br J Ophthalmol* (1996) **80**:246–51.
9. Bloodworth JMB, Diabetic retinopathy, *Diabetes* (1962) **11**:1–22.
10. Bloodworth JMB, Molitor DL, Ultrastructural aspects of human and canine diabetic retinopathy, *Invest Ophthalmol Vis Sci* (1965) **4**:1037–48.
11. Nork TM, Wallow IHL, Sramed SJ, Anderson G, Müller's cell involvement in proliferative diabetic retinopathy, *Arch Ophthalmol* (1987) **105**: 1424–9.
12. Malecaze F, Clamens S, Simorre-Pinatel V et al, Detection of vascular endothelial growth factor messenger RNA and vascular endothelial growth factor-like activity in proliferative diabetic retinopathy, *Arch Ophthalmol* (1994) **112**: 1476–82.
13. Bek T, Jensen PK, Three-dimensional structure of human retinal vessels studied by vascular casting, *Acta Ophthalmol* (1993) **71**:506–13.
14. Lutty GA, McLeod DS, A new technique for visualization of the human retinal vasculature, *Arch Ophthalmol* (1992) **110**:267–76.
15. Bek T, Glial cell involvement in vascular occlusion of diabetic retinopathy, *Acta Ophthalmol* (1997) **75**:239–43.
16. Bek T, Immunohistochemical characterization of retinal glial cell changes in areas of vascular occlusion secondary to diabetic retinopathy, *Acta Ophthalmol* (1997) **75**:388–92.
17. Kuwabara T, Cogan DG, Retinal glycogen, *Arch Ophthalmol* (1961) **66**:96–104.
18. Speiser P, Gittelsohn AM, Patz A, Studies on diabetic retinopathy. III. Influence of diabetes on intramural pericytes, *Arch Ophthalmol* (1968) **80**:332–7.
19. Martinez-Hernandez A, Amenta PS, The basement membrane in pathology, *Lab Invest* (1983) **48**:656–77.
20. Hogan MJ, Feeney L, The ultrastructure of the retinal blood vessels, II. The small vessels, *J Ultrastruct Res* (1963) **9**:29–46.
21. Friedenwald JS, Diabetic retinopathy, *Am J Ophthalmol* (1950) **33**:1187–9.

22. Bek T, Ledet T, Glycoprotein deposition in vascular walls of diabetic retinopathy, a histopathological and immunohistochemical study, *Acta Ophthalmol* (1996) **74**:385–90.
23. Stitt AW, Anderson HR, Gardiner TA, Archer DB, Diabetic retinopathy: quantitative variation in capillary basement membrane thickening in arterial or venous environments, *Br J Ophthalmol* (1994) **78**:133–7.
24. Anderson HR, Stitt AW, Archer DB, Diabetic retinopathy. Morphometric analysis of basement membrane thickening of capillaries in different retinal layers within arterial and venous environments, *Br J Ophthalmol* (1995) **79**:1120–3.
25. Toussaint D, Dustin P, Electron microscopy of normal and diabetic retinal capillaries, *Arch Ophthalmol* (1963) **70**:96–108.
26. Ashton N, Vascular basement membrane changes in diabetic retinopathy, *Br J Ophthalmol* (1974) **58**:344–66.
27. Bek T, Ledet T, Vascular occlusion in diabetic retinopathy. A qualitative and quantitative histopathological study, *Acta Ophthalmol* (1996) **74**:36–40.
28. Shakib M, de Oliveira LF, Studies on developing retinal vessels. X. Formation of the basement membrane and differentiation of intramural pericytes, *Br J Ophthalmol* (1966) **50**:124–33.
29. Cogan DG, Toussaint D, Kuwabara T, Retinal vascular patterns IV. Diabetic retinopathy, *Arch Ophthalmol* (1961) **66**:366–78.
30. Addison DJ, Garner A, Ashton N, Degeneration of intramural pericytes in diabetic retinopathy, *BMJ* (1970) **1**:264–6.
31. Hohmann TC, Nishimura C, Robison WG, Aldose reductase and polyol in cultured pericytes of human retinal capillaries, *Exp Eye Res* (1989) **48**:586–93.
32. Hogan MJ, Feeney L, The ultrastructure of the retinal blood vessels, III. Vascular-glial relationships, *J Ultrastruct Res* (1963) **9**:47–64.
33. Wolter JR, The astroglia of the human retina and other glial elements of the retina under normal and pathologic conditions, *Am J Ophthalmol* (1955) **40**:88–100.
34. Newman E, Reichenbach A, The Müller cell: a functional element of the retina, *Trends Neurosci* (1996) **19**:307–12.
35. Mizutani M, Gerhardinger C, Lorenzi M, Müller cell changes in human diabetic retinopathy, *Diabetes* (1998) **47**:445–9.
36. Wolter JR, Perivascular glia of the blood vessels of the human retina, *Am J Ophthalmol* (1957) **44**:766–73.
37. Bek T, Transretinal histopathological changes in capillary-free areas of diabetic retinopathy, *Acta Ophthalmol* (1994) **72**:409–15.
38. Rodrigues MM, Currier CA, Histopathology of argon laser photocoagulation in juvenile diabetic retinopathy, *Ophthalmology* (1983) **90**:1023–7.
39. Bresnick GH, Diabetic retinopathy viewed as a neurosensory disorder, *Arch Ophthalmol* (1986) **104**:989–90.
40. de Venecia G, Davis M, Engerman R, Clinicopathologic correlations in diabetic retinopathy I. Histology and fluorescein angiography of microaneurysms, *Arch Ophthalmol* (1976) **94**:1766–73.
41. Stitt AW, Gardiner TA, Archer DB, Histological and ultrastructural investigation of retinal microaneurysm development in diabetic patients, *Br J Ophthalmol* (1995) **70**:362–7.
42. Ashton N, Diabetic retinopathy. A new approach, *Lancet* (1959) 625–30.
43. Peyman GA, Bok D, Peroxidase diffusion in the normal and laser-coagulated primate retina, *Invest Ophthalmol Vis Sci* (1972) **11**:35–45.
44. Wallow IHL, Engerman RL, Permeability and patency of retinal blood vessels in experimental diabetes, *Invest Ophthalmol Vis Sci* (1977) **16**:447–61.
45. Raviola G, Butler JM, Unidirectional vesicular transport mechanism in retinal vessels, *Invest Ophthalmol Vis Sci* (1983) **24**:1465–74.
46. Taniguchi Y, Ultrastructure of newly formed blood vessels in diabetic retinopathy. *Jap J Ophthalmol* (1976) **20**:19–31.
47. Wallow IHL, Geldner PS, Endothelial fenestrae in proliferative diabetic retinopathy, *Invest Ophthalmol Vis Sci* (1980) **19**:1176–83.

48. Tout S, Chan-Ling T, Holländer H, Stone J, The role of Müller cells in the formation of the blood–retinal barrier, *Neuroscience* (1993) **55**:291–301.
49. Bek T, Lund-Andersen H, Localised blood–retina barrier leakage and retinal light sensitivity in diabetic retinopathy, *Br J Ophthalmol* (1990) **74**:388–92.
50. Diezel PB, Willert HG, Morphologie und Histochemie der harten und weichen Exsudate der Retina bei Diabetes mellitus und essentieller Hypertonie, *Klin Monatsbl Augenheilkd* (1961) **139**:475–91.
51. Toussaint D, Cogan DG, Kuwabara T, Extravascular lesions of diabetic retinopathy, *Arch Ophthalmol* (1962) **67**:42–7.
52. Murata T, Ishibashi T, Inomata H, Immunohistochemical detection of extravasated fibrinogen (fibrin) in human diabetic retina, *Graefes Arch Exp Clin Ophthalmol* (1992) **230**:428–31.
53. Dobree JH, Simple diabetic retinopathy. Evolution of the lesions and therapeutic considerations, *Br J Ophthalmol* (1970) **54**:1–10.
54. Kishi S, Numaga T, Yamazaki S, Structure of the inner retinal surface on simple diabetic retinopathy, *Jpn J Ophthalmol* (1982) **26**:141–9.
55. Sigurdsson R, Begg IS, Organised macular plaques in exudative diabetic maculopathy, *Br J Ophthalmol* (1980) **64**:392–7.
56. Bresnick GH, Diabetic maculopathy. A critical review highlighting diffuse macular edema, *Ophthalmology* (1983) **90**:1301–17.
57. Tso MOM, Pathology and pathogenesis of cystoid macular edema, *Ophthalmologica* (1981) **183**:46–54.
58. Fine BS, Brucker AJ, Macular edema and cystoid macular edema, *Am J Ophthalmol* (1981) **92**:466–81.
59. Heymann, Ueber Amaurose bei Brightischer Krankheit, und Fettdegeneration der Netzhaut, *Arch f Ophthalmol* (1856) **2**:137–50.
60. Brown GC, Brown MM, Hiller T et al, Cotton-wool spots, *Retina* (1985) **5**:206–14.
61. Wolter JR, Pathology of a cotton-wool spot, *Am J Ophthalmol* (1959) **48**:473–85.
62. Ashton N, Harry J, The pathology of cotton wool spots and cytoid bodies in hypertensive retinopathy and other diseases, *Am J Ophthalmol* (1963) **83**:91–114.
63. Ashton N, Pathophysiology of retinal cotton-wool spots, *Br Med Bull* (1970) **26**:143–50.
64. Kohner EM, Dollery MB, Bulpitt CJ, Cotton-wool spots in diabetic retinopathy, *Diabetes* (1969) **18**:691–704.
65. McLeod D, Marshall J, Kohner EM, Bird AC, The role of axoplasmic transport in the pathogenesis of retinal cotton-wool spots, *Br J Ophthalmol* (1977) **61**:177–91.
66. Roy MS, Rick ME, Higgins KE, McCulloch JC, Retinal cotton-wool spots: an early finding in diabetic retinopathy? *Br J Ophthalmol* (1986) **70**:772–8.
67. Williams DK, Drance SM, Harris GS, Fairclough M, Diabetic cotton-wool spots: An evaluation using perimetric and angiographic techniques, *Can J Ophthalmol* (1970) **5**:68–77.
68. Bek T, Lund-Andersen H, Cotton wool spots and retinal light sensitivity in diabetic retinopathy, *Br J Ophthalmol* (1991) **75**:13–17.
69. Ashton N, Arteriolar involvement in diabetic retinopathy, *Br J Ophthalmol* (1953) **37**:282–92.
70. Kohner EM, Henkind P, Correlation of fluorescein angiogram and retinal digest in diabetic retinopathy, *Am J Ophthalmol* (1970) **69**:403–14.
71. Bek T, Localized scotomata and types of vascular occlusion in diabetic retinopathy, *Acta Ophthalmol* (1991) **69**:11–18.
72. Ashton N, Pathogenesis of diabetic retinopathy. In: Little HL Jack RL, Patz A, Forsham PH, eds, *Diabetic Retinopathy* (Thieme Stratton: New York, 1983) 85–106.
73. Imesch PD, Bindley CD, Wallow IHL. Clinicopathologic correlation of intraretinal microvascular abnormalities. *RETINA* (1997) **17**:321–9.
74. O'Brien CS, Allen JH, Unusual changes in the retinal veins in diabetes, *Arch Ophthalmol* (1940) **24**:742–57.
75. Bek T. Venous loops in diabetic retinopathy. Prevalence, distribution, and pattern of development. *Acta Ophthalmol* (1999) **77**:130–4.

76. D'Amore PA, Mechanisms of retinal and choroidal neovascularization, *Invest Ophthalmol Vis Sci* (1994) **35**:3974–9.
77. Adamis AP, Miller JW, Bernal MT et al, Increased vascular endothelial growth factor levels in the vitreous of eyes with proliferative diabetic retinopathy, *Am J Ophthalmol* (1994) **118**:445–50.
78. Amin RH, Frank RN, Kennedy A et al, Vascular endothelial growth factor is present in glial cells of the retina and optic nerve of human subjects with nonproliferative diabetic retinopathy, *Invest Ophthalmol Vis Sci* (1997) **38**:36–47.
79. Okamoto N, Tobe T, Hackett SF et al, Transgenic mice with increased expression of vascular endothelial growth factor in the retina. A new model of intraretinal and subretinal neovascularisation, *Am J Pathol* (1997) **151**:281–91.
80. Stefánsson E, Machemer R, de Juan E et al, Retinal oxygenation and laser treatment in patients with diabetic retinopathy, *Am J Ophthalmol* (1992) **113**:36–8.

14 Aldose reductase and tissue damage in diabetes

David R Tomlinson

INTRODUCTION

Aldose reductase is one member of a superfamily of NADPH-dependent aldo-keto reductases, which has over 40 members with diverse physiological properties and roles.[1] The aldo-keto reductases are present in eukaryotes and prokaryotes and metabolize a wide range of substrates, including aliphatic aldehydes, monosaccharides, steroids, prostaglandins and xenobiotics. The companion members of the superfamily that are of practical importance in this context are aldehyde reductase, present largely in liver, and prostaglandin synthase (a component of the cyclooxygenase complex). This is because certain inhibitors of aldose reductase also have the capacity to inhibit these enzymes, with consequent effects on detoxification in the liver and on prostanoid syntheses, especially in the stomach. Abbreviated nomenclature is in use, coding aldehyde reductase as AR1 and aldose reductase as AR2.[1]

STRUCTURE AND ACTION

Although aldose reductase will act on a range of substrates, the primary action in diabetes is the conversion of glucose to sorbitol, with NADPH as the proton donor. Generally present at the same site is the enzyme sorbitol dehydrogenase, which further converts the sorbitol to fructose, using NAD^+ as its proton acceptor. This pair of reactions comprises the sorbitol pathway, which is illustrated in *Fig. 14.1*.

X-ray crystallography and protein analysis have been used to establish three-dimensional structures for aldose reductase[2,3] and the active site has been characterized.[4,5]

Aldose reductase has an affinity for glucose which is much lower than that of hexokinase. Under physiological conditions most intracellular glucose is converted to glucose 6-phosphate and only trace amounts of sorbitol are present in nerve.[6] The steady state levels give no clue about flux of glucose through the system, but

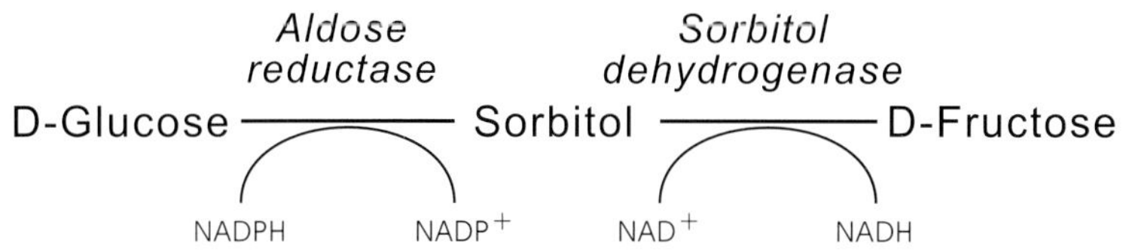

Figure 14.1
The sorbitol (polyol) pathway.

studies on relative affinity of aldose reductase in vitro indicate that little sorbitol is formed in normal nerve. Those tissues which are central to the development of diabetes complications can take up appreciable amounts of glucose in the absence of insulin, so that in diabetes, hexokinase is almost certainly saturated and glucose levels rise to bring its concentration towards the K_m of aldose reductase. Under these conditions appreciable amounts of sorbitol are formed. Attainment of steady state, when clearance of metabolites matches their production, is associated with marked accumulations of both sorbitol and fructose.[7–9] This presumably reflects low diffusibility of the metabolites and relatively low affinities of sorbitol dehydrogenase and fructokinase for sorbitol and fructose respectively.

TISSUE DISTRIBUTION

The tissue distribution of aldose reductase has been elucidated in a stop–start manner with the evolution of technology. The early histochemical studies localized aldose reductase activity to the lens, retina, kidney and peripheral nerve.[10–15] Subsequently, more refined methods based on immunocytochemistry or in situ hybridization showed that aldose reductase is concentrated in cells that form boundaries between fluid compartments. Thus, endothelial, epithelial and renal tubular cells are classic foci. Furthermore, in these cells aldose reductase expression is induced by hypertonicity at the interface.[16–20]

Significantly, aldose reductase is not expressed at functional levels in normal liver, where aldehyde reductase is present in substantial amounts.[21] However, an aldose reductase-like protein has been found in several hepatoma cell lines, hepatocarcinomas and livers with hepatitis.[22–24] It is important that these characterizations are completed to show, without doubt, that the induced protein is aldose (rather than aldehyde) reductase and that differentiation is made between a general induction of proteins as part of a hyperplastic disease response and a protective induction of a specific enzyme. One other observation suggests a protective effect. Elevated expression of aldose reductase-like immunoreactivity was observed in cancerous lesions of 3'-methyl-4-dimethyl-aminoazobenzene-induced hepatocarcinomas. Increased aldose reductase mRNA was confirmed in these cells by Northern blot analysis, indicating specificity, but aldehyde reductase-like activity did not change in cancerous tissue or in the cell lines. The viability of hepatoma cells in the presence of 3-deoxyglucosone and glyceraldehyde was decreased by the aldose reductase inhibitor epalrestat.[25] Before concluding that aldose reductase—rather than or as well as aldehyde reductase—is involved in hepatic protection against toxic carbonyl compounds, these experiments must be repeated with a range of inhibitors, varying in selectivity for aldose over aldehyde reductase. This is especially true because epalrestat is one of the least selective (aldose versus aldehyde reductase) inhibitors; it would be useful to repeat these studies with really selective inhibitors such as zopolrestat or IDD 676 (Sredy, personal communication).

REGULATION OF EXPRESSION AND PHYSIOLOGICAL PROPERTIES

Renal tubular cells at the medullary extremity of the loop of Henle are bathed in hypertonic interstitial fluid. Compensation for this osmotic stress involves production of sorbitol from glucose by aldose reductase.[26] Exposure of kidney cells in culture to increments in tonicity of their culture medium stimulates transcription of the mRNA for aldose reductase, with increased enzyme activity—signalled by the accumulation of sorbitol; this increased transcription is arrested once the sorbitol levels have achieved a new steady state appropriate to the extracellular osmolality.[27] The accumulated sorbitol provides the intracellular offsetting of the extracellular tonicity. Other osmolytes also contribute, in particular *myo*-inositol, betaine and glycerophosphorylcholine; the amino acids taurine and aspartate may also be increased intracellularly on exposure to hypertonic extracellular fluid.[28–30] This phenomenon is not restricted to kidney cells—similar changes in vitro are seen in lens epithelium[31] and the retinal pigmented epithelium.[29] It is, therefore, possible that the capacity to increase aldose reductase expression and produce graded amounts of sorbitol in response to hypertonicity is a highly conserved and a fundamental property of all nucleated cells.

The identity of the osmosensor initiating these changes has provoked recent interest in renal physiology, but also has a bearing on the involvement of aldose reductase in diabetes-induced changes in extrarenal tissues. Yeast (*Saccharomyces cerevisiae*) responds to osmotic stress by autophosphorylation of at least two cell-surface osmosensors. These then activate a signal cascade upstream of a mitogen-activated protein kinase (MAPK) called HOG1 (high-osmolarity glycerol), which, as the name implies, results in reduction of glycerol-3-phosphate to produce glycerol as an intracellular osmolyte.[32–34] This sequence of events is analogous to activation of a mammalian MAPK, known as p38, though the mammalian osmosensors have not been characterized. Osmotic challenge of kidney cells induces p38 with follow-on activation of immediate early genes. These almost certainly include some of the transcription-dependent osmoprotective events triggered by hypertonicity,[35] but this pathway does not appear to induce aldose reductase.[36] It is likely, therefore, that osmotic stress can activate more than one MAPK in susceptible tissues.

The capacity to generate sorbitol also confers cryoprotection. There are examples of poikilotherms whose capacity to survive environments with seasonal subzero temperatures depends upon generation of sorbitol via aldose reductase as an intracellular 'antifreeze'.[37] Interestingly this property is being exploited for cryoprotection of erythrocytes[38] and, via transfection of the enzyme gene, for the freezing of plant tissues without distortion.[39] Thus, aldose reductase may be considered as an inducible enzyme whose physiological role appears to be the production of electrically neutral solute with osmo- and cryoprotective properties in cells exposed to marked increases in the osmolality of their extracellular fluid or to ambient freezing conditions.

The discussion of aldose reductase expression in the liver (see above) indicates a possible role in detoxification of noxious xenobiotics and metabolites. However, since aldose and aldehyde reductase have overlap in substrate selectivity and since aldehyde reductase is expressed in the normal liver,[40] detailed studies are necessary to ensure that a detoxifying role exists for aldose reductase. This is, of course, very important in view of the therapeutic possibilities of its inhibition in diabetes.

Not all detoxification reactions occur in the liver and it is entirely possible that aldose reductase in other tissues acts to remove toxic moieties. Of particular interest in this context are the observations that aldose reductase can act on toxic products of glucose, such as methylglyoxal[41] or 3-deoxyglucosone,[42] both of which are increased in the circulation in badly controlled diabetes and are implicated in the post-translational glycosylation of proteins,[43,44] which may be involved in the development of complications of diabetes.

Thus, the effects of selective (see above) inhibitors of aldose reductase on the levels of these metabolites and their incorporation into glycosylated macromolecules would give valuable information on their clinical potential.

ALDOSE REDUCTASE IN THE EYE

Early studies with polyclonal antibodies located aldose reductase-like immunoreactivity (ARLI) to several ocular structures in the rat.[45] These include the corneal endothelium, the lens epithelium and its cortical fibres, the inner non-pigmented layer of the ciliary body epithelium plus its extension as the posterior surface of the iris and the Müller cells of the retina. Subsequent studies revealed ARLI in blood vessels of the human retina[46] and in ganglion cells, Müller cell processes, retinal pigmented epithelium and in the pericytes and endothelial cells of retinal capillaries in the BB (Bio-Breeding) spontaneously diabetic rat.[47]

Aldose reductase-like immunoreactivity is increased in expression with osmotic challenge of human retinal pigmented epithelium cells in culture.[48] Nevertheless, a detailed study of human eyes[49] showed that aldose reductase was immunohistochemically undetectable in the retinal pigmented epithelia and neural retinas of eyes from non-diabetic human subjects. Weak, focal staining for aldose reductase was present unilaterally in the retinal pigmented epithelium of 1 of 11 diabetic patients without retinopathy. A small majority (55%) of patients with background retinopathy demonstrated aldose reductase positivity in the retinal pigmented epithelium, and half of these expressed aldose reductase in the retinal pigmented epithelium of both eyes. The majority (88%) of patients with proliferative diabetic retinopathy showed bilateral staining in the retinal pigmented epithelium. Retinal positivity was present in 36% of background retinopathy and 75% of proliferative retinopathy cases, demonstrating a positive correlation between aldose reductase expression and the severity of the disorder. In weakly staining retinas, only the ganglion cell bodies, nerve fibres and Müller cells were positive, whereas in intensely staining cases, virtually the entire retina, except for the rod outer segments, was positive. These observations indicate clearly that aldose reductase is induced in the retinas of human diabetic patients in association with retinopathy, though the roles of 'chicken' and 'egg' are not defined. Furthermore, the distribution is extensive through neural, glial and vascular components of the retina.

ALDOSE REDUCTASE IN DIABETIC COMPLICATIONS

The extent to which osmotic stress participates in the pathophysiology of diabetes will vary with control of glycaemia and the involvement of the sorbitol pathway in diabetes is not simple. Under certain conditions the pathway may be driven by both osmotic stress and exaggerated concentrations of substrate—raised intracellular glucose resulting from exposure to hyperglycaemia of cells whose glucose uptake is independent of insulin. This latter feature may confer the degree of selectivity of cell type required for a real involvement in the development of complications, because there is coincidence between insulin-independent glucose uptake and susceptibility to complications.[40] Thus, the situation that pertains in the lens, where the pathway was first studied,[50] probably exemplifies its most extreme manifestation in diabetes. The lens can contain extremely high concentrations of glucose, to which the lenticular epithelium (the site of aldose reductase) is permeable. In diabetes this is associated with accumulation of sorbitol, which leaks out into the aqueous and vitreous, contributing to an osmotic stress of the lenticular epithelium and increasing expression of aldose reductase.[51,52] Thus, these combined influences induce aldose reductase and drive a large flux of substrate through its pathway. In other tissues, such as peripheral nerve or kidney, where the cells containing aldose reductase are exposed to interstitial fluid in equilibrium with plasma, which is normotonic even in severe hyperglycaemia,[53] the major force driving flux is the high glucose concentration, though hypertonic transients must occur during hyperglycaemic peaks and/or dehydration. Under these conditions, the cell is forced to produce sorbitol without extracellular hypertonic stress and the generation of such an intracellular osmolyte provokes an inappropriate osmotic response. This might be termed intracellular osmotic stress. That this occurs is demonstrated by the fact that such tissues reduce their content of *myo*-inositol, by reducing expression of its carrier protein.[54,55] This must compensate for the intracellular stress imposed by the accumulated sorbitol, but it is not possible to judge the efficacy of this compensation.

It was argued earlier in this review that activation of MAPKs forms a precursive step in the transduction of extracellular osmotic stress to those cells in which aldose reductase is transcriptionally induced. It is also possible that intracellular osmotic stress, as defined above, is also capable of activating MAPKs and such an event is likely to occur wherever depletion of *myo*-inositol is associated with sorbitol accumulation in nerve,[56,57] kidney[58,59] and retina.[60–62] Differential examination of the influences of dehydration and glucose in the kidney reveals some of the complexity of interaction, shows different pathways signalling the two stimuli and indicates multiple activation of MAPKs.[63,64]

ALDOSE REDUCTASE AND DIABETIC RETINOPATHY

At the time of writing there are no published studies which explore activation of MAPKs in the retina in either clinical or experimental diabetes. However, another approach to the aetiology of diabetic retinopathy connects the polyol pathway and MAPKs to the disease. Ten years ago it was reported that exposure of renal glomeruli[65] or endothelial cells[66] to high glucose activates protein kinase C (PKC). These observations were refined to show activation of multiple subtypes of PKC in retinas of diabetic rats, together with raised levels of diacylglycerol; these changes were normalized by insulin treatment.[67] The mechanism linking raised glucose to PKC activation may involve oxidative stress because treatment with either vitamin E or probucol prevents activation.[68] Vitamin E also prevents the retinal hyperaemia which is associated with activation of PKC and increased diacylglycerol production.[69] The important link between these phenomena in retinal vasculature and the proliferative phase of retinopathy came with the demonstration that the activated PKC is involved in the generation of vascular endothelial growth factor (VEGF) and its effects on capillary permeability.[69]

The next important step in the development of understanding of these processes came with the observation that calphostin C, a PKC inhibitor, prevented activation of MAPK and phospholipase A_2 (PLA_2) in mesangial cells cultured in high glucose.[70] The polyol pathway was also tied into these phenomena with the observation that an aldose reductase inhibitor prevented the activation of PLA_2 in glomeruli from diabetic rats.[71] More directly still, an aldose reductase inhibitor was shown to inhibit the activation of PKC and the increase in transforming growth factor (TGF) production in human mesangial cells cultured in high glucose.[72] The co-activation of PKC and MAPKs in vascular cells maintained in high glucose[73] reinforces the notion that the two are linked. There is a growing literature outside of diabetes research showing that PKC can activate MAPKs and that PKC inhibitors can prevent their activation by a range of stimuli.[74–76] Thus, assembly of the observations cited above suggests that, in vascular tissue, activation of PKC (possibly amplified by increases in its expression) occurs in diabetes via oxidative stress and exaggerated flux through the polyol pathway. These latter phenomena are, in any case, linked as described earlier. PKC and diacylglycerol provide haemodynamic abnormalities via impairment of prostanoid and nitric oxide production. The production of VEGF is stimulated synergistically by activated PKC and hypoxia derived from the haemodynamic disturbance. Increased TGF provokes increased synthesis of extracellular matrix materials. The activation of MAPKs via PKC—as well as via the other pathways described earlier—is implicated in the transcription-dependent changes and phenotypic switches underlying these and probably other undisclosed phenomena. Although some of these phenomena have been tracked only in renal cells and others in non-ocular endothelial cells, there is no reason why they should not be extrapolated to the retina. Such considerations support the exploration of the potential benefits of a selective inhibitor of PKC subforms as agents targeted at diabetic retinopathy.[77]

Direct evidence of involvement of aldose reductase and the sorbitol pathway in diabetic retinopathy is pragmatically based on effects of aldose reductase inhibitors. The issue has been somewhat clouded by the use of galactose feeding instead of diabetes to produce a 'diabetes-like experimental retinopathy'.[78–80] The predictive value of this model is contentious;[81] certainly it could be argued that the step from humans to rats is a big enough remove from clinical reality, without dispensing with diabetes altogether. However, there were early demonstrations that aldose reductase inhibitors prevent retinal pathology derived from galactose feeding in different animal species[82–84] and, in parallel, similar observations in diabetic rats.[85,86] Functional studies in diabetic models also indicated beneficial effects of aldose reductase inhibitors.[87–89] In longer-term diabetic and galactosaemic models the effects of aldose reductase inhibition were less convincing,[90] though in this study the dose of inhibitor may not have been adequate. Clinically, there are studies which claim significant efficacy for aldose reductase inhibitors against diabetic retinopathy,[91–93] balanced by others which do not.[94,95] The fact that none of these drugs has yet been licensed with diabetic retinopathy as a primary target perhaps tells us something, in spite of the overwhelming evidence of efficacy against morphological and some functional defects in the retinas of diabetic animals. However, the message may inform more about trial design than about genuine therapeutic potential. *Figure 14.2* illustrates this point for drugs targeted at diabetes complications in general. The first line of defence against complications is insulin, but we know that even the best-motivated patients with the best health care will sustain poor glycaemic control at times—so that first line of defence will be breached and, in the worst-controlled patients, this will be a regular event. It follows that the second line of defence should give protection which approximates as closely as possible to the broad spectrum offered by insulin. It has been outside the realms of this review, but there is strong evidence implicating protein glycation and oxidative stress, in addition to flux through aldose reductase, in the development of diabetes complications. This evidence encompasses or can be extrapolated to retinopathy.[96–98] Thus, drugs giving specific pharmacological protection against glycation, oxidative

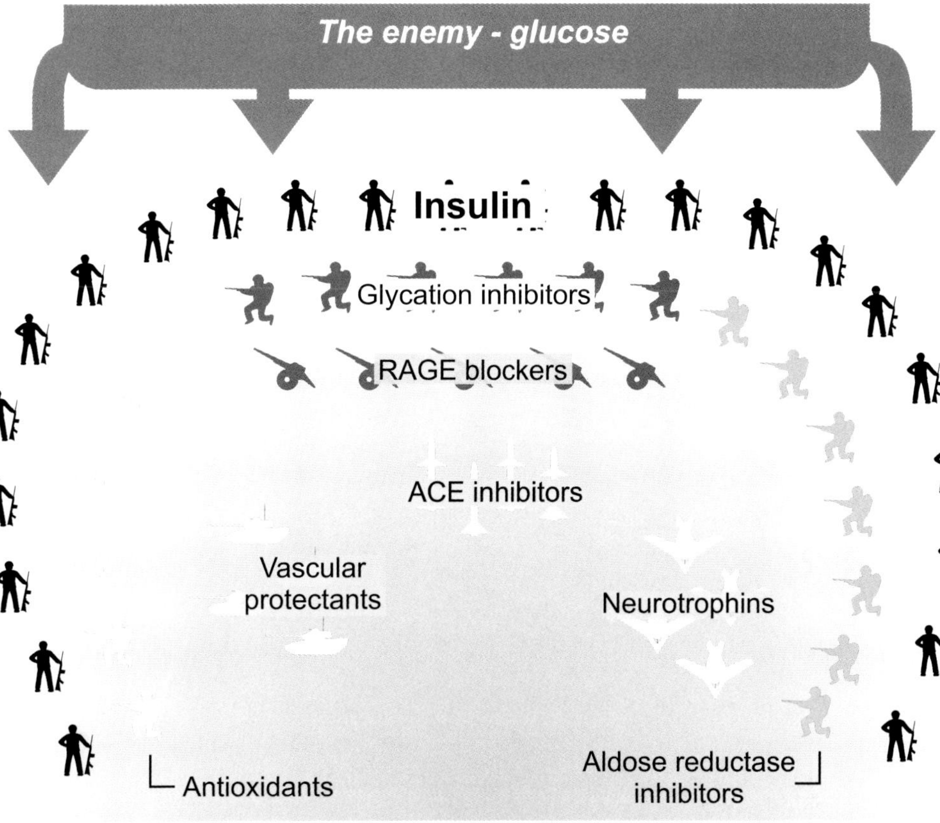

Figure 14.2
Defence against diabetes complications.

stress and flux through aldose reductase probably have little overlap and would give a narrower spectrum of protection than perfect glycaemic control. Indeed, as represented in *Fig.14.2*, the placement of one of these three forms of defence on the field of battle without the other two would be military suicide. Yet, this is exactly what is done in a clinical trial of an aldose reductase inhibitor. It follows, therefore, that even a significant degree of protection by such drugs may never be realized in isolation. We may need to rethink the way that we organize such trials and the demands made by the drug licensing bodies to demonstrate efficacy against diabetic retinopathy.

REFERENCES

1. Jez JM, Flynn TG, Penning TM, A new nomenclature for the aldo-keto reductase superfamily, *Biochem Pharmacol* (1997) 54:639–47.
2. Wilson DK, Bohren KM, Gabbay KH, Quiocho FA, An unlikely sugar substrate site in the 1.65 Å structure of the human aldose reductase holoenzyme implicated in diabetic complications, *Science* (1992) 257:81–4.
3. Wilson DK, Tarle I, Petrash JM, Quiocho FA, Refined 1.8 Å structure of human aldose reductase complexed with the potent inhibitor zopolrestat, *Proc Natl Acad Sci USA* (1993) 90:9847–51.

4. Tarle I, Borhani DW, Wilson DK et al, Probing the active site of human aldose reductase. Site-directed mutagenesis of Asp-43, Tyr-48, Lys-77, and His-110, *J Biol Chem* (1993) **268**:25687–93.
5. Wermuth B, Burgisser H, Bohren KM, Von Wartburg JP, Purification and characterization of human-brain aldose reductase, *Eur J Biochem* (1982) **127**:279–84.
6. Holcomb GN, Klemm LA, Dulin WE, The polyol pathway for glucose metabolism in tissues from normal, diabetic, and ketotic Chinese hamsters, *Diabetologia* (1974) **10**:549–53.
7. Gabbay KH, Merola LO, Field RA, Sorbitol pathway: presence in nerve and cord with substrate accumulation in diabetes, *Science* (1966) **151**:209–10.
8. Gabbay KH, O'Sullivan JB, The sorbitol pathway in diabetes and galactosemia: enzyme and substrate localization and changes in kidney, *Diabetes* (1968) **17**:239–43.
9. Hutton JC, Schofield PJ, Williams JF, Hollows FC, Sorbitol metabolism in the retina: accumulation of pathway intermediates in streptozotocin induced diabetes in the rat, *Aust J Exp Biol Med Sci* (1974) **52**:361–73.
10. Collins JG, Corder CN, Aldose reductase and sorbitol dehydrogenase distribution in substructures of normal and diabetic rat lens, *Invest Ophthalmol Vis Sci* (1977) **16**:242–3.
11. Corder CN, Collins JG, Brannan TS, Sharma J, Aldose reductase and sorbitol dehydrogenase distribution in rat kidney, *J Histochem Cytochem* (1977) **25**:1–8.
12. Corder CN, Braughler JM, Culp PA, Quantitative histochemistry of the sorbitol pathway in glomeruli and small arteries of human diabetic kidney, *Folia Histochem Cytochem* (1979) **17**:137–45.
13. Ludvigson MA, Sorenson RL, Immunohistochemical localization of aldose reductase. II. Rat eye and kidney, *Diabetes* (1980) **29**:450–9.
14. Ludvigson MA, Sorenson RL, Immunohistochemical localization of aldose reductase. I. Enzyme purification and antibody preparation—localization in peripheral nerve, artery and testis, *Diabetes* (1980) **29**:438–49.
15. Orosz SE, Townsend SF, Tornheim PA, Brownscheidle CM, Localization of aldose reductase and sorbitol dehydrogenase in the nervous system of normal and diabetic rats, *Acta Diabetol* (1981) **18**:373–81.
16. Bondy CA, Lightman SL, Developmental and physiological regulation of aldose reductase mRNA expression in renal medulla, *Mol Endocrinol* (1989) **3**:1409–16.
17. Bondy CA, Lightman SL, Developmental and physiological pattern of aldose reductase mRNA expression in lens and retina, *Mol Endocrinol* (1989) **3**:1417–25.
18. Carper D, Kaneko M, Stark H, Hohman T, Increase in aldose reductase mRNA in dog lens epithelial cells under hypertonic conditions, *Exp Eye Res* (1990) **50**:743–9.
19. Cowley BD Jr, Ferraris JD, Carper DA, Burg MB, In vivo osmoregulation of aldose reductase mRNA, protein, and sorbitol in renal medulla, *Am J Physiol* (1990) **258**:F154–61.
20. Hohman TC, Carper D, Dasgupta S, Kaneko M, Osmotic stress induces aldose reductase in glomerular endothelial cells, *Adv Exp Med Biol* (1991) **284**:139–52.
21. Dvornik D, *Aldose Reductase Inhibition* (McGraw-Hill: New York,1987).
22. Zeindl EE, Jungblut PR, Otto A et al, Further characterization of a rat hepatoma-derived aldose-reductase-like protein—organ distribution and modulation in vitro, *Eur J Biochem* (1997) **247**:792–800.
23. Zeindl EE, Jungblut PR, Otto A, Rabes HM, Identification of tumor-associated protein variants during rat hepatocarcinogenesis. Aldose reductase, *J Biol Chem* (1994) **269**:14589–94.
24. Takahashi M, Hoshi A, Fujii J, et al, Induction of aldose reductase gene expression in LEC rats during the development of the hereditary hepatitis and hepatoma, *Jpn J Cancer Res* (1996) **87**:337–41.
25. Takahashi M, Fujii J, Miyoshi E et al, Elevation of aldose reductase gene expression in rat

primary hepatoma and hepatoma cell lines: implication in detoxification of cytotoxic aldehydes, *Int J Cancer* (1995) **62**:749–54.
26. Bagnasco SM, Balaban R, Fales HM et al, Predominant osmotically active solutes in rat and rabbit renal medullas, *J Biol Chem* (1986) **261**:5872–77.
27. Smardo FL Jr, Burg MB, Garcia-Perez A, Kidney aldose reductase gene transcription is osmotically regulated, *Am J Physiol* (1992) **262**:C776–82.
28. Edmands S, Yancey PH, Effects on rat renal osmolytes of extended treatment with an aldose reductase inhibitor, *Comp Biochem Physiol* (1992) **103C**:499–502.
29. Lin L-R, Carper D, Yokoyama T, Reddy VN, The effect of hypertonicity on aldose reductase, $alpha_B$- crystallin, and organic osmolytes in the retinal pigment epithelium, *Invest Ophthalmol Vis Sci* (1993) **34**:2352–9.
30. Stevens MJ, Lattimer SA, Kamijo M et al, Osmotically-induced nerve taurine depletion and the compatible osmolyte hypothesis in experimental diabetic neuropathy in the rat, *Diabetologia* (1993) **36**:608–14.
31. Bondy CA, Lightman SL, Developmental and physiological pattern of aldose reductase mRNA expression in lens and retina, *Mol Endocrinol* (1989) **3**:1417–25.
32. Posas F, Wurgler MS, Maeda T et al, Yeast HOG1 MAP kinase cascade is regulated by a multistep phosphorelay mechanism in the SLN1–YPD1–SSK1 'two-component' osmosensor, *Cell* (1996) **86**:865–75.
33. Maeda T, Takekawa M, Saito H, Activation of yeast PBS2 MAPKK by MAPKKKs or by binding of an SH3–containing osmosensor, *Science* (1995) **269**:554–8.
34. Maeda T, Wurgler MS, Saito H, A two-component system that regulates an osmosensing MAP kinase cascade in yeast [see comments], *Nature* (1994) **369**:242–5.
35. Sheikh-Hamad D, Di Mari J, Suki WN et al, p38 kinase activity is essential for osmotic induction of mRNAs for HSP70 and transporter for organic solute betaine in Madin-Darby canine kidney cells, *J Biol Chem* (1998) **273**:1832–37.
36. Kultz D, Garcia-Perez A, Ferraris JD, Burg MB, Distinct regulation of osmoprotective genes in yeast and mammals. Aldose reductase osmotic response element is induced independent of p38 and stress-activated protein kinase/Jun N- terminal kinase in rabbit kidney cells, *J Biol Chem* (1997) **272**:13165–70.
37. Storey KB, Miceli M, Butler KW et al, 31P-NMR studies of the freeze-tolerant larvae of the gall fly, *Eurosta solidaginis*, *Eur J Biochem* (1984) **142**:591–5.
38. Behr W, Doukas K, Lang H et al, Is preservation of erythrocyte concentrates with added solutions an alternative to deep freezing in heart surgery autologous blood donation? *Beitr Infusionsther* (1990) **26**:252–6.
39. Tao R, Uratsu SL, Dandekar AM, Sorbitol synthesis in transgenic tobacco with apple cDNA encoding NADP-dependent sorbitol-6-phosphate dehydrogenase, *Plant Cell Physiol* (1995) **36**:525–32.
40. Dvornik D, *Aldose Reductase Inhibition* (McGraw-Hill: New York,1987).
41. Vander Jagt DL, Robinson B, Taylor KK, Hunsaker LA, Reduction of trioses by NADPH-dependent aldo-keto reductases. Aldose reductase, methylglyoxal, and diabetic complications, *J Biol Chem* (1992) **267**:4364–9.
42. Sato K, Inazu A, Yamaguchi S et al, Monkey 3-deoxyglucosone reductase: tissue distribution and purification of three multiple forms of the kidney enzyme that are identical with dihydrodiol dehydrogenase, aldehyde reductase, and aldose reductase, *Arch Biochem Biophys* (1993) **307**:286–94.
43. McCance DR, Dyer DG, Dunn JA et al, Maillard reaction products and their relation to complications in insulin-dependent diabetes mellitus, *J Clin Invest* (1993) **91**:2470–8.
44. Selwood T, Thornalley PJ, Binding of methylglyoxal to albumin and formation of fluorescent adducts. Inhibition by arginine, *N*-alpha-acetyl-arginine and aminoguanidine, *Biochem Soc Trans* (1993) **21**:170S.

45. Ludvigson MA, Sorenson RL, Immunohistochemical localization of aldose reductase. II. Rat eye and kidney, *Diabetes* (1980) **29**:450–9.
46. Akagi Y, Yajima Y, Kador PF et al, Localization of aldose reductase in the human eye, *Diabetes* (1984) **33**:562–6.
47. Chakrabarti S, Sima AAF, Nakajima T et al, Aldose reductase in the BB rat: isolation, immunological identification and localization in the retina and peripheral nerve, *Diabetologia* (1987) **30**:244–51.
48. Stevens MJ, Henry DN, Thomas TP et al, Aldose reductase gene expression and osmotic dysregulation in cultured human retinal pigment epithelial cells, *Am J Physiol* (1993) **265**:E428–38.
49. Vinores SA, Campochiaro PA, Williams EH et al, Aldose reductase expression in human diabetic retina and retinal pigment epithelium, *Diabetes* (1988) **37**:1658–64.
50. van Heyningen R, Formation of polyols by the lens of the rat with 'sugar' cataracts, *Nature* (1959) **184**:194–5.
51. Iwata T, Sato S, Jimenez J et al, Osmotic response element is required for the induction of aldose reductase by tumor necrosis factor-α, *J Biol Chem* (1999) **274**:7993–8001.
52. Xiong H, Cheng HM, Aqueous/vitreous tonicity in 'sugar' cataracts, *Ophthalmic Res* (1989) **21**:292–6.
53. Willars GB, Lambourne JE, Tomlinson DR, Does galactose feeding provide a valid model of the consequences of exaggerated polyol-pathway flux in peripheral nerve in experimental diabetes? *Diabetes* (1987) **36**:1425–31.
54. Burger-Kentischer A, Müller E, Neuhofer W et al, Expression of Na^+/Cl^-/betaine and Na^+/*myo*-inositol transporters, aldose reductase and sorbitol dehydrogenase in macula densa cells of the kidney, *Pflugers Arch* (1998) **436**:807–9.
55. Burger-Kentischer A, Müller E, Neuhofer W et al, Expression of aldose reductase, sorbitol dehydrogenase and Na^+/*myo*-inositol and Na^+/Cl^-/betaine transporter mRNAs in individual cells of the kidney during changes in the diuretic state, *Pflugers Arch* (1999) **437**:248–54.
56. Finegold D, Lattimer SA, Nolle S et al, Polyol pathway activity and myo-inositol metabolism. A suggested relationship in the pathogenesis of diabetic neuropathy, *Diabetes* (1983) **32**:988–92.
57. Mayer JH, Tomlinson DR, Prevention of defects of axonal transport and nerve conduction velocity by oral administration of myo-inositol or an aldose reductase inhibitor in streptozotocin-diabetic rats, *Diabetologia* (1983) **25**:433–8.
58. Cohen MP, Aldose reductase, glomerular metabolism, and diabetic nephropathy, *Metabolism* (1986) **35**:55–9.
59. Cohen MP, Klepser H, Glomerular Na^+-K^+-ATPase activity in acute and chronic diabetes and with aldose reductase inhibition, *Diabetes* (1988) **37**:558–62.
60. MacGregor LC, Rosecan LR, Laties AM, Matschinsky FM, Altered retinal metabolism in diabetes I. Microanalysis of lipid, glucose, sorbitol and myo-inositol in the choroid and in the individual layers of the rabbit retina, *J Biol Chem* (1986) **261**:4046–51.
61. Li WY, Zhou Q, Tang L et al, Intramural pericyte degeneration in early diabetic retinopathy study in vitro, *Chin Med J Engl* (1990) **103**:7–13.
62. Kern TS, Engerman RL, Retinal polyol and myo-inositol in galactosemic dogs given an aldose-reductase inhibitor, *Invest Ophthalmol Vis Sci* (1991) **32**:3175–7.
63. Nakanishi T, Uyama O, Sugita M, Osmotically regulated taurine content in rat renal inner medulla, *Am J Physiol* (1991) **261**:F957–62.
64. Nakanishi T, Yamauchi A, Sugita M, Takamitsu Y, Aldose reductase and myo-inositol transporter mRNA are independently regulated in rat renal medulla, *J Am Soc Nephrol* (1996) **7**:283–9.
65. Craven PA, De Rubertis FR, Protein kinase C is activated in glomeruli from streptozotocin diabetic rats. Possible mediation by glucose, *J Clin Invest* (1989) **83**:1667–75.
66. Lee T-S, Saltsman KA, Ohashi H, King GL, Activation of protein kinase C by elevation of glucose concentration: proposal for a mechanism in the development of diabetic vascular complications, *Proc Natl Acad Sci USA* (1989) **86**:5141–5.

67. Shiba T, Inoguchi T, Sportsman JR et al, Correlation of diacylglycerol level and protein kinase C activity in rat retina to retinal circulation, *Am J Physiol* (1993) **265**:E783–93.
68. Kunisaki M, Bursell S-E, Umeda F et al, Normalization of diacylglycerol-protein kinase C activation by vitamin E in aorta of diabetic rats and cultured rat smooth muscle cells exposed to elevated glucose levels, *Diabetes* (1994) **43**:1372–7.
69. Kunisaki M, Bursell S-E, Clermont AC et al, Vitamin E prevents diabetes-induced abnormal retinal blood flow via the diacylglycerol–protein kinase C pathway, *Am J Physiol* (1995) **269**:E239–46.
70. Haneda M, Araki S, Togawa M et al, Mitogen-activated protein kinase cascade is activated in glomeruli of diabetic rats and glomerular mesangial cells cultured under high glucose conditions, *Diabetes* (1997) **46**:847–53.
71. Keogh RJ, Dunlop ME, Larkins RG, Effect of inhibition of aldose reductase on glucose flux, diacylglycerol formation, protein kinase C, and phospholipase A_2 activation, *Metabolism* (1997) **46**:41–7.
72. Ishii H, Tada H, Isogai S, An aldose reductase inhibitor prevents glucose-induced increase in transforming growth factor- and protein kinase C activity in cultured human mesangial cells, *Diabetologia* (1998) **41**:362–4.
73. Haneda M, Kikkawa R, Sugimoto T et al, Abnormalities in protein kinase C and MAP kinase cascade in mesangial cells cultured under high glucose conditions, *J Diabetes Comp.* (1995) **9**:246–8.
74. Wood KW, Sarnecki C, Roberts TM, Blenis J, *ras* mediates nerve growth factor receptor modulation of three signal-transducing protein kinases: MAP kinase, Raf-1, and RSK, *Cell* (1992) **68**:1041–50.
75. Clerk A, Michael A, Sugden PH, Stimulation of multiple mitogen-activated protein kinase subfamilies by oxidative stress and phosphorylation of the small heat shock protein, HSP25/27, in neonatal ventricular myocytes, *Biochem J* (1998) **333**:581–9.
76. Dent P, Jarvis WD, Birrer MJ et al, The roles of signaling by the p42/p44 mitogen-activated protein (MAP) kinase pathway; a potential route to radio- and chemo-sensitization of tumor cells resulting in the induction of apoptosis and loss of clonogenicity, *Leukemia* (1998) **12**:1843–50.
77. Bursell SE, Takagi C, Clermont AC et al, Specific retinal diacylglycerol and protein kinase C beta isoform modulation mimics abnormal retinal hemodynamics in diabetic rats, *Invest Ophthalmol Vis Sci* (1997) **38**:2711–20.
78. Robison WG Jr, Kador PF, Kinoshita JH, Retinal capillaries: basement membrane thickening by galactosemia prevented with aldose reductase inhibitor, *Science* (1983) **221**:1177–9.
79. Cogan DG, Kinoshita JH, Kador PF et al, Aldose reductase and complications of diabetes, *Ann Intern Med* (1984) **101**:82–91.
80. Engerman RL, Kern TS, Experimental galactosemia produces diabetic-like retinopathy, *Diabetes* (1984) **33**:97–100.
81. Willars GB, Lambourne JE, Tomlinson DR, Does galactose feeding provide a valid model of the consequences of exaggerated polyol-pathway flux in peripheral nerve in experimental diabetes? *Diabetes* (1987) **36**:1425–31.
82. Lou MF, Dickerson JEJ, Chandler ML et al, The prevention of biochemical changes in lens, retina, and nerve of galactosemic dogs by the aldose reductase inhibitor AL01576, *J Ocul Pharmacol* (1989) **5**:233–40.
83. Robison WG Jr, Nagata M, Laver N et al, Diabetic-like retinopathy in rats prevented with an aldose reductase inhibitor, *Invest Ophthalmol Vis Sci* (1989) **30**:2285–92.
84. Vinores SA, Campochiaro PA, Prevention or moderation of some ultrastructural changes in the RPE and retina of galactosemic rats by aldose reductase inhibition, *Exp Eye Res* (1989) **49**:495–510.
85. Chandler ML, Shannon WA, Desantis L, Prevention of retinal capillary basement membrane thickening in diabetic rats by aldose reductase inhibitors, *Invest Ophthalmol Vis Sci* (1984) **25**:159–9.

86. Robison WG Jr, Tillis TN, Laver N, Kinoshita JH, Diabetes-related histopathologies of the rat retina prevented with an aldose reductase inhibitor, *Exp Eye Res* (1990) **50**:355–66.
87. MacGregor LC, Matschinsky FM, Treatment with aldose reductase inhibitor or with myo-inositol arrests deterioration of the electroretinogram of diabetic rats, *J Clin Invest* (1985) **76**:887–9.
88. Hotta N, Kakuta H, Koh N et al, Aldose reductase inhibitor can improve diabetic retinopathy in experimental and clinical studies, *Diabetes* (1988) **37**:123A.
89. Hotta N, Koh N, Sakakibara F et al, An aldose reductase inhibitor, TAT, prevents electroretinographic abnormalities and ADP-induced hyperaggregability in streptozotocin-induced diabetic rats, *Eur J Clin Invest* (1995) **25**:948–54.
90. Engerman RL, Kern TS, Aldose reductase inhibition fails to prevent retinopathy in diabetic and galactosemic dogs, *Diabetes* (1993) **42**:820–5.
91. Pitts NE, Vreeland F, Shaw GL et al, Clinical experience with sorbinil—an aldose reductase inhibitor, *Metabolism* (1986) **35**:96–100.
92. Hotta N, Kakuta H, Ando F, Sakamoto N, Clinical trial of the aldose reductase inhibitor ONO 2235: effect in diabetic retinopathy. In: Sakamoto N, Kinoshita JH, Kador PF, Hotta N, eds, *Polyol Pathway and its Role in Diabetic Complications* (Exerpta Medica: Amsterdam, 1988) 253–66.
93. Sorbinil Retinopathy Trial Research Group, A randomized trial of sorbinil, an aldose reductase inhibitor, in diabetic retinopathy, *Arch Ophthalmol* (1990) **108**:1234–44.
94. Christensen JEJ, Varnek L, Gregersen G, The effect of an aldose reductase inhibitor (sorbinil) on diabetic neuropathy and neural function of the retina: a double-blind study, *Acta Neurol Scand* (1985) **71**:164–7.
95. Van Gerven JMA, Boot JP, Lemkes HHPJ, Van Best JA, Effects of aldose reductase inhibition with tolrestat on diabetic retinopathy in a six months double blind trial, *Doc Ophthalmol* (1994) **87**:355–65.
96. Armstrong D, Al-Awadi F, Lipid peroxidation and retinopathy in streptozotocin-induced diabetes, *Free Radic Biol Med* (1991) **11**:433–6.
97. Grattagliano I, Vendemiale G, Boscia F et al, Oxidative retinal products and ocular damages in diabetic patients, *Free Radic Biol Med* (1998) **25**:369–72.
98. Paget C, Lecomte M, Ruggiero D et al, Modification of enzymatic antioxidants in retinal microvascular cells by glucose or advanced glycation end products, *Free Radic Biol Med* (1998) **25**:121–9.

15 Blood coagulation and haemostasis: alterations in diabetes and their role in diabetic vascular disease

Michael Greaves and Isobel Ford

THE PHYSIOLOGY OF HAEMOSTASIS

The physiology of haemostasis can be considered according to its component parts, although there are numerous points of interaction in a complex mechanism. It is initiated by a rapid and early response to vessel injury and involves vasoconstriction, adhesion of platelets to the site and platelet aggregation–'primary haemostasis'. The platelet plug is then consolidated by the deposition of fibrin, the insoluble product of the interaction of the plasma components of the fluid phase of coagulation. Platelet activation and fibrin formation are both modulated by inhibitors to prevent inappropriate thrombosis. In addition, a separate mechanism exists for the generation of the enzyme plasmin, which rapidly digests fibrin–the fibrinolytic system.

Primary haemostasis

Damage to the wall, or transection, of an arteriole or larger-calibre vessel results in immediate vasoconstriction, which serves to slow the flow of blood. The role of blood platelets is to seal the vascular breach. Platelets are anucleate structured fragments generated from the cytoplasm of the polyploid megakaryocyte. Megakaryocytes are haemopoietic cells which mature in the red bone marrow under the stimulus of cytokines including interleukin-6 and thrombopoietin. The precise site of platelet production is debated, there being some evidence for egress of megakaryocytes into the bone marrow circulation with transit to the lungs and platelet generation in the pulmonary vasculature.

There are between 150 and 400 $\times$ 10^9 platelets per litre of blood. They are highly reactive, contractile and secretory cells, with four main functions:

1. To adhere to sites of vessel injury, through surface receptors.
2. To interact with adjacent platelets, through additional receptors using fibrinogen, the plasma precursor of fibrin, as an intercellular binding protein.
3. To deliver vasoactive, haemostatic and tissue repair components to the site.
4. To catalyse the local generation of fibrin through provision of a phospholipid surface. This acts as a template for the interaction of the components of the fluid phase of coagulation.

Average platelet life span is around 10 days and this may be shortened by activation at sites of vessel injury. Newly formed platelets tend to be larger with a higher average mean platelet volume.

*Platelet adhesion (*Fig. 15.1a*)*

Resting platelets are disc-shaped cells, their configuration being maintained by a peripheral arrangement of intracellular microtubules. They rapidly transform to a 'spiny sphere' shape when stimulated. Adhesion of platelets to the intact unactivated vascular endothelium does not occur, but loss of endothelial continuity exposes subendothelial fibrillar components including collagen. Binding of platelets to subendothelium requires von Willebrand factor (vWF), a macromolecular plasma protein. vWF is synthesized by megakaryocytes and vascular endothelial cells and undergoes a conformational change when it binds to subendothelial components. This exposes a binding site for platelet membrane receptors, principally glycoprotein Ib/IX, a dimeric transmembrane receptor for vWF which mediates platelet adhesion. In addition to its role in platelet function vWF is also the carrier protein for coagulation factor VIII in the circulation.

*Platelet aggregation (*Fig. 15.1b*)*

The platelet plasma membrane has additional receptors for agonists which induce platelet to platelet interaction and aggregate formation. These agonists include thrombin – the final enzyme of the fluid phase system of coagulation; adenosine diphosphate (ADP) – which may be released from erythrocytes damaged by shear forces at sites of vessel injury; and platelet activating factor (PAF) – a lipid mediator of platelet activation, adrenaline, serotonin and collagen. Platelet aggregation begins within seconds of the interaction of an agonist with its receptor.

Agonist–receptor binding triggers intracellular reactions comparable to those mechanisms of stimulus–response coupling in other secretory

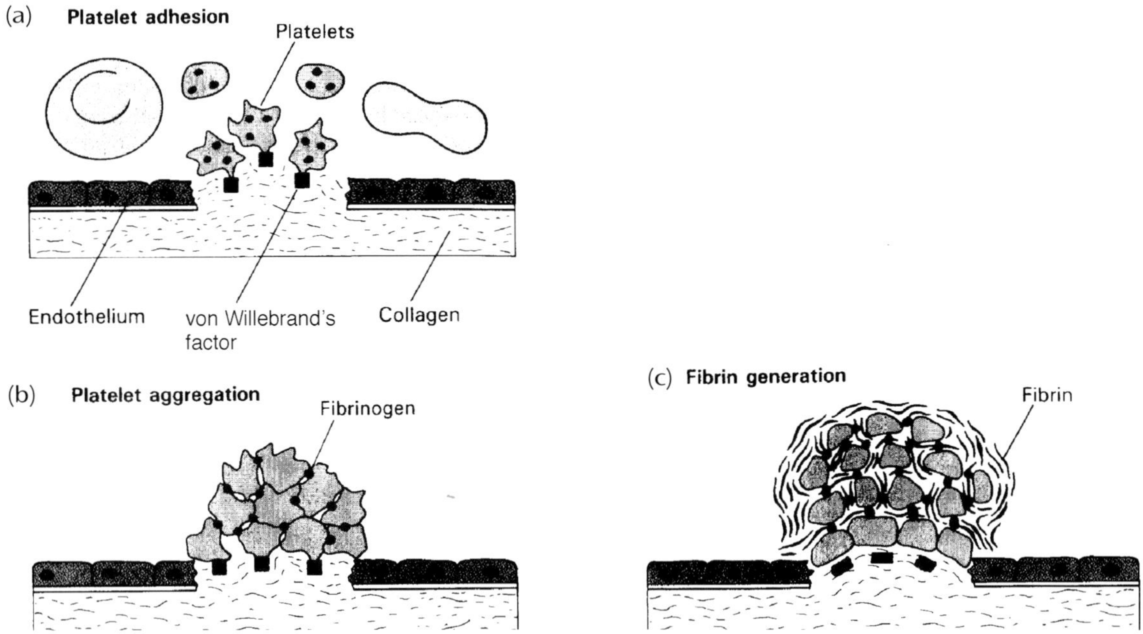

Figure 15.1
A simplified diagram of the process of primary haemostasis.

cells. In platelets activation of these pathways leads to the exposure of a binding site for fibrinogen and stimulation of contractile elements of the platelet. The principal fibrinogen receptor is the transmembrane integrin glycoprotein IIb/IIIa. The contractile components include actin and myosin, stimulation of which initiates shape change and the secretion of intracellular granules into the extracellular environment. This secretory response is referred to as the release reaction.

Stimulus–response coupling within the platelet is mediated by G-proteins (guanine nucleotide binding proteins), which control the metabolism of platelet membrane phosphatidylinositol from which the second messengers diacylglycerol and inositol triphosphate (IP-3) are generated. Mobilization of calcium ions from intracellular stores, particularly the dense tubular system of the platelet, by inositol triphosphate is an essential mechanism in stimulus–response coupling. There is also synthesis of thromboxane A_2, a potent vasoconstrictor and proaggregatory short-lived prostanoid, from membrane arachidonic acid. Thromboxane A_2 is secreted into the plasma, binds to its own platelet receptor and amplifies the aggregation response by recruiting passing platelets into the forming thrombus.

Platelet release

Alpha granules are intraplatelet organelles which serve as repositories for peptides and proteins. They are delivered to the site of platelet aggregation during the release reaction. The released proteins include coagulation factors, a fibrinolytic inhibitor (PAI 1), ligands for platelet receptors, such as fibrinogen, vWF and thrombospondin, and cytokines which stimulate fibroblasts and smooth muscle cells and therefore assist tissue repair. Platelet factor 4 and β-thromboglobulin are alpha granule components. Measurement of their plasma concentration has been used as a marker of in vivo platelet activation. P-selectin is a member of the selectin adhesion molecule family and is located on the membrane of platelet alpha granules. On stimulation, alpha granules are translocated to the surface and membrane fusion leads to expression of P-selectin on the cytoplasmic membrane.

Dense bodies are calcium-rich granules which serve as a store for ADP and serotonin, both of which are platelet agonists. Platelets also contain lysosomes; these are mobilized relatively late during release and the function of the lysosomal enzymes thus made available is unclear. A lysosomal glycoprotein, CD63, can be detected on the platelet surface after activation.

Leukocytes may also play a role in the haemostatic response. They are a potent source of PAF. Platelets interact with leukocytes through adhesion molecules which include P-selectin released from alpha granules.

Platelet function can be assessed in the laboratory by aggregometry, in which the interaction of platelets stirred in plasma or buffer is monitored by changes in the transmission of light through the suspension. The response to physiological agonists such as ADP, collagen and thrombin can be investigated. Flow cytometry is a sensitive tool which allows study of events at the platelet's surface, including fibrinogen receptor activation and expression of P-selectin and CD63. By careful blood sample collection and preparation, the presence of circulating activated platelets can be deduced. In vivo, primary haemostasis is best assessed using the skin bleeding time in which a standardized skin incision is made under controlled conditions and the duration of bleeding is measured.

The fluid phase of coagulation (secondary haemostasis)

The components of the coagulation network are illustrated in *Fig. 15.2*. All are synthesized in the liver. Vitamin K catalyses the γ-carboxylation of

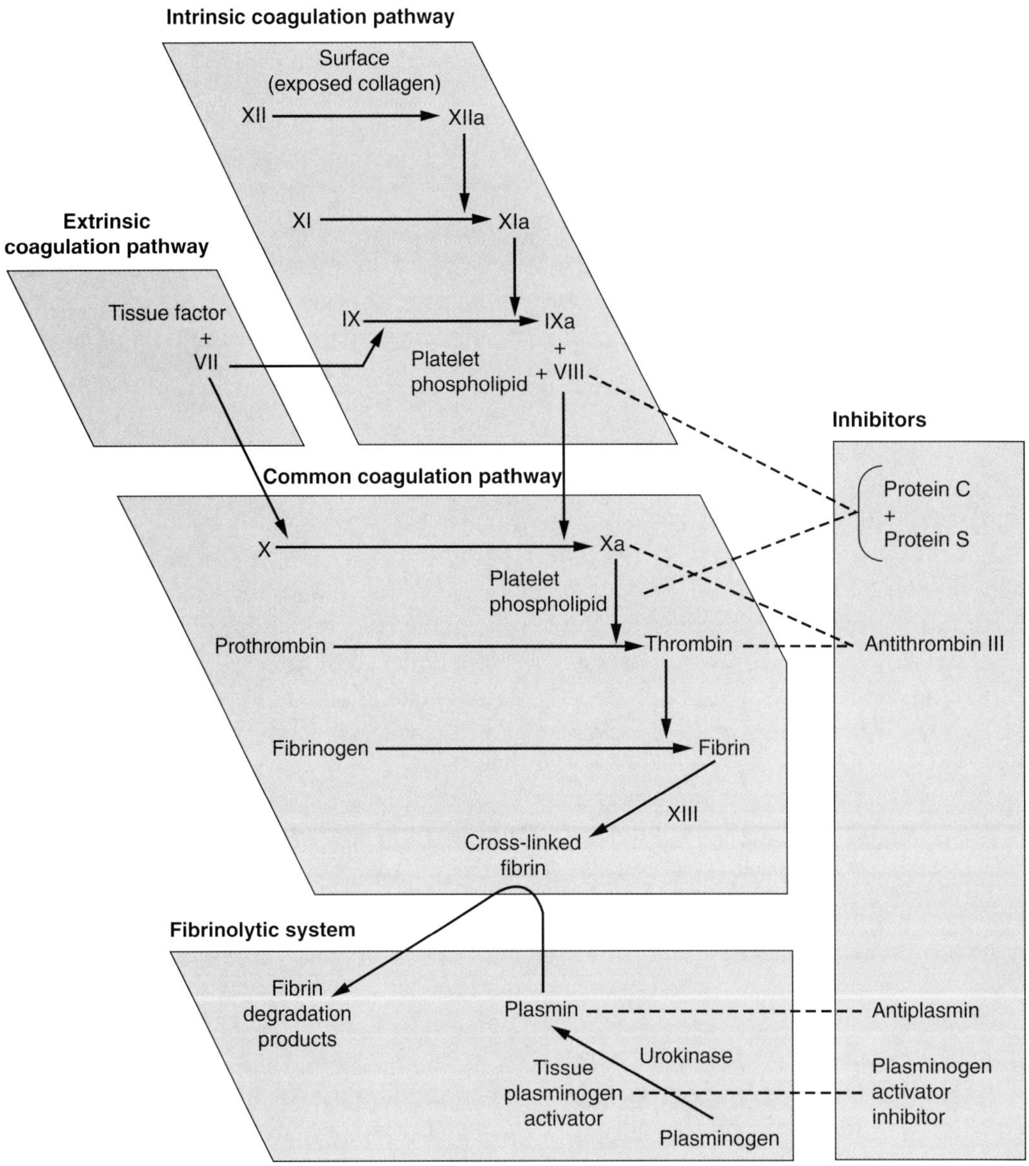

Figure 15.2
The principal components of the coagulation and fibrinolytic systems and their inhibitors.

glutamic acid residues in factors II, VII, IX and X. This γ-carboxylation is essential for calcium-binding and interaction with phospholipid, which are crucial to their role in thrombin generation. These glutamic acid residues are also needed for the binding of factor VII to tissue factor.

Plasma contains around 3 g/litre of soluble fibrinogen, the precursor of fibrin. As well as being the substrate for fibrin generation, fibrinogen is essential for normal platelet to platelet interaction and is a principal determinant of the viscosity of plasma. Blood viscosity is therefore also dependent on the fibrinogen concentration, with a major contribution from the red cell concentration as well as the membrane characteristics of red cells which determine their deformability and tendency to form aggregates. Fibrin is generated from fibrinogen when two peptides–fibrinopeptides A and B–are cleaved from the fibrinogen molecule by thrombin. Fibrin is rapidly cross-linked through the action of factor XIII, rendering it insoluble.

The coagulation network is composed of a series of serine protease proenzymes and cofactors which interact. Calcium ions are essential for several reactions, as is negatively charged phospholipid, which is provided by exposure of the inner leaflet of the platelet plasma membrane through platelet activation. This acts as a template for the interaction of factors VIIIa, IXa and X (the tenase complex) in the generation of factor Xa, and of factors Va, Xa and prothrombin (the prothrombinase complex) in the generation of thrombin.

Activation of the coagulation cascade occurs through two routes. Factors XII and XI can be activated by surface contact, for example, when blood is exposed to subendothelial components (or in the laboratory, a wettable surface such as glass or plastic). Thrombin generation through this route is relatively slow. It has been historically termed the 'intrinsic pathway' of blood coagulation because all the components necessary for clot formation through this route are present in the blood.

In contrast, the 'extrinsic pathway' requires an additional component–tissue factor–and is rapid, clotting occurring within seconds. Tissue factor is an integral membrane molecule with protein and phospholipid components and is present in many tissues but not normally in the blood nor on resting vascular endothelium. It becomes available through tissue trauma and can be expressed on activated monocytes and endothelial cells. When tissue factor combines with factor VII, the latter becomes activated and the complex of VIIa–tissue factor catalyses the conversion of factor X to Xa and factor IX to IXa, thus bypassing the intrinsic pathway. Recent evidence indicates that normal haemostasis depends predominantly upon the extrinsic system, the intrinsic pathway perhaps acting in an amplifying role. This explains the absence of a bleeding tendency in congenital deficiency of factor XII, although factor XI deficiency is associated with a bleeding tendency. Factor XII may have a more important role in the generation of kinins in the inflammatory response and, possibly, in the activation of fibrinolysis.

The efficiency of the coagulation cascade can be roughly assessed in the laboratory using standardized coagulation time tests. In the estimation of the prothrombin time, tissue factor is added to recalcified plasma. This measures the efficiency of the extrinsic and common pathways. In the activated partial thromboplastin time (APTT), the extrinsic pathway is activated by the provision of surface (usually kaolin) and phospholipid without tissue factor (usually a rabbit brain extract) to recalcified plasma. The test is, therefore, also referred to as the kaolin cephalin clotting time (KCCT) and it interrogates the function of the extrinsic and common pathways. In testing the thrombin time, thrombin is added to recalcified plasma, thus bypassing all stages proximal to fibrinogen digestion.

Over recent years a number of techniques have been developed for the assessment of in vivo activation of coagulation on carefully collected venous blood samples. Thrombin itself is rapidly bound and of short half-life and cannot be measured in plasma. However, assays for thrombin bound to its inhibitor antithrombin (thrombin–antithrombin complex–see below), and a fragment generated from prothrombin during thrombin generation (prothrombin fragment 1.2), are useful markers of coagulation activation. Assays for fibrinopeptide A and B are also available and the plasma levels also reflect thrombin generation.

Inhibitors of haemostasis and coagulation

The potent procoagulant mechanism must be closely controlled to prevent unwanted and potentially lethal clot formation–that is, thrombosis. Mechanisms have been identified that are additional to the avoidance of stasis by the maintenance of blood flow. The normal function of the vascular endothelium is crucial in the prevention of inappropriate platelet and coagulation activation, through:

- synthesis of antiaggregatory and vasodilator metabolites–prostaglandin I_2 and nitric oxide
- anticoagulant components–heparans, thrombomodulin, tissue factor pathway inhibitor
- fibrinolytic components–tissue plasminogen activator.

Inhibitors of primary haemostasis

An intact vascular endothelium is antagonistic to platelet activation. Interaction with subendothelium is prevented by the continuous endothelial barrier, and endothelium is the major source of prostaglandin I_2 (prostacyclin), a potent inhibitory and vasodilator prostanoid. This is a short-lived metabolite of arachidonic acid. As in the platelet, arachidonic acid is mobilized from the endothelial cell membrane phospholipid by a phospholipase and is converted to endoperoxide intermediaries by cyclo-oxygenase; thromboxane synthetase is active in platelets, whereas the activity of prostacyclin synthetase results in high local concentrations of prostaglandin I_2 in the vicinity of the endothelium. Prostaglandin I_2 causes an increase in intraplatelet cyclic AMP by stimulation of adenyl cyclase. Cyclic AMP is an inhibitor of platelet adhesion and aggregation. Prostaglandin I_2 and thromboxane A_2 are rapidly degraded to their inactive metabolites, 6–keto-prostaglandin $F_{1\alpha}$ and thromboxane B_2, respectively. It has been suggested that the maintenance of the appropriate balance between the synthesis of pro- and antiaggregatory prostanoids is essential for normal homeostasis. Aspirin results in acetylation of the cyclo-oxygenase enzyme and therefore inhibits synthesis of thromboxane A_2 by the platelet and prostaglandin I_2 by the endothelial cell. Anucleate platelets cannot resynthesize the enzyme and the inhibitory effect therefore persists for the life span of the affected platelet.

Nitric oxide, once known as endothelium-derived relaxing factor, is a second potent, short-lived, endothelium-dependent inhibitor of platelet activation and is also a vasodilator. In contrast to prostacyclin, it inhibits platelets by stimulating a guanylate cyclase, thus increasing the intraplatelet concentration of cyclic GMP.

Coagulation inhibitors (Fig. 15.2)

The uncontrolled generation of thrombin is potentially catastrophic and a series of checks and balances exists, often utilizing negative feedback and involving the vascular endothelium.

Thrombomodulin is an endothelial surface membrane protein through which the activity of thrombin can be locally redirected from a prothrombotic to an anticoagulant pathway. The combination of thrombin–thrombomodulin activates a coagulation inhibitor–protein C. Protein C is a vitamin K-dependent protein which, when activated, inhibits activated factors

V and VIII in the coagulation pathway, thus damping down further thrombin generation. A second vitamin K dependent factor, protein S, is needed for the full expression of this inhibitory function.

Thrombin is also inhibited by antithrombin III, a plasma protein that is synthesized in the liver. Its capacity to inhibit thrombin is increased several thousandfold by interaction with glycosaminoglycan components of the endothelial plasma membrane–the heparans. Heparin cofactor II is a second potent thrombin inhibitor but its physiological role is less well defined.

Tissue factor pathway inhibitor (TFPI) is a plasma protein inhibitor of coagulation activation by means of the factor VIIa–tissue factor complex. It binds avidly to vascular endothelium.

Although it provides an antithrombotic surface, vascular endothelium does manifest some prothrombotic properties, including synthesis and secretion of vWF, factor V and plasminogen activator inhibitor (the major inhibitor of fibrinolysis–see below). When stimulated, endothelial cells can express tissue factor. This response is mediated by inflammatory cytokines including interleukin-1 and tumour necrosis factor.

The fibrinolytic system (*Fig. 15.2*)

Vascular patency is preserved by the lysis of excess fibrin by the serine protease plasmin. Plasmin circulates as an inert precursor, plasminogen. This is converted to plasmin by plasminogen activators. As in the case of thrombin the generation of plasmin must be tightly controlled because free plasmin in the circulation can digest fibrinogen, factor V and factor VIII, thus producing a haemorrhagic state.

Tissue plasminogen activator (t-PA) appears to be the most physiologically important activator of plasminogen. It is synthesized and released by vascular endothelium and has a high affinity for, and binds to, fibrin. Plasminogen also binds to fibrin through lysine binding sites. This arrangement serves to localize fibrinolysis to the clot and, at the same time, limits systemic fibrinolytic activity. A second plasminogen activator is urokinase-type plasminogen activator (u-PA). It was originally isolated from urine as it is synthesized by urothelium. It is also expressed by monocytes and activated endothelial cells and appears to be present in plasma in trace amounts; its physiological role is, however, unclear. Factor XII and plasma prekallikrein can also activate plasminogen but, again, the physiological role of these 'intrinsic' activators is unknown.

Control of fibrinolysis is achieved through plasma inhibitors of plasmin and plasminogen activators. Of these, α_2–antiplasmin acts rapidly by forming a stable complex and blocks the adsorption of plasminogen on to fibrin. Furthermore, α_2–antiplasmin is itself cross-linked to fibrin through the action of activated factor XIII. Plasminogen activator inhibitor 1 (PAI 1) is another inhibitor synthesized by vascular endothelium. It is also present in platelet alpha granules. PAI 1 rapidly inactivates t-PA and urokinase.

Clearly, the system is ideally constructed for the localization of plasmin generation and activity at the site of fibrin clot. A series of fragments known as fibrin(ogen) degradation products (FDP) is generated when fibrin or fibrinogen is digested by plasma. Their appearance in plasma indicates active clot lysis. The D-dimer fragment reflects digestion of cross-linked fibrin by plasmin.

ALTERATIONS OF HAEMOSTASIS IN DIABETES

Abnormalities in all components of the haemostatic mechanism, as well as in blood rheology and endothelial function, have been described in experimental and human diabetes.

Platelets

The key role of platelets in the maintenance of blood vessel integrity in health and in response to injury, and in the development of thrombosis and atherosclerosis, suggests their importance in the pathogenesis of diabetic vascular disease. Platelet function in diabetes has been extensively investigated using both in vitro and in vivo methods. Platelets from diabetic subjects show enhanced adhesiveness to vessel wall sections and to artificial surfaces, which is more marked in the presence of vascular disease,[1] or in patients with proteinuria.[2]

One of the most widely applied tests of haemostasis in studies of diabetes is that of platelet aggregation. Hypersensitivity to a range of aggregating agents, including ADP, collagen, adrenaline and arachidonic acid, is a common finding.[3,4] The presence of microvascular complications or macrovascular disease in diabetes appears to enhance further the platelet aggregation response.[5–7] Increased platelet sensitivity has also been demonstrated, however, in young subjects without complications,[8] in 'prediabetic' subjects and in people with impaired glucose tolerance.[9] Other studies found that there was greater sensitivity to low doses of agonists in patients with complications than in those without.[10] Diabetic platelets also synthesize more thromboxane A_2 (TxA_2) in response to in vitro stimulation, and this too is related to the presence of complications, including neuropathy.[11] Synthesis of thromboxane is apparently normal in insulin-dependent patients without complications. Interestingly, aggregation appears to be more readily influenced by changes in glycaemic control in the early stages of diabetes, whereas later in the course of the disease, increased aggregation was not reversible by improved control.[12,13]

The phenomenon of 'spontaneous aggregation' (SPA) refers to the occurrence of in vitro aggregation on stirring of platelet-rich plasma without exogenous agonists, and has been demonstrated in diabetic patients with and without complications, as well as in non-diabetic subjects with macrovascular disease. In a large prospective study by Breddin et al, SPA was demonstrated to be a risk factor for new arterial occlusions in diabetic men.[14,15] SPA is not predictive of deterioration in diabetic retinopathy, however,[16] and may therefore be related to the presence of large vessel disease and atherosclerosis. SPA has also been found in diabetic patients without complications[17] and even in a high proportion of diabetic children and adolescents.[18] Increased SPA is a feature on stirring of anticoagulated whole blood from insulin-dependent diabetic patients without complications, and SPA is enhanced further in the presence of microvascular[19] or macrovascular disease.[20] There is some evidence that enhanced aggregation in diabetic whole blood may relate to changes in erythrocyte deformability.[21,22]

Increased amounts of fibrinogen are bound by diabetic platelets after stimulation.[23] It appears that fibrinogen binding is similar in subjects with and without retinopathy although, in patients with diabetic retinopathy, binding is more resistant to inhibition by aspirin.[23]

Alterations in platelet metabolic pathways

There have been numerous investigations into the mechanisms of increased platelet reactivity in diabetes, but no clear pattern has emerged. In view of the increased synthesis of thromboxane A_2, attempts have been made to measure levels of arachidonic acid (AA) and other fatty acids in diabetic platelet membranes. AA has been reported to be increased, decreased, or normal! Takahashi et al[24] reported increased incorporation of AA, but not oleic or linoleic acid, into diabetic platelets. Increased uptake of AA in platelets of insulin-dependent patients may be due to increased utilization of AA through the cyclo-oxygenase pathway.[25] Loss of platelet sensitivity to aspirin, found principally in patients with proliferative retinopathy,[26] suggests that alternative pathways of platelet activation which bypass the cyclo-oxygenase pathway may be operative. This has been confirmed in experimental models.

A range of metabolic abnormalities in diabetic platelets has been described. For example, platelets are deficient in vitamin E,[27,28] a finding related to increased thromboxane synthesis.[29] A defect in δ_6–desaturase, the rate-limiting enzyme in the conversion of dietary linoleic acid into γ-linolenic acid, has been described in diabetic platelets.[30] The δ_5–desaturase enzyme may also be less active. The central role of phosphoinositide and the second messengers diacylglycerol and inositol triphosphate in stimulus–response coupling has been described above. Paradoxically, in view of the increased platelet reactivity, phosphoinositide turnover was reported to be decreased in platelets from insulin-dependent patients[31] and inositol triphosphate (IP-3)-induced calcium ion release can be reduced by hyperglycaemia or hypoinsulinaemia in experimental models.[32] Platelet calcium ion influx and uptake appears normal, however.[32] Adenylate cyclase activity is apparently increased, with greatest levels being found in patients with severe retinopathy, another seemingly paradoxical observation.[33] It is clear that no single mechanism has so far been identified which accounts for the increased platelet aggregability found in diabetes.

Evidence for platelet activation in vivo

Platelet aggregometry does not necessarily reflect events in vivo. Also, it is unclear from the in vitro studies of platelet function whether abnormalities precede or are a consequence of vascular disease in diabetes. Where there is existing vascular disease, platelets could be activated by areas of vascular damage, or consumed in atherosclerotic or thrombotic lesions, thus leading to increased turnover and a relatively 'young' population of platelets which are larger and more haemostatically active.[34] In support of this theory, there have been reports of increased numbers of circulating large platelets,[33] and there was an association between mean platelet volume and diabetic retinopathy in one study.[36] Other groups have found no difference in platelet volume in diabetes.[37] It appears, though, that both production and consumption of platelets are indeed accelerated in diabetes, leading to a net increase in turnover.[38,39]

Direct evidence for enhanced platelet activity in diabetes comes from the finding of microthrombi, made up of aggregated platelets, in the small vessels of the brain after fatal diabetic ketoacidosis,[40] in endoneurial vessels from biopsy of sural nerve in patients with diabetic neuropathy,[41] and in the retina of diabetic rats.[42] Platelet microaggregates have been observed in the conjunctival vessels of diabetic patients with and without vascular disease.[43] Circulating platelet aggregates are found in blood from diabetic patients without complications, including newly diagnosed patients,[44] and also in non-diabetic subjects with severe vascular disease.[45]

The measurement of urinary metabolites of arachidonic acid metabolism has been used as a marker of in vivo platelet activation. No differences were found between patients with and without complications, and there was no correlation with blood glucose, in a small study by Alessandrini et al.[46] Davi et al found urinary excretion of the 11-dehydro-metabolite of thromboxane B_2 to be increased in type II diabetic patients with normal renal function.[47]

The development of flow cytometry as a tool for the study of platelets in whole blood has added greatly to our knowledge of platelet activity in diabetic patients. Using this approach it has been demonstrated that the major platelet membrane glycoprotein receptors for adhesive proteins, GPIb/IX and GPIIb/IIIa, are present in greater numbers on the surface of diabetic compared with normal platelets.[48] The increase is thought to be determined during the maturation of megakaryocytes in bone marrow. Total platelet content of GPIIb/IIIa is reduced in diabetic patients, but a greater proportion appears to be expressed on the surface membrane of unstimulated platelets.[49] This may be due to in vivo stimulation of circulating platelets. Using flow cytometry, secretion from platelet granules can also be accurately measured in whole blood samples, with the possibility of ex vivo activation kept to a minimum. This overcomes difficulties of many earlier studies which attempted to measure circulating platelet release products such as β-thromboglobulin and platelet factor 4, in which artefactual activation of samples was often a confounding factor. Surface expression of P-selectin (CD62P), which is secreted from the alpha granules and involved in platelet to leukocyte adhesion, is increased in unstimulated platelets from recent-onset type I diabetic patients, and the institution of near normoglycaemia did not correct this abnormality.[50] The same authors also showed that platelet P-selectin expression is even increased in first-degree relatives of type I patients, as is surface expression of GPIIIa, and the lysosomal glycoprotein CD63.[51] In the presence of retinopathy or neuropathy, the percentage of circulating activated platelets, measured by surface expression of P-selectin, CD63, thrombospondin and the ligand-induced binding site on GPIIb/IIIa (LIBS-1), was not as high as in diabetic patients without complications.[52] Whether this is evidence against the role of platelets in the pathogenesis of vascular complications, or is due to the consumption of activated platelets at sites of vascular disease, is unclear. The formation of platelet–leukocyte aggregates does appear to be related to the presence and severity of diabetic microangiopathy.[53] Several cellular adhesion molecules which mediate platelet–leukocyte adhesion are recognized, including selectins and ICAM-1 (intercellular adhesion molecule 1). E-selectin levels in plasma are increased in type I[54] and type II diabetes,[55,56] and elevated levels of ICAM-1 and L-selectin were found in patients with insulin-dependent diabetes of recent onset.[57] Increases in plasma ICAM-1, P-selectin and E-selectin have been found to correlate with deterioration in peripheral nerve function in diabetic patients,[58] further supporting a role for platelet activation and platelet–leukocyte interaction.

The fluid phase of coagulation

Plasma concentrations of fibrinogen and factor VIII in diabetes have been extensively studied. In the Northwick Park Heart Study,[2] there was no difference in factor VIII levels when all subjects with diabetes were compared to non-diabetics without heart disease. Men with non-insulin-dependent diabetes, however, had elevated factor VIII. Most of the larger studies have demonstrated increased plasma factor VIII in diabetic subjects, with or without retinopathy or other complications.[1,59,60] The exception is that of Christe et al, who found that factor VIII was significantly abnormal only in patients with nephropathy.[61]

Fibrinogen is of particular interest, as, in addition to being the substrate for thrombin in coagulation, it makes a major contribution to the viscosity of blood and is essential for platelet–platelet interaction. Plasma levels of clottable and antigenic fibrinogen are increased in subjects with diabetes[2,62,63] and may be increased further in those with complications. Fibrinogen is higher in patients with proliferative retinopathy,[64] and was associated with retinopathy and neuropathy in the Eurodiab study.[65] Associations also exist with proteinuria[2, 61,65,66] and/or hypertension.[67] We have demonstrated a correlation between plasma fibrinogen levels and thickening of vessel wall in the endoneurial capillaries of diabetic patients,[10] this being further evidence for a role of fibrinogen in the pathogenesis of diabetic microvascular disease.

Factor VII is also relevant to the pathogenesis of thrombotic and vascular disease as it has a central role in the extrinsic coagulation pathway through its interaction with tissue factor. Plasma factor VII levels in the general population are associated with lipid status, and with age. Factor VII is increased in diabetic subjects with retinopathy and nephropathy.[2,61] Ford et al found increased plasma factor VII in young (less than 30 years old) diabetic subjects with or without complications, when compared to age-matched normal subjects.[62] Interestingly, factor VII levels in these young diabetic patients were similar to normals in an older age group, and the usual correlation with age was absent in type I diabetes.[62] In one report a good correlation between factor VII and blood glucose was obtained in diabetic and normal subjects,[68] but this is not evident from other studies. Our group showed that factor VII in type II patients is significantly lowered by a period on a reduced-fat diet without improvement in glycaemic control, but not by intensified insulin treatment, which significantly reduces the fasting blood glucose levels and glycosylated haemoglobin.[69] The institution of near-normoglycaemia does not alter factor VII levels in insulin-dependent diabetes either.[70]

Thrombin cannot be measured directly in plasma but its generation can be inferred through measurement of fibrinopeptide A (FPA) or prothrombin fragment f1.2 peptide, the levels of which are considered to be more indicative of ongoing in vivo coagulation than assays of individual coagulation factors. Their accurate measurement is dependent on the avoidance of ex vivo activation during sampling and processing. Elevated levels of plasma FPA are found in type I and II diabetes, with and without vascular disease.[71–73] f1.2 was also elevated in a group of non-insulin-dependent patients.[56] FPA concentration is related to glycaemic control. Near-normalization of blood glucose is associated with a fall in FPA levels,[71,73] but both hyper- and hypoglycaemia are able to induce a rise in thrombin activity, which is particularly marked in patients with complications, including retinopathy.[71,74] Urinary excretion of FPA, assay of which may avoid some of the artefacts associated with blood sampling, is also increased in type I and II diabetes, and is correlated with age and duration of diabetes in type I patients.[62,71] Turnover of fibrinogen is also enhanced in diabetes, even in the absence of vascular disease.[75] Its catabolism was accelerated in male insulin-dependent patients with background retinopathy compared to those with no retinopathy, or with proliferative retinopathy.[76] The coexistence of impaired renal function with proliferative retinopathy, leading to reduced clearance of fibrinogen, might explain the findings in those patients. Overall, these data are consistent with a state of enhanced blood coagulation in diabetes.

Natural inhibitors of coagulation

Although conflicting results have been reported, plasma levels of the natural inhibitors of coagulation, protein C,[77] protein S[70] and antithrombin III,[2,61,78] may be increased in diabetes. Using an assay which measures activated protein C in complex with its inhibitor PCI, Gabazzo et al reported increased in vivo activation of protein C in non-insulin-dependent diabetic patients.[56] In the general population, inherited or acquired deficiencies of PC, PS or ATIII are more commonly associated with venous thromboembolism, which is not a common feature of diabetes. The seemingly paradoxical finding of increased levels of coagulation inhibitors in diabetes, where a hypercoagulable state is present, might be accounted for by a response to enhanced thrombin activity. In support of this explanation, increased levels of coagulation inhibitors are also found in non-diabetic patients with arterial disease.[15,79]

Fibrinolysis

Decreased fibrinolytic activity in plasma has been found in some studies of diabetic subjects but this has not been a consistent finding. There are differences between type I and II diabetes.[2] Thus, basal fibrinolytic activity appears to be reduced in male and female non-insulin-dependent patients, as well as in female insulin-dependent but not in male insulin-dependent patients. Plasma lytic activity is principally determined by the balance between tissue plasminogen activator (t-PA) and its main inhibitor, plasminogen activator inhibitor (PAI 1). Increases in both t-PA and PAI 1 have been reported, which were again more marked in type II patients,[80] and were also related to age, obesity and hypertension. In a study by Sundkvist et al the increment in PAI 1 after exercise was greater in patients who had, or who went on to develop, diabetic retinopathy,[81] but the exercise-induced decrease in fibrinolytic activity was not observed when autonomic neuropathy was also present.[82] t-PA activity appears to be negatively correlated with duration of diabetes, perhaps reflecting diminishing endothelial cell function.[83,84]

The B-β 15–42 peptide is cleaved from fibrin by plasmin and therefore serves as a plasma marker for in vivo fibrinolytic activity. Plasma B-beta 15–42 has been found to be elevated in type II compared with type I patients or with age-matched controls,[85] despite diminished fibrinolytic activity measured by global in vitro tests. B-β 15–42 was increased in both type I and type II male patients in another study[72,73] but was not significantly different from normal in female patients, although their fibrinopeptide A concentration was elevated.[73] Levels of the fibrin degradation product, D-dimer, are increased in diabetes and correlated with age,[86,87] although abnormally raised D-dimer was also found in the younger diabetic subjects. In the study of van Wersch et al, there was a negative correlation between HbA_1 and D-dimer[87] and, in that of Small et al,[73] a negative relationship between HbA_1 and B-beta 15–42 peptide. Consistent with this, intensive insulin treatment of type II patients was associated with an increase in B-beta 15–42 levels,[72] and with enhanced[88] or unchanged[69] basal fibrinolytic capacity, measured by the resting euglobulin clot lysis time. Interestingly, the effect of insulin treatment on B-beta 15–42 levels occurred independently of any change in glycaemic control.[72]

In summary, current evidence is consistent with a reduced fibrinolytic capacity in plasma in diabetes, but also enhanced in vivo fibrinolysis, presumably focally at sites of pathological fibrin deposition.

Rheology

There is general agreement that rheological abnormalities are found in diabetic patients and that these may contribute to disturbed haemostasis and vascular insufficiency. The changes include increased viscosity of plasma or whole blood,[89,90] due to an increase in plasma proteins, particularly fibrinogen and the macroglobulins, and reduced deformability of erythrocytes.[91,92] There is also enhanced formation of red cell aggregates which are, in addition, abnormally resistant to disruption.[93] Enhanced adhesion of erythrocytes to other cells, notably to endothelial cells, is also found.[94] Erythrocyte pathology in diabetes is discussed in detail elsewhere in this volume. There is some evidence that elevated blood viscosity may precede the development of complications in type I and type II patients,[90,95] and deterioration in blood flow properties has been found to be associated with the presence of vascular disease, and particularly with proliferative retinopathy.[63,96]

Endothelium

Reference has already been made to enhanced thromboxane synthesis by platelets in diabetes. The resulting proaggregatory effect is possibly augmented by diminished endothelial synthesis of prostaglandin I_2. Thus, production of prostaglandin I_2 by vessel sections is reduced, although uptake of arachidonic acid is normal. Diabetic serum inhibits prostaglandin I_2 synthesis by normal human umbilical vein endothelial cells, whereas normal serum stimulates synthesis of the vessel relaxant.[97] The phenomenon appears unrelated to abnormalities in concentrations of glucose, insulin or lipids. EDRF activity (nitric oxide) may also be diminished in diabetes.[98] On the other hand, plasma levels of endothelin-1, a potent vasoconstrictor, are reported to be increased.[99]

Plasma vWF is a marker of endothelial cell activation. This multimeric glycoprotein is particularly important in platelet adhesion to damaged endothelium at the high shear rates found in small arterial vessels. Increases in vWF, both antigenic and activity levels, have been reported in many studies of diabetes. Thus, raised vWF levels have been found in diabetic children without complications[100] and vWF is increased in non-insulin-dependent diabetic subjects, with or without retinopathy or macrovascular disease, in 'newly diagnosed' type II patients,[101] and in prediabetes.[9] There is a relationship between vWF and duration of diabetes.[102,103] In some studies, however, increased vWF has been noted only in patients with existing complications, and especially severe retinopathy.[104,105] Indeed, an association between fluorescein leakage from retinal vessels and increased vWF antigen and activity has been reported and the well-described exercise-induced release of vWF into the circulation appears to be enhanced in insulin-dependent patients with diabetic retinopathy.[84] In contrast, in patients with long-standing diabetes who remained free of retinopathy, the exercise-induced rise was absent.[81]

It seems likely that vWF is important in the progression of vascular lesions in diabetes.[14,65,106,107] Thus, vWF was associated with the occurrence of new arterial lesions in type I and II diabetes, in a large prospective study (the PARD study).[14] Furthermore, endothelial cell dysfunction appears to be present at an early stage in the development of diabetic nephropathy, and there is an association between vWF and urinary albumin excretion rate, but not with HbA_1, serum creatinine or blood pressure.[107] Stehouwer and colleagues[106,108] noted that a rise in vWF levels over 3 years was predictive of the development of nephropathy, and rises in the marker of endothelial activation may even precede the detection of microalbuminuria. It has been suggested that vWF might be a contributing factor to the excess cardiovascular mortality in diabetic patients with albuminuria.[109] The Eurodiab study,[65] which examined over 2000 diabetic patients, reported higher levels of vWF, when adjusted for age and glycaemic control, in subjects with increased albumin excretion or neuropathy. There was a positive relationship between both fibrinogen and vWF concentration and albumin excretion rate in the patients who also had retinopathy, but not in those without this complication.[65] Furthermore, vWF levels were found to be predictive of deteriorating peripheral nerve function in a prospective study of type I diabetic patients carried out in Sheffield.[110] However, in another prospective study of type I patients with no retinopathy or albuminuria at the entry to the study, patients in whom there was an increase in vWF over 42 months were no more likely to develop retinopathy than patients in whom vWF levels remained stable.[111]

On balance the evidence points toward altered endothelial function in diabetes in a direction which could be of pathogenic significance in diabetic vascular disease.

CONCLUSION

Changes in platelets, coagulation, fibrinolytic activity, rheology and endothelial function, associated with diabetes, all seem to point towards the existence of a prothrombotic state. The balance between formation and removal of fibrin is altered in the direction of increased thrombus formation. The haemostatic abnormalities are not entirely accounted for by hyperglycaemia or other metabolic changes in diabetes. It is still unclear, however, despite a wealth of experimental data, whether the abnormalities precede or are a consequence of vascular complications. Disturbances of platelet aggregation, for example, appear to be strongly related to existing vascular disease, but there is evidence to indicate that some of the abnormalities, such as increased vWF and blood viscosity, are present from an early stage, and that these may be involved in the pathogenesis of microangiopathy or large vessel disease in diabetes. There is sufficient evidence to warrant the design and execution of studies of the effects of therapies which modulate haemostatic and endothelial function on the development and progression of vascular disease in diabetes mellitus.

REFERENCES

1. Mayne EE, Bridges JM, Weaver JA, Platelet adhesiveness, plasma fibrinogen and factor VIII levels in diabetes mellitus, *Diabetologia* (1970) **6**: 436–40.
2. Fuller JH, Keen H, Jarrett RJ et al, Haemostatic variables associated with diabetes mellitus and its complications, *BMJ* (1979) **2**:964–6.
3. Colwell JA, Halushka PV, Annotation: platelet function in diabetes mellitus, *Br J Haematol* (1980) **44**:521–6.
4. Winocour PD, The role of platelets in the pathogenesis of diabetic vascular disease. In: Draznin B, Melmed S, LeRoith D, eds, *Molecular and Cellular Biology of Diabetes Mellitus*, vol 3 (AR Liss: New York, 1989) 37–47.
5. Agardh CD, Agardh E, Bauer B, Platelet aggregation in type 1 diabetics with and without proliferative retinopathy, *Acta Ophthalmol* (1987) **65**:358-62.
6. Fritschi J, Christe M, Lammle B et al, Platelet aggregation, beta-thromboglobulin and platelet factor 4 in diabetes mellitus and in patients with vasculopathy, *Thromb Haemost* (1984) **52**: 236-9.
7. Kwaan HC, Colwell JA, Suwanwela N, Increased platelet aggregation in diabetes mellitus, *J Lab Clin Med* (1972) **80**:236.
8. Colwell JA, Sagel J, Crook L et al, Correlation of platelet aggregation, plasma factor activity and megathrombocytes in diabetic subjects with and without vascular disease, *Metabolism* (1977) **26**:279-85.
9. Gensini GF, Abbate R, Favilla S, Neri-Serneri GG, Changes of platelet function and blood clotting in diabetes mellitus, *Thromb Haemost* (1979) **42**:983–93.
10. Ford I, Malik RA, Newrick PG et al, Relationships between haemostatic factors and capillary morphology in human diabetic neuropathy, *Thromb Haemost* (1992) **68**:628–33.
11. Cartwright I, Pickering C, Galloway J et al, Relationship between fatty acid composition of platelet membrane phospholipid and prostaglandin biosynthesis in diabetes mellitus, *Thromb Res* (1986) Suppl **VI**:3.
12. Jackson CA, Greaves M, Boulton AJM et al, Near-normal glycaemic control does not correct abnor-

mal platelet reactivity in diabetes mellitus, *Clin Sci* (1984) **67**:574–9.

13. Colwell JA, Gonzalez J, Sarji KE et al, Effect of metabolic control with insulin on plasma von Willebrand factor activity, growth hormone and platelet aggregation in diabetes mellitus, *Thromb Haemost* (1979) **42**:382 (abstract).
14. Breddin HK, Kryzywanek HJ, Althoff P et al, PARD: Platelet aggregation as a risk factor in diabetes: results of a prospective study, *Horm Metab Res* (1985) Suppl **15**:63–7.
15. Breddin K, Detection of prethrombotic states in patients with atherosclerotic lesions, *Sem Thromb Hemost* (1986) **12**:110–23.
16. Plu G, Lecrubier C, Scarabin PY et al (the Damad Study Group), Does increased platelet aggregation have a diagnostic value in the deterioration of background diabetic retinopathy? *Thromb Haemost* (1990) **64**:202–5.
17. O'Malley BC, Timperley WR, Ward JD et al, Platelet abnormalities in diabetic peripheral neuropathy, *Lancet* (1975) **ii**:1274–6.
18. Krzywanek HJ, Breddin K, Platelet aggregation as a risk factor in diabetic subjects, *Horm Metab Res* (1981) Suppl **11**:11–14.
19. Hendra TJ, Yudkin JS, 'Spontaneous' platelet aggregation in whole blood in diabetic patients with and without microvascular disease, *Diabet Med* (1992) **9**:247–51.
20. Cho NH, Becker D, Dorman JS et al, Spontaneous whole blood platelet aggregation in insulin-dependent diabetes mellitus: an evaluation in an epidemiological study, *Thromb Haemost* (1989) **61**:127–30.
21. Juhan I, Vague P, Buonocore M et al, Effects of insulin on erythrocyte deformability in diabetics–relationship between erythrocyte deformability and platelet aggregation, *Scand J Clin Lab Invest* (1981) **41** (Suppl 156):159–64.
22. Hendra TJ, Britton ME, Roper DR et al, Effects of fish oil supplements in NIDDM subjects–a controlled study, *Diabetes Care* (1990) **13**: 821–30.
23. Di Minno G, Silver MJ, Cerbone AM et al, Platelet fibrinogen binding in diabetes mellitus: differences between binding to platelets from non-retinopathic and retinopathic diabetic patients, *Diabetes* (1986) **35**:182–5.
24. Takahashi R, Morita I, Saito Y et al, Increased arachidonic acid incorporation into platelet phospholipids in type 2 (non-insulin-dependent) diabetes, *Diabetologia* (1990) **33**:306–10.
25. Perez C, Ramiro JJM, Campillo JE, Increased arachidonic acid uptake by platelets from insulin-dependent diabetics and diabetic rats, *Diab Res Clin Pract* (1989) **7**:69-73.
26. Watanabe J, Umeda F, Wasada T, Ibayashi H, Effect of prostaglandin synthetase inhibitors on platelet aggregation and thromboxane production in diabetes mellitus, *Tokohu J Exp Med* (1984) **144**:143–50.
27. Karpen CW, Cataland S, O'Dorisio TM, Panganamala RV, Interrelation of platelet vitamin E and thromboxane synthesis in type I diabetes mellitus, *Diabetes* (1984) **33**:239–43.
28. Watanabe J, Umeda F, Wakasugi H, Ibayashi H, Effect of vitamin E on platelet aggregation in diabetes mellitus, *Thromb Haemost* (1984) **51**: 313–16.
29. Karpen CW, Pritchard KA, Arnold JH et al, Restoration of prostacyclin/thromboxane A2 balance in the diabetic rat: influence of dietary vitamin E, *Diabetes* (1982) **31**:947–51.
30. Jamal GA, Pathogenesis of diabetic neuropathy: the role of the n-6 essential fatty acids and their derivatives, *Diabet Med* (1990) **7**:574–9.
31. Bastyr EJ III, Kadrofske MM, Dershimer RC, Vinik AI, Decreased platelet phosphoinositide turnover and enhanced platelet activation in IDDM, *Diabetes* (1989) **38**:1097–102.
32. Bergh CH, Hjalmarson A, Holm G et al, Calcium exchange in platelets in human diabetes. In: Jamieson JA, ed, *Platelet Membrane Receptors: Molecular Biology, Immunology, Biochemistry and Pathology* (AR Liss: New York, 1988) 437–40.
33. Janka HV, Standl E, Mehnert H, Increased platelet adenylate cyclase activity in diabetic patients with microangiopathy, *Horm Metab Res* (1981) Suppl **11**:26–9.

34. Greaves M, Preston FE, The laboratory investigation of acquired and congenital platelet disorders. In: Thomson JM, ed, *Blood Coagulation and Haemostasis: A Practical Guide*, 3rd edn (Churchill Livingstone: Edinburgh, 1985) 56–134.
35. Colwell JA, Sagel J, Crook L et al, Correlation of platelet aggregation, plasma factor activity and megathrombocytes in diabetic subjects with and without vascular disease, *Metabolism* (1977) **26**:279–85.
36. Cagliero E, Porta M, Cousins S, Kohner EM, Increased platelet volume in diabetic retinopathy, *Haemostasis* (1982) **12**:293–9.
37. Brooks AMV, Hussein S, Chesterman CN et al, Platelets, coagulation and fibrinolysis in patients with diabetic retinopathy, *Thromb Haemost* (1983) **49**:123–7.
38. Paton RC, Platelet survival in diabetes mellitus using an aspirin-labelling technique, *Thromb Res* (1979) **15**:793–802.
39. Jones RL, Peterson CM, Hematologic alterations in diabetes mellitus, *Am J Med* (1981) **70**: 339–52.
40. Timperley WR, Preston FE, Ward JD, Cerebral intravascular coagulation in diabetic ketoacidosis, *Lancet* (1974) **i**:952–6.
41. Timperley WR, Ward JD, Preston FE et al, A reassessment of vascular factors in relation to intravascular coagulation. Clinical and histological studies in diabetic neuropathy, *Diabetologia* (1976) **12**:237–43.
42. Ishibashi T, Tanaka K, Taniguchi Y, Platelet aggregation and coagulation in the pathogenesis of diabetic retinopathy in rats, *Diabetes* (1981) **30**:601–6.
43. Colwell J, Sagel J, Pennington R et al, Effect of therapy on platelet aggregation in diabetes, *Clin Res* (1973) **21**:884.
44. Preston FE, Ward JD, Marcola BH et al, Elevated beta-thromboglobulin levels and circulating platelet aggregates in diabetic microangiopathy, *Lancet* (1978) **i**:238–9.
45. Wu K, Hoak JC, A new method for the quantitative detection of platelet aggregation in patients with arterial insufficiency, *Lancet* (1974) **ii**:924–6.
46. Alessandrini P, McRae J, Feman S, Fitzgerald GA, Thromboxane biosynthesis and platelet function in type 1 diabetes mellitus, *N Engl J Med* (1988) **319**:208–12.
47. Davi G, Catalano I, Avena M et al, Thromboxane biosynthesis and platelet function in type 2 diabetes mellitus, *N Engl J Med* (1990) **322**:1769–74.
48. Tschoepe D, Roesen P, Kaufmann L et al, Evidence for abnormal platelet glycoprotein expression in diabetes mellitus, *Eur J Clin Invest* (1990) **20**:166–70.
49. Watala C, Golanski J, Walkowiak B et al, Does reduced membrane fluidity underlie the altered thrombin-induced expression of integrin $\alpha_{IIb}\beta_3$ and PADGEM-140 in membranes of platelets from diabetic juveniles? *Platelets* (1996) **7**:173–80.
50. Tschoepe D, Driesch E, Schwippert B et al, Exposure of adhesion molecules on activated platelets in patients with newly-diagnosed IDDM is not normalised by near-normoglycaemia, *Diabetes* (1995) **44**:890–4.
51. Tschoepe D, Driesch E, Schwippert B, Lampeter EF (on behalf of the DENIS Study Group), Activated platelets in subjects at increased risk of IDDM, *Diabetologia* (1997) **40**:573–7.
52. Rauch U, Schwippert B, Schultheiss H-P, Tschoepe D, Platelet activation in diabetic microangiopathy, *Platelets* (1998) **9**:238–40.
53. Tschoepe D, Rauch U, Schwippert B, Platelet–leukocyte cross-talk in diabetes mellitus, *Horm Metabol Res* (1997) **29**:631–5.
54. Cominacini L, Fratta Pascini A, Garbin U et al, Elevated levels of soluble E-selectin in patients with IDDM and NIDDM: relation to metabolic control, *Diabetologia* (1995) **38**:1122–4.
55. Steiner M, Reinhardt KM, Blann AD, Soluble adhesion molecules in NIDDM: increased concentration, relation to glycometabolic control, and possible pathophysiological significance, *Diabetologia* (1996) **39**:868–72 (letter).
56. Gabazza EC, Takeya H, Deguchi H et al, Protein

C activation in NIDDM patients, *Diabetologia* (1996) **39**:1455–61.

57. Lampeter ER, Kishimoto TK, Rothlein R et al, Elevated levels of circulating adhesion molecules in IDDM patients and in subjects at risk for IDDM, *Diabetes* (1992) **41**:1668–71.
58. Jude EB, Abbott CA, Young MJ et al, The potential role of cell adhesion molecules in the pathogenesis of diabetic neuropathy, *Diabetologia* (1998) **41**:330–6.
59. Elder GE, Mayne EE, Daly JG et al, Antithrombin III activity and other coagulation changes in proliferative diabetic retinopathy, *Haemostasis* (1980) **9**:288–96.
60. Pandolfi M, Almer LO, Holmberg L, Increased von Willebrand-antihaemophilic factor in diabetic retinopathy, *Acta Opthalmol* (1974) **52**:822–8.
61. Christe M, Fritschi J, Lammle B et al, Fifteen coagulation and fibrinolysis parameters in diabetes mellitus and in patients with vasculopathy, *Thromb Haemost* (1984) **52**:138–43.
62. Ford I, Singh TP Kitchen S et al, Activation of coagulation in diabetes mellitus in relation to the presence of vascular complications, *Diabet Med* (1991) **8**:322–9.
63. Lowe GDO, Ghafour IM, Belch JJF et al, Increased blood viscosity in diabetic proliferative retinopathy, *Diabetes Res* (1986) **3**:67–70.
64. Almer LO, Pandolfi M, Nilsson IM, Diabetic retinopathy and the fibrinolytic system, Diabetes 1975; 24:529-34.
65. Greaves M, Malia RG, Goodfellow K et al, and the Eurodiab IDDM Complications Study Group, Fibrinogen and von Willebrand factor in IDDM: relationships to lipid vascular risk factors, blood pressure, glycaemic control and urinary albumin excretion rate: the Eurodiab IDDM complications study, *Diabetologia* (1997) **40**:698–705.
66. Jones SL, Close CF, Mattock MB et al, Plasma lipid and coagulation factor concentrations in insulin-dependent diabetics with microalbuminuria, *BMJ* (1989) **298**:487–90.
67. Rampling MW, Feher MD, Sever PS, Elkeles RS, Haemorheological disturbances in non-insulin-dependent diabetes and the effects of concomitant hypertension, *Clin Hemorheol* (1989) **9**:101–7.
68. Ceriello A, Giugliano D, Quatraro A et al, Blood glucose may condition factor VIIc levels in diabetic and normal subjects, *Diabetologia* (1988) **31**:889–92.
69. Jennings AM, Ford I, Murdoch S et al, The effects of diet and insulin therapy on coagulation factor VII, blood viscosity and platelet release proteins in diabetic patients with secondary sulphonylurea failure, *Diabet Med* (1991) **8**:346–53.
70. Schernthaner G, Vukovich T, Knobl P et al, The effect of near-normoglycaemic control on plasma levels of coagulation factor VII and the anticoagulant proteins C and S in insulin-dependent diabetic patients, *Br J Haematol* (1989) **73**: 356–9.
71. Jones RL, Fibrinopeptide A in diabetes mellitus. Relation to levels of blood glucose, fibrinogen disappearance and haemodynamic changes, *Diabetes* (1985) **34**:836–43.
72. Small M, Paterson KR, Flannigan P et al, Enhancement of fibrinolysis after insulin administration in NIDDM, *Diabetes Care* (1986) **9**:216–17.
73. Small M, Lowe GDO, MacCuish AC, Forbes CD, Thrombin and plasmin activity in diabetes mellitus and their association with glycaemic control, *Q J Med* (1987) **65**:1025–31.
74. Ishii M, Kameyama M, Inokuchi T, Isogai S, Plasma fibrinopeptide A levels during insulin-induced plasma glucose falls in diabetics, *Diab Res Clin Pract* (1987) **4**:45–50.
75. Jones RL, Peterson CM, Reduced fibrinogen survival in diabetes mellitus: a reversible phenomenon, *J Clin Invest* (1979) **63**:485–93.
76. Cederholme-Williams SA, Dornan TL, Turner RC, The metabolism of fibrinogen and plasminogen related to diabetic retinopathy, *Eur J Clin Invest* (1981) **11**:133–8.
77. Vigano S, Mannucci PM, D'Angelo A et al, Protein C antigen is not an acute phase protein and is often high in ischaemic heart disease and diabetes, *Thromb Haemost* (1984) **52**:263–6.

78. Masperi R, Mussoni L, Bini A et al, Haemostatic variables in uncomplicated diabetic children, *Thromb Haemost* (1980) **43**:227.
79. Mettinger KL, A study of haemostasis in ischaemic cerebrovascular disease. V, A multivariate evaluation of risk indicators and predictors. Early results of a longitudinal study, *Thromb Res* (1982) **28**:521–32.
80. Auwerx J, Bouillon R, Collen D, Geboers J, Tissue-type plasminogen activator antigen and plasminogen activator inhibitor in diabetes mellitus, *Arteriosclerosis* (1988) **8**:68–72.
81. Sundkvist G, Lilja B, Almer LO, Absent elevations in growth hormone, factor VIII related antigen, and plasminogen activator activity during exercise in diabetic patients resistant to retinopathy, *Diabetes Res* (1988) **7**:25–30.
82. Almer LO, Sundkvist G, Lilja B, Fibrinolytic activity, autonomic neuropathy and circulation in diabetes mellitus, *Diabetes* (1983) **32** (Suppl 2):4–13.
83. Nilsson TK, Lithner F, Glycaemic control, smoking habits and diabetes duration affect the extrinsic fibrinolytic system in type I diabetic patients but microangiopathy does not, *Acta Med Scand* (1988) **224**:123–9.
84. Sundkvist G, Almer LO, Lilja B, Pandolfi M, Growth hormone and endothelial function during exercise in diabetics with and without retinopathy, *Acta Med Scand* (1984) **215**:55–61.
85. Walmsley D, Hampton KK, Grant PJ, Contrasting fibrinolytic responses in type 1 (insulin-dependent) and type 2 (non-insulin-dependent) diabetes, *Diabet Med* (1991) **8**:954–9.
86. Vukovich TC, Schernthaner G, Knobl PN, Hay V, The effect of near-normoglycemic control on plasma factor VIII/von Willebrand factor and fibrin degradation products in insulin-dependent diabetic patients, *J Clin Endocrinol Metab* (1989) **69**:84–9.
87. Van Wersch JWJ, Westerhuis LWJJM, Venekamp WJRR, Coagulation activation in diabetes mellitus, *Haemostasis* (1990) **20**:263–9.
88. Greaves M, Preston FE, Jackson CA et al, Changes in fibrinolytic activity and fibrinogen concentration in response to improved glycaemic control in diabetic subjects. In: Jesperson J, Kluft C, Korsgaard O, eds, *Clinical Aspects of Fibrinolysis and Thrombolysis* (South Jutland University Press: Esberg, Denmark, 1993).
89. Lowe GDO, Blood rheology in general medicine and surgery, In: Lowe GDO, ed, *Baillière's Clinical Haematology*, vol 1, *Blood Rheology and Hyperviscosity Syndromes* (Baillière Tindall: London, 1987) 597–636.
90. McMillan DE, Plasma protein changes, blood viscosity and diabetic microangiopathy, *Diabetes* (1976) **25** (Suppl 2):858–901.
91. McMillan DE, Utterback NG, LaPuma J, Reduced erythrocyte deformability in diabetes, *Diabetes* (1978) **27**:895–901.
92. Juhan I, Vague P, Buonocore M et al, Effects of insulin on erythrocyte deformability in diabetics–relationship between erythrocyte deformability and platelet aggregation, *Scand J Clin Lab Invest* (1981) **41** (Suppl 156):159–64.
93. LeDevehat C, Vimeux M, Bondoux G, Bertrand A, Red blood cell aggregation and disaggregation in diabetes mellitus, *Clin Hemorheol* (1989) **9**:845–54.
94. Wautier JL, Paton RC, Wautier MP et al, Increased adhesion of erythrocytes to endothelial cells in diabetes mellitus and its relation to vascular complications, *N Engl J Med* (1981) **305**:237–42.
95. Lowe GDO, Lowe JM, Drummond MM et al, Blood viscosity in young male diabetics with and without retinopathy, *Diabetologia* (1980) **18**:359–63.
96. Barnes AJ, Oughton J, Kohner EM, Blood rheology and the progression of diabetic retinopathy: a prospective study, *Clin Hemorheol* (1986) **7**:460.
97. Aanderud S, Krane H, Nordoy A, Influence of glucose, insulin, and sera from diabetic patients on the prostacyclin synthesis in vitro in cultured human endothelial cells, *Diabetologia* (1985) **28**:641–4.
98. Harris KH, MacLeod KM, Influence of the endothelium on contractile responses of arteries

from diabetic rats, *Eur J Pharmacol* (1988) **153**:55–64.

99. Takahashi K, Ghatei MA, Lam HC et al, Elevated plasma endothelin in patients with diabetes mellitus, *Diabetologia* (1990) **33**:306–10.
100. Muntean WE, Borkenstein MH, Haas J, Elevation of factor VIII coagulant activity over factor VIII coagulant antigen in diabetic children without vascular disease, *Diabetes* (1985) **34**:140–4.
101. Paton RC, Passa PL, Canivet J, Von Willebrand factor, diabetes mellitus and retinopathy, *Horm Metab Res* (1981) **Suppl 11**:55–8.
102. Borkenstein MH, Muntean WE, Elevated factor VIII activity and factor VIII-related antigen in diabetic children without vascular disease, *Diabetes* (1982) **31**:1006–9.
103. Porta M, Townsend C, Clover GM et al, Evidence for functional endothelial cell damage in early diabetic retinopathy, *Diabetologia* (1981) **20**: 597–601.
104. Coller BS, Frank RN, Milton RC, Gralnick HR, Plasma cofactors of platelet function: correlation with diabetic retinopathy and haemoglobins A1a-c, *Ann Intern Med* (1978) **88**:311–16.
105. Porta M, Kohner EM, Molinatti GM, In vivo studies of endothelial cell function in diabetic microangiopathy, *Frontiers in Diabetes* (1987) **8**:16–28.
106. Stehouwer CDA, Stroes ESG, Hackeng WHL et al, Von Willebrand factor and development of diabetic nephropathy in IDDM, *Diabetes* (1991) **40**:971–6.
107. Jensen T, Bjerre-Knudsen J, Feldt-Rasmussen B, Deckert T, Features of endothelial dysfunction in early diabetic nephropathy, *Lancet* (1989) **i**: 461–3.
108. Stehouwer CDA, Andreas Fischer HR, VanKuijk AWR et al, Endothelial dysfunction precedes development of microalbuminuria in IDDM, *Diabetes* (1995) **44**:561–4.
109. Jensen T, Borch-Johnsen K, Kofoed-Enevoldsen A, Deckert T, Coronary heart disease in young type I diabetic patients with and without diabetic nephropathy: incidence and risk factors, *Diabetologia* (1987) **30**:144–8.
110. Plater ME, Ford I, Dent MT et al, Elevated von Willebrand factor antigen predicts deterioration in diabetic peripheral nerve function, *Diabetologia* (1996) **39**:336–43.
111. Stehouwer CDA, Zellenrath P, Polack BCP et al, Von Willebrand factor and early diabetic retinopathy: no evidence for a relationship in patients with Type 1 (insulin-dependent) diabetes mellitus and normal urinary albumin excretion, *Diabetologia* (1992) **35**:555–9.

16 Erythrocyte pathology in relation to diabetic retinopathy

Jan D Banga and Philip G de Groot

INTRODUCTION

Blood is a suspension of blood cells in a protein solution called plasma. By far the most abundant cells in blood are red cells: these occupy approximately 40% of the blood volume. The behaviour of blood as a fluid is highly dependent upon the presence of the red cells. Pathological alterations of the red cell will result in changes in the rheological properties of blood and these alterations appear to play a pivotal role in the generation of retinopathy.[1] Diabetes mellitus results in stiffening of the red cells and this creates microcirculatory flow disturbances in the retina. Subsequently, these flow disturbances can cause functional and structural abnormalities in the microvessels which result in damage to the retina. These mechanisms appear not to be unique to diabetes, but represent common pathways in the pathogenesis of retinopathy, in which different aetiological factors characteristic to a particular disease may be involved. To appreciate the apparently essential role of erythrocyte pathology in the genesis of retinopathy, a general overview of the unique features of the red cells and of factors that contribute to blood flow disturbances, especially in the microcirculation, is necessary.[2,3] It is thought that physicochemical alterations in the red cell membrane, induced by the diabetic milieu, render the red cells less deformable. This decreased deformability leads to mechanical obstruction of vessel branches in the microcirculation and subsequent flow disturbances and imbalances in the distribution of nutrients to the tissue. The stiffening of red cells is apparent from a doubling of the resistance of the erythrocyte to membrane curvature change.[4] This creates an increase in the peak arteriolar wall force causing high tangential forces generated by flow over local endothelial cells.[4,5] This presumably induces endothelial cell perturbation and loss of endothelial cell functions, and even endothelial cell anchoring. In an apparent response to these higher tangential forces, local deposition of collagen type IV is increased, which is visualized as local hyalinization of the basement membrane.[5] In addition, increased plasma viscosity may further contribute to both flow disturbances and increased aggregability of red cells.

Hyperglycaemia also results in non-enzymatic glycation and oxidation of proteins and lipids, resulting in accumulation of irreversibly formed advanced glycation end products (AGEs). These AGEs also accumulate on the surface of red cells.[6] The AGEs bind to a specific receptor present on vessel wall cells, thereby inducing oxidant stress in the vasculature.[7] The oxidant stress may result in the development of vascular lesions which may also contribute to the retinopathy. This mechanism will not be included in this review.

The microcirculation has specific rheological characteristics as opposed to the macrocirculation. The rheological properties that determine flow in the microcirculation are two separate entities: the deformability of red cells and the vicosity of plasma. The viscosity of plasma is determined by fibrinogen and total globulin levels. In the macrocirculation, increased red cell stiffness also has consequences for the rheological properties of blood. But here, blood flow is determined by vessel radius in the first place, and by perfusion pressure and blood rheological properties in the second and third place, respectively.[8] The rheological properties of blood in the macrocirculation are determined largely by the viscosity of whole blood.[8] At low shear rates (as present in the largest vessels), whole blood viscosity may increase by 15–25%, at high shear rates (as present in smaller arteries) by 5–10%. In diabetes it is thought that high plasma levels of fibrinogen and of α_2-macroglobulin are mainly responsible for this increase, and that deformability of red cells is less important in the macrocirculation.

Diabetic retinopathy may be described as a disease resulting from a haemorrheological derangement. For this assumption there is no direct proof, but circumstantial evidence suggests that both red cell stiffness and aggregability (and also white cell rigidity and adhesiveness) and hyperviscosity are involved in the aetiology of diabetic retinopathy, and probably in all forms of retinopathy. The different forms of retinopathy all have features in common, such as retinal microaneurysms, haemorrhages, distended veins, and neovascularization. Among these conditions are sickle cell disease, leukaemia, myeloma and macroglobulinaemia.[9] An essential feature of these conditions is retinal hypoxia leading to ocular neovascularization. Increased blood viscosity may also be found in retinal vein occlusion with associated capillary non-perfusion. Hyperviscosity appears a potent stimulus for occlusion of capillaries. In patients with diabetic retinopathy fibrinogen and total globulin levels were higher and fibrinogen was both cross-sectionally and predictively related to retinopathy.[10] Expression was blocked by good metabolic control, without lowering plasma protein levels.[1]

It has been postulated that in the early phase of retinopathy there is an initial state of hyperperfusion,[11] concurring with elevation of plasma and blood viscosity and an increase in rigidity of red cells. It appears that in this phase the increased shear stress on the vessel wall locally induces the first thickening of basement.[12,13]

The increase in shear stress and the abnormal composition of the thickened basement membrane may permit increased transduction of plasma components into the extravascular space.[14] Later on there is a decrease in retinal blood flow. Red cells express increased adhesion to the endothelium and platelets become subject to enhanced aggregability. This leads to a predisposition to capillary occlusion.[14]

THE ERYTHROCYTE

Red blood cells transport oxygen towards the tissues. The mature red cell has no nucleus or other organelles and is made up of a cell membrane with a cytoskeleton, and haemoglobulin with a concentration of about 0.35 g/ml.[15] The red cell has a typical biconcave shape as a consequence of the excess surface in relation to its content as compared to a sphere with the same volume. The normal red cell volume is about 90 μm^3, its diameter 8 μm, with a surface area of about 164 μm^2. Two main components make up the cell membrane: a lipid bilayer and an underlying cytoskeleton. The bilayer contains several phospholipids, uncharged species at the outer leaflet and anionic species at the inner leaflet.[15,16] Phospholipids move freely within the plane of the membrane. Several proteins are located in the bilayer, some of them with domains on the inside and outside of the bilayer (transmembrane proteins). Glycophorin is one of the main glycoproteins and contributes largely to the negative surface charge of the red cell due to its sialic acid groups on the outer side. The cytoskeleton beneath the lipid bilayer is made up among others of spectrin and actin and is anchored to the lipid bilayer by membrane proteins 3 and 4 and actin. The red cell does not have a fixed shape: the biconcavity (dimple) may move through the membrane. Both the cytoskeleton and the lipid bilayer contribute to the biconcave shape and the ability of the dimple to migrate over the cell. This phenomenon has been coined tank-treading, in reference to the movement of the tracks of a tank or bulldozer.[17] Apart from the migration of the biconcavity, red cells are also capable of deformation into bullet- or slipper-like shapes. Whereas the dimple migration (tank-treading) occurs in larger vessels, the bullet- or slipper-like shape changes typically take place in the microcirculation.

During the life of the red cell both the lipids and proteins present in the membrane and the haemoglobulin content undergo glycosylation, and this process is accelerated in diabetes. The red cell volume decreases and the haemoglobulin concentration increases, which results in a higher internal viscosity. Old cells become less deformable and this reduction in deformability is thought to play a principal role in the trapping (removal) of old cells from the circulation by the spleen.[18,19] In a life span of about 120 days, a red cell has circulated 200 000 times. Its excess surface, flexible membrane, and lack of internal structures make the red cell highly deformable. Both elastic and viscous properties contribute to the ability to change shape. Elasticity determines the force needed to deform the cell and the ability to regain its original shape. Elasticity is solely determined by the red cell membrane. Components within the membrane are capable of constant rearrangement, while area and curvature are kept constant. This prevents local area dilatation of the membrane which would otherwise lead to membrane rupture. The resultant membrane dilatation is called shear or extensional deformation. Shear elasticity is the concomitant elasticity and is within the plane of the membrane. The cytoskeleton as the only solid element in the membrane plane is considered the principal source of the shear elasticity. Within the cytoskeleton, spectrin with its network of cross-linked filaments, elastic in itself, presumably plays the major role. Perpendicular to the membrane plane is the bending elasticity, determined mainly by the bending resistance of the lipid bilayer, and somewhat by that of the cytoskeleton.[15,20] Red blood cells strongly resist membrane area dilatation and shape change only within the restrictions of surface area and volume (geometrical limitations). Elasticity resists deformation and determines the forces needed to keep a cell deformed.

The speed at which the shape changes take place is determined by the maximum speed in energy dissipation within the cell structures, which depends on the viscous components. Viscosity of red cells is made up of a membrane viscosity and internal viscosity. Membrane viscosity is determined by the solid membrane bilayer which behaves as a two-dimensional fluid as a result of the mobility within the membrane plane of its constituents. The internal viscosity is much higher than the plasma viscosity (mean value, 14 mPa; plasma viscosity is only about 1.3 mPa) and increases with the ageing of the red cell (9 mPa in young cells and 54 mPa in old cells).[21]

BLOOD RHEOLOGY

Rheology is the study of the deformation and flow of a material. Blood rheology is the study of the interrelationships of the forces acting on blood and its constituents, the deformation and flow produced in blood, and the relation with time.[22,23] The flow behaviour of blood is determined by the flow properties and flow conditions of blood. The flow properties of blood depend on whole blood viscosity (determined by haematocrit), plasma viscosity (which depends on plasma protein concentrations), erythrocyte aggregation, and erythrocyte deformability. The inverse of deformability is rigidity. Flow conditions depend on the haemodynamic and angioarchitectonic parameters that determine or facilitate blood flow, such as blood pressure, pressure gradient, vessel diameter, and branching. Shear rate (velocity gradient, shear velocity, shear gradient, shear rate, dimensions s-1) is the unit for the shear of a fluid between two layers. It is the quotient of the differentials of velocity v and distance x (dv/dx). The shear stress (shear force, dimension N/m^2 is the tangential force that produces a mutual displacement of the fluid layers. Viscosity (internal friction, toughness, shear stress/shear rate) is the force per unit area required to maintain unit gradient in velocity and is the physical property of fluid that mainly determines the flow behaviour of that fluid. This is expressed as pascal (Pa) or millipascals (mPa) (formerly: centipoise cP; 1 cP = 1 mPa). The apparent viscosity is flow resistance of blood due to friction, that is, the resultants of flow conditions and flow properties. Newtonian fluids are fluids in which the viscosity behaves according to Newton's law, wherein the quotient of shear stress and shear rate is a constant. Blood behaves like a non-Newtonian fluid and acts like ketchup that has to be shaken out of the bottle. At first, a large force is needed to set blood in motion; once in motion, the resistance to flow appears greatly diminished. The Fahraeus–Lindqvist effect is the reduction of the blood viscosity in narrow capillaries with a rapid flow rate. This effect is only important in capillary diameters less than 0.3 mm. In vivo measurements with intravital microscopy of the rat mesentery showed that in small microvessels a high flow resistance exists that may be related to interactions between blood components and the inner vessel surface that do not occur in vitro models with smooth-walled tubes.[24]

Erythrocyte deformability (flexibility, fluidity) is the ability of erythrocytes to adapt to blood flow passively and to change their shape in the process. This enables the cells to pass through capillaries with diameters smaller than that of resting erythrocytes. Deformation of erythrocytes is determined by: (a) intracellular viscosity (which is a function of mean corpuscular haemoglobulin concentration); (b) membrane material properties (including elasticity and viscosity); (c) cellular geometry (surface area to volume ratio, and morphology); and (d) the shear stresses acting on the cell surface. Erythrocyte aggregation is the side to side attachment of erythrocytes as rouleaux-type structures. This may yield a three-dimensional net-like structure. Clump aggregation has been described as a disorganized aggregation of erythrocytes that may occur in diabetes mellitus. Aggregation represents an algebraic balance of energies: the bridging energy due to fibrinogen and the globulins, the electrostatic repulsive energy at the cell surface, and the mechanical shear energy due to cell deformability and cell membrane bending.

RED CELL DEFORMABILITY

The deformability of red cells can be assessed by several methods.[2,3] Guidelines for measurements of blood viscosity and erythrocyte deformability were published by the International Committee for Standardization in Haematology (Expert Panel on Blood Rheology) in 1986.[25] But a clear overview of the field and comparisons are impossible, owing to ongoing development of techniques. In static experiments the extent of deformation is measured at a known deformation force, in dynamic experiments the ability to change shape in time is measured. A population of cells can be studied by viscometry, filtration techniques, ektacytometry and the flow channel photometric monolayer technique.[26] Individual cell deformability can be measured by micropipette, rheoscope, and microscopic flow channel techniques. Techniques that measure individual cell properties yield the best information but are very cumbersome to use.

The elliptical deformations with tank-treading occur in the larger vessels and have physiological relevance, as they constitute an important determinant of whole blood viscosity. These deformations can be measured by rheoscopy, ectocytometry, and viscometry. In capillaries red cells change shape into bullets or slippers[27] but display no tank-treading. From in vitro and in vivo studies it is apparent that the flow properties (including the transit time through the microcirculation) or erythrocytes as well as granulocytes are dependent upon the viscoelastic characteristics of these cells. Micropipette aspiration techniques make it possible to quantify these properties.[28,29] The microcirculation is designed in modules consisting of feeding arterioles, capillaries, and postcapillary collecting venules. Architecture and topography of the microcirculation may show local characteristics, depending on the respective tissue or organ, with maintenance of certain common anatomic and physiological features. These, together with blood rheological factors, influence the distribution of pressure–flow values within a module. The microcirculation in these modules has an autonomic behaviour. These factors also determine the local apportionment of erythrocytes and their overall flux through various tissues. Thus, there may be local differences in rheological conditions and this may also affect leukocyte–endothelial cell interactions. This process, mediated by adhesion molecules expressed in the arteriolar and venular bed, may in turn influence the distribution of flow. Leukocyte adhesion to endothelial cells in vivo occurs almost exclusively in postcapillary venules.[23] Their significance in processes such as local and haemorrhage-induced ischaemia, as well as ischaemia-reperfusion, is becoming more and more apparent.[10,30–32] Furthermore, the plugging of a vessel branch at a dichotomous branch point by a white cell may have a firm impact on the distribution of red cells in that microcirculatory unit.[23,33,34] At branch points, cells are always pulled into the branch vessel with the lesser resistance. This is determined by the diameter ratio of cells and vessels, shape and deformability of the cells, haematocrit in the parent vessel, pressure and shear stress distribution at the branch point, and the ratio of flow velocities in the offspring vessels downstream.[35,36] The entrance of a red cell or leukocyte into a branch vessel at a bifurcation causes an increase in local resistance and decreases the flow in that vessel, such that the next cell enters the other branch vessel. Alternation of entrance into branch vessels leads to adjustment of distribution. An entering leukocyte causes a more substantial increase in the local resistance than the red cell because of high coefficient of viscosity, lower deformability, and larger effective volume. The entry and distribution of leukocytes into the capillary network can exert a considerably larger effect on the distribution of red cells than red cells proper. Entrance of a leukocyte into one branch vessel will cause 20–30 red cells to go the other way. Dynamic studies of the microcirculation (videomicroscopy) show apparent dominance of white cells in regulating flow. Granulocytes lodge at capillary constrictions near endothelial cell nuclei and hold up an accumulating mass of red cells. The moment a white cell moves downstream, it is followed by a swift passage of red cells without apparent resistance to flow.[37] A high white cell count, as described in subjects with diabetes with proliferative retinopathy as compared to diabetic controls, may therefore have significance as an important flow determinant.[38] White cells mainly pass through shunts between arterioles and venules and preferentially reside in venules. The passage along the endothelium of a vessel wall has been termed 'cartwheeling'.[1] In this process, white cells roll along the endothelium by temporary attachment to cellular endothelial ligands. Subsequently, they either become adherent and may enter the vessel wall (inflammation) or they become dislodged again. The phenomena discussed above contribute to continuous non-homogeneity of blood flow in the microcirculation, with temporal and spatial fluctuations and heterogeneity in the number of capillaries with active red cell flow. This leads to fluctuations in oxygen delivery to the tissue. Most tissues regulate own rates of perfusion by mechanisms intrinsic to the tissues involved. In kidney and brain there is autoregulation of blood flow, so that a relatively constant flow can be maintained despite changes in perfusion pressure. The vascularity of most tissues is directly regulated to the local metabolism.[23] Collateral vessels may develop to facilitate continual tissue perfusion when the parent vessel is blocked. Opening of collateral vessels is initiated by vascular occlusion at proximal sites. In the hypoxic retina (and other hypoxic tissues), this process appears to be mediated by vascular endothelial growth factor (VEGF).[39] This factor induces growth and proliferation of new haemovascular networks in several tissues that exhibit excessive metabolic activity. Lack of oxygen or excessive metabolic activity are primary stimuli for the synthesis of this angiogenesis factor.[40] The factor may be significant in the angiogenesis found in proliferative retinopathy of haemoglobulinopathies and diabetes mellitus.

RHEOLOGY AND RED CELL ALTERATIONS IN DIABETES

The rheological properties of plasma, erythrocytes, leukocytes, and whole blood in subjects with diabetes and microvascular or macrovascular disease have been the subject of intensive study. Data come from in vitro and in vivo observations, and are collected with a host of different measuring techniques. The lack of a uniform standard of rheological measurements may make interpretation difficult. Moreover, in addition to specific alterations as a consequence of diabetes, countless clinical variables may affect blood rheology as well, temporarily or permanently. Despite these shortcomings, it is generally accepted that whole blood viscosity is often increased in diabetes, especially in subjects in poor metabolic control[41] and with vascular complications.[42] Subjects with diabetes mellitus and high plasma levels of glucose have less deformable red cells.[43] Rheological abnormalities in diabetes are greater in hypertensive subjects than in non-hypertensive subjects.[44] Increased aggregability of red cells[45] and increased adhesion of red cells to cultured endothelium[7] have also been described in relation to glycaemic control. In patients with diabetic retinopathy plasma viscosity was increased as a result of elevated plasma levels of fibrinogen and total globulin. These were both cross-sectionally and predictively related to retinopathy.[10] Elevation of fibrinogen and plasma globulins predisposed conventionally treated subjects with type I diabetes to earlier development of retinopathy. Expression of retinopathy was blocked by good metabolic control, actually without lowering plasma protein levels.[1] Thus, the increase in plasma viscosity in diabetes may not be sufficient to explain the predisposition to retinopathy. It appears that a reduced red cell deformability and a concomitant increased tendency to aggregation under poor metabolic control and mediated by plasma protein composition is fundamental.[1] Rigid red cells and red cell aggregates may block capillaries and arterioles, thereby increasing wall shear stress.[1] The higher peak load mediated by reduced deformability and increased aggregation of red cells stimulates endothelial cells to increase their anchoring. The thickness of the underlying intima is increased and arteriolar flexibility falls. With progression, the flexibility of the vessel to increase diameter to compensate for pressure diminishes. The distribution and delivery of blood become compromised. In vulnerable areas such as the retina, the loss of balance between pressure and flow in arterioles and capillaries may become evident as damage, whereas in less vulnerable tissues such as skeletal muscle this may not lead to apparent tissue damage.

The lipid composition of the red cell membrane, especially the cholesterol/phospholipid ratio, is probably a major determinant of its membrane deformability and hence of whole-cell deformability.[46–49] In addition the phospholipid composition of erythrocytes, platelets, and polymorphonuclear cells may be altered in diabetes, with an overall increased abundance of phosphatidylethanolamine (PE) and loss of phosphatidylserine (PS).[50] Rheological parameters correlated with the alteration of the PE/PS ratio in the red cell membrane. Insulin deficiency in poorly controlled type I (insulin-dependent) diabetes is associated with an increased ratio of cholesterol to phospholipid in the red cell membrane, and an increased ratio of saturated to unsaturated fatty acids: these abnormalities may explain the decreased membrane deformability in these patients.[49,51,52] Administration of insulin significantly corrected all these abnormalities within 24 hours.[49,51,52] Poor metabolic control, rheological abnormalities, and retinopathy appear to be interrelated. Improved metabolic control in type I (insulin-dependent) diabetes correlates with improved blood rheology.[53,54]

In subjects with type II diabetes, a high level of erythrocyte aldose reductase may affect the prognosis of diabetic retinopathy. An elevated level of erythrocyte aldose reductase was independently associated with active proliferative retinopathy compared to lower levels in those with non-proliferative or quiescent proliferative retinopathy.[55] The specificity of this relationship remains unclear, and a relation with haemorrheological alterations has not been described. The same authors described elevated levels of erythrocyte aldose reductase protein (AR-p) in subjects with type II diabetes with neuropathy, compared to type II diabetes without neuropathy.

An association of erythrocyte polyamine content of spermine and spermidine with microangiography has been suggsted. Erythrocyte content of polyamines was found to be increased in type I diabetics with microalbuminuria, suggesting that these polyamines when elevated could be associated with angiopathy. The erythrocyte content of the polyamines spermine and spermidine can be measured by high-performance liquid chromatography. It was also found that both spermine and spermidine levels were elevated in subjects with type II diabetes with both microalbuminuria and macroangiography, while spermidine was on average increased in patients with retinopathy.[56]

High levels of malondialdehyde (MDA) indicate increased lipid peroxidation, which could be involved in vessel damage. In patients with retinopathy, erythrocyte content of MDA was reported to be elevated.[57] The cause and effect relation of this observation is as yet not clear, but it could mean that increased lipid peroxidation as evident from a high erythrocyte MDA content plays a role in the generation of retinopathy.

TREATMENT

The contribution of haemorrheological treatment to prevention and treatment of retinopathy has not been established.[1] Improvement of haemorrheological conditions may be achieved by: (a) improved metabolic control, and (b) pharmacological interventions specifically aimed at improving haemorrheology.[1]

Improvement of metabolic control is the first logical strategy to improve overall prognosis in diabetes. In several large-scale trials, improved metabolic control is associated with better outcome of retinopathy in terms of prevention and retardation of progression, both in type I diabetes[58–60] and type II diabetes.[61,62]

Pharmacological means of improving blood rheology aim at reducing the peak tangential force acting on arteriolar endothelial cells. These treatments comprise three categories. A first approach is to restore red cell deformability. This approach has not been successful so far, despite the availability of so-called haemorrheological drugs and indications of a favourable effect of such drugs on red cell deformability in in vitro experiments.[63]

A second approach would be to reduce the increased aggregability of red cells. Compounds such as aspirin[64] and dietary supplements (including fish oil[65,66]) could directly reduce aggregation. Indeed, the use of aspirin by patients with diabetes had not led to unwanted side effects such as vitreous bleeding,[67] but rather had a stabilizing influence on diabetic retinopathy, with reduction of the number of newly developed microaneurysms.[68]

The third approach would aim at lowering the level of plasma proteins that enhance the aggregation of red cells. This includes treatments aimed at lowering the plasma fibrinogen level as the dominant globulin. No long-term drug regimens to this purpose are available. Non-pharmacological measures, however, such as giving up smoking[69] and taking regular exercise[70,71] lower the plasma fibrinogen level. Correction of dyslipidaemia, especially the lowering of plasma triglycerides, also brings down the fibrinogen level.[72] Lipid-lowering drugs belonging to the class of fibrates such as clofibrate[73] and bezafibrate[74] but not gemfibrozil[75] can accomplish a fibrinogen reduction of at least 15% in diabetes.

An increase of haematocrit in patients with end-stage renal disease by administration of erythropoietin may also have beneficial effects on retinopathy.[76,77] Diabetic retinopathy improved in three patients with renal insufficiency and chronic anaemia after a rise in haematocrit induced by administration of recombinant human erythropoietin. The change involved significant resorption of hard exudates in patients who were not eligible to receive laser treatment. Within 6 months of initiation of erythropoietin treatment, a substantial reduction of exudate was observed in all three patients, the haematocrit having increased from 21% to 33%. Visual acuity improved in two patients and stabilized in the other. There was no change in the leaking pattern. Although no direct cause and effect relationship can be derived from this observation, it appears that improvement of the haematocrit (leading to restoration of rheological parameters by beating hypoxia, or by a direct antihypoxic effect on the vessel wall) may serve as adjunctive treatment of diabetic retinopathy in patients with diabetic renal insufficiency.

REFERENCES

1. McMillan DE, Development of vascular complications in diabetes, *Vas Med* (1997) **2**:132–42.
2. Bronkhorst PJH, Red cell deformability (Thesis Utrecht University: Utrecht, 1966).
3. Turitto VT, Goldsmith HL, Rheology, transport and thrombosis in the circulation. In: Loscalzo J, Creager MA, Dzau VJ, eds, *Vascular Medicine. A Textbook of Vascular Biology and Diseases*, 2nd edn (Little, Brown: Boston, 1996) 141–84.

4. McMillan DE, Utterback NG, Mitchell TP, Doublet formation of diabetic erythrocytes as a model of impaired membrane viscous deformation, *Microvasc Res* (1983) **26**:205–20.
5. Sobin SS, Lindal RG, Bernick S, The pulmonary arteriole, *Microvasc Res* (1977) **14**:227–39.
6. Wautier J-L, Wautier M-P, Schmidt A-M et al, Advanced glycation end products (AGEs) on the surface of diabetic erythrocytes bind to vessel wall via a specific receptor inducing oxidant stress in the vasculature: a link between surface-associated AGEs and diabetic complications, *Proc Natl Acad Sci USA* (1994) **91**:7742–6.
7. Wautier J-L, Zoukourian C, Chappey O et al, Receptor-mediated endothelial cell dysfunction in diabetic vasculopathy–soluble receptor advanced glycation end products block hyperpermeability in diabetic rats, *J Clin Invest* (1996) **97**:238–43.
8. Gaehtgens P, Pries AR, Ley K, Structural, hemodynamic and rheological characteristics of blood flow in the circulation. In: Chien S, Dormandy J, Ernst E, Matrai A, eds, *Clinical Hemorrheology, Applications in Cardiovascular and Hematological Disease, Diabetes, Surgery and Gynecology* (Martinus Nijhoff: Dordrecht, 1987) 97–124.
9. Lowe GDO, Foulds WS, Rheology in retinal disorders. In: Lowe GDO, ed, *Clinical Blood Rheology* (CRC Press: Boca Raton, FL, 1988) 189–202.
10. McMillan DE, Malone JI, Rand LI, Progression of diabetic retinopathy is linked to rheologic plasma proteins in the DCCT, *Diabetes* (1995) **44**:54A.
11. Tooke JE, Microvascular function in human diabetes. A physiological perspective, *Diabetes* (1995) **44**:721–6.
12. Williamson JR, Kilo C, Current status of capillary basement membrane disease in diabetes mellitus, *Diabetes* (1977) **26**:65–73.
13. Longhurst J, Capone JR, Zelis R, Evaluation of skeletal muscle capillary basement membrane thickness in congestive cardiac failure, *Chest* (1975) **67**:195–8.
14. Simpson LO, Intrinsic stiffening of red blood cells as the fundamental cause of diabetic nephropathy and microangiography: a new hypothesis, *Nephron* (1985) **39**:344–51.
15. Steck TL, Red cell shape. In: Stein W, Donner F, eds, *Cell Shape: Determinants, Regulation and Regulatory Role* (Academic Press: New York, 1989) 205–46.
16. Op den Kamp JAF, Lipid asymmetry in membranes, *Annu Rev Biochem* (1979) **48**:47–71.
17. Sutera SP, Zahalak GI, Deduction of intrinsic mechanical properties of the erythrocyte membrane from observations of tank-treading in the rheoscope, *Biorheology* (1989) **26**:177–97.
18. Weed RI, Reed CF, Alterations leading to red cell destruction, *Am J Med* (1996) **41**:681–90.
19. Sutera SP, Gardner RA, Poylan CW et al, Age-related changes in deformability of human erythrocytes, *Blood* (1985) **65**:275–82.
20. Svoboda K, Schmidt CF, Branton D, Block SM, Conformation and elasticity of the isolated red blood cell membrane skeleton, *Biophys J* (1992) **63**:784–93.
21. Williams AR, MOrris DR, The internal viscosity of the human erythrocyte may determine its lifespan in vivo, *Scand J Haematol* (1980) **24**:57–62.
22. Ehrly AM, *Therapeutic Hemorrheology* (Springer Verlag: Berlin, 1991).
23. Kurantsin-Mills J, Blood rheology and the microcirculation. In: Sidawy AN, Sumpio BE, DePalma RG, eds, *The Basic Science of Vascular Disease* (Futura: Armonk, NY, 1997) 503–33.
24. Pries AR, Secomb TW, Gessner T et al, Resistance to blood flow in microvessels in vivo, *Circ Res* (1994) **75**:904–15.
25. International Committee for Standardization in Haematology (Expert Panel on Blood Rheology), Guidelines for measurements of blood viscosity and erythrocyte deformability, *Clin Hemoorheol* (1986) **6**:439–53.
26. Artmann G, A microscopic photometric method for measuring erythrocyte deformability, *Clin Hemorheol* (1986) **6**:617–21.
27. Gaehtgens P, Duhrssen C, Albrecht KH, Motion, deformation, and interaction of blood cells and plasma during flow through narrow capillary tubes, *Blood Cells* (1980) **6**:799–812.
28. Bronkhorst PJH, Berends HG, Nijhof EJ, Sixma JJ, Red cell deformability (RCD) in plasma as

compared with phosphate-buffered saline, *Int J Microcir Clin Exp* (1994) **14**:235–6.
29. Chien S, Sung KLP, Skalak R et al, Theoretical and experimental studies on viscoelastic properties of erythrocyte membrane, *Biophys J* (1978) **24**:463–87.
30. McMillan DE, Development of vascular complications in diabetes, *Vasc Med* (1997) **2**:132–42.
31. Harlan JM, Leukocyte-endothelial interactions, *Blood* (1985) **65**:513–25.
32. Williamson JR, Grisham JW, Electron microscopy of leukocyte margination and emigration in acute inflammation in dog pancreas, *Am J Pathol* (1961) **39**:239–56.
33. House SD, Lipowsky HH, Microvascular hematocrit and red cell flux in rat cremaster muscle, *Am J Physiol* (1987) **252**:H211–H222.
34. Lipowski HH, Usami S, Chien S, In vivo measurements of hematocrit and apparent viscosity in the microvasculature of cat mesentery, *Mircovasc Res* (1980) **19**:297–319.
35. Yen RT, Fung YC, Effect of velocity distribution on red cell distribution in capillary blood vessels, *Am J Physiol* (1978) **235**:H251–259.
36. Schmid-Schoenbein GW, Usami S, Skalak R et al, Cell distribution in capillary networks, *Microvasc Res* (1980) **19**:18–44.
37. Chien S, White blood cell rheology. In: Lowe GDO, ed, *Clinical Blood Rheology*, Vol 1 (CRC Press: Boca Raton, FL, 1988) 87–109.
38. Lowe GDO, Ghafour M, Belch JJF et al, Increased blood viscosity in diabetic proliferative retinopathy, *Diabetes Res* (1986) **3**:67–70.
39. Schlingemann RO, van Hinsbergh VWM, Role of vascular permeability factor/vascular endothelial growth factor in eye disease, *Br J Ophthalmol* (1997) **81**: 501–12.
40. Folkman J, Angiogenesis in cancer, vascular, rheumatoid and other disease, *Nat Med* (1995) **1**:27–31.
41. Barnes AJ, Rheology of diabetes mellitus. In: Lowe GDO, ed, *Clinical Blood Rheology*, Vol 2 (CRC Press: Boca Raton, FL, 1988) 163–88.
42. McRury SM, Lowe GDO, Blood rheology in diabetes mellitus, *Diabet Med* (1990) **7**:285–91.
43. Schmid Schoenbein H, Volger E, Red-cell aggregation and red-cell deformability in diabetes, *Diabetes* (1976) **25** (Suppl 2):897–902.
44. McRury SM, Lennie SE, McColl P et al, Increased red cell aggregation in diabetes mellitus: association with cardiovascular risk factors, *Diabet Med* (1993) **10**:21–6.
45. Satoh M, Imaizumi K, Bessho T et al, Increased erythrocyte aggregation in diabetes mellitus and its relationship to glycosylated haemoglobulin and retinopathy, *Diabetologia* (1984) **27**:517–21.
46. Shiga T, Maeda N, Suda T et al, Influences of cholesterol on red cell deformability, *Clin Hemorheol* (1982) **2**:77–84.
47. Garnier M, Hanss M, Paraf A, Erythrocytes filterability reduction and membrane lipids in liver cirrhosis, *Clin Hemorheol* (1983) **3**:45–52.
48. Garnier M, Koutsouris D, Hanss M, On the membrane determinant of the erythrocyte deformability, *Clin Hemorheol* (1983) **5**:401–4.
49. Juhan I, Vague P, Buonocore M et al, Abnormalities of erythrocyte deformability and platelet aggregation in insulin-dependent diabetes corrected by insulin in vivo and in vitro, *Lancet* (1982) **i**:535–7.
50. Labrouche S, Freyburger G, Gin H et al, Changes in phospholipid composition of blood cell membranes (erythrocyte, platelet, and polymorphonuclear) in different types of diabetes–clinical and biological correlations, *Metabolism* (1996) **45**:57–62.
51. Juhan-Vague I, Driss F, Roul C et al, Abnormalities of erythrocyte membrane lipids in insulin-dependent diabetes are improved by short term strict control of diabetes, *Clin Hemorheol* (1984) **4**:455–9.
52. Juhan-Vague I, Rahmani-Jourdheuil D, Mourayre Y et al, Study of red blood cell (RBC) membrane fluidity in insulin-dependent diabetics using fluoresecence polarization, *Clin Hemorheol* (1985) **5**:670–76
53. Holman RR, Dorman TL, Mayon-White V et al, Prevention of deterioration of renal and sensory-nerve function by more intensive management of insulin-dependent diabetic patients, *Lancet* (1983) **i**:204–8.

54. Leiper JM, Lowe GDO, Anderson J et al, Effects of diabetic control and biosynthetic human insulin on blood rheology in established diabetics, *Diabetes Res* (1984) 1:27–30
55. Nishimura C, Hotta Y, Gui T et al, The level of erythrocyte aldose reductase is associated with the severity of diabetic retinopathy, *Diabetes Res Clin Pract* (1997) **37**:173–77.
56. Seghieri G, Anichini R, Ciuti M et al, Raused erythrocyte polyamine levels in non-insulin-dependent diabetes mellitus with great vessel disease and albuminuria, *Diabetes Res Clin Pract* (1997) **37**:15–20.
57. Rud'ko IA, Balashova TS, Golega EN et al, The results of a comparative study of the lipid peroxidation process and of the malondialdehyde level of the blood cells in patients with diabetic angiopathies and during insulin therapy, *Ter Arkh* (1994) **66**:27–9.
58. Hanssen KF, Bangstad H-J, Brinchmann-Hansen, Dahl-Jorgensen K, Blood glucose control and diabetic microvascular complications. Long-term effects of near-normoglycaemia, *Diabet Med* (1992) **9**:697–705.
59. Reichard P, Nilsson B-Y, Rosenqvist U, The effect of long-term intensified insulin treatment on the development of microvascular complications in diabetes mellitus, *N Engl J Med* (1993) **329**:304–9.
60. DCCT Research Group, The effect of intensive treatment of diabetes on the development and progression of long-term complications in insulin-dependent diabetes mellitus, *N Engl J Med* (1993) **329**:977–86.
61. UK Prospective Diabetes Study Group, Intensive blood glucose control with sulfonylureas or insulin compared with conventional treatment and risk of complications in patients with type 2 diabetes (UKPDS 33), *Lancet* (1998) **352**:837–53.
62. UK Prospective Diabetes Study Group, Effect of intensive blood glucose control policy with metformin on complications in type 2 diabetes patients (UKPDS 34), *Lancet* (1998) **352**:837–53.
63. Aarts PAMM, Banga JD, van Houwelingen HC et al, Increased red blood cell deformability due to isoxsuprine administration decreases platelet adherence in a perfusion chamber: a double blind crossover study in patients with intermittent claudication, *Blood* (1986) **67**:1474–81.
64. McMillan DE, Utterback NG, Wujek JJ, Effect of anionic amphophiles on erythrocyte properties, *Ann N Y Acad Sci* (1983) **416**:633–41.
65. Popp-Snijders C, Schouten JA, Van der Meer J et al, Fatty fish-induced changes in membrane lipid composition and viscosity of human erythrocyte suspensions, *Scand J Clin Lab Invest* (1986) **46**:253–8.
66. Westerveld HE, De Graaf JC, Van Breugel HHFI et al, Effects of low-dose EPA-E on glycemic control, lipid profile, lipoprotein (a), platelet aggregation, viscosity, and platelet and vessel wall interaction in NIDDM, *Diabetes Care* (1993) **16**:683–8.
67. ETDRS Investigations, Aspirin effects on mortality and morbidity in patients with diabetes mellitus. ETDRS Report no. 14, *JAMA* (1992) **268**:1292–300.
68. The DAMAD Study Group, Effect of aspirin alone and aspirin plus dipyridamole in early diabetic retinopathy: a randomized controlled clinical trial, *Diabetes* (1989) **38**:491–8.
69. Meade TW, Imeson J, Stirling Y, Effects of changes in smoking and other characteristics on clotting factors and the risk of ischemic heart disease, *Lancet* (1987) **ii**:986–8.
70. Hornsby G, Boggess K, Lyons T et al, Exercise conditioning reduces plasma fibrinogen in non-insulin dependent diabetes mellitus, *Diabetes* (1988) **37** (Suppl 1):240a.
71. Volger E, Pfafferot C, Effects of acute physical effort versus endurance training on blood rheology in coronary heart disease patients, *Clin Hemorheol* (1990) **10**:423–30.
72. Simpson HCR, Meade TW, Stirling Y et al, Hypertriglyceridaemia and hypercoagulability, *Lancet* (1983) **i**:786–90.
73. Calvert GD, Blight L, Franklin J et al, The effects of clofibrate on plasma glucose, lipoproteins, fibrinogen and other biochemical and haematological variables in patients with mature onset diabetes mellitus, *Eur J Clin Pharmacol* (1980) **17**:355–62.

74. Durrington PN, Winocour PH, Bhatnagar D, Bezafibrate retard in patients with insulin-dependent diabetes–effect on serum lipoproteins, fibrinogen anf glycemic control, *J Cardiovasc Pharmacol* (1990) **16**:S30–S34.
75. Stringer MD, Rampling MW, Kakkar W, Rheological effects of gemfibrozil in occlusive arterial disease, *Clin Hemorheol* (1990) **10**:339–46.
76. Berman DH, Friedman EA, Partial absorption of hard exudates in patients with diabetic end-stage renal disease and severe anemia after treatment with erytropoietin, *Retina* (1994) **14**:1–5.
77. Friedman EA, Brown CD, Berman DH, Erythropoietin in diabetic macular edema and renal insufficiency, *Am J Kidney Dis* (1995) **26**:202–8.

Index